Children's Well-Being: Indicators and Research

Volume 13

This series focuses on the subject of measurements and indicators of children's well being and their usage, within multiple domains and in diverse cultures. More specifically, the series seeks to present measures and data resources, analysis of data, exploration of theoretical issues, and information about the status of children, as well as the implementation of this information in policy and practice. By doing so it aims to explore how child indicators can be used to improve the development and the well being of children.

With an international perspective the series will provide a unique applied perspective, by bringing in a variety of analytical models, varied perspectives, and a variety of social policy regimes.

Children's Well-Being: Indicators and Research will be unique and exclusive in the field of measures and indicators of children's lives and will be a source of high quality, policy impact and rigorous scientific papers.

More information about this series at http://www.springer.com/series/8162

Cory Shulman

Research and Practice in Infant and Early Childhood Mental Health

Springer

Cory Shulman
The Paul Baerwald School of Social Work
and Social Welfare
The Hebrew University of Jerusalem
Jerusalem, Israel

ISSN 1879-5196 ISSN 1879-520X (electronic)
Children's Well-Being: Indicators and Research
ISBN 978-3-319-31179-1 ISBN 978-3-319-31181-4 (eBook)
DOI 10.1007/978-3-319-31181-4

Library of Congress Control Number: 2016940192

Printed on acid-free paper

This Springer imprint is published by Springer Nature
The registered company is Springer International Publishing AG Switzerland

Preface

We live in a world which is both technologically sophisticated and globally connected to an extent which could not have been imagined a century, or even half a century, ago. In spite of the remarkable achievements of the twentieth century, however, there are still a great many children living in conditions which place them at an enormous disadvantage, not only in the developing world but even in the most advanced and prosperous Western societies. We, as individuals and as societies, have a profound responsibility to the weakest and most disadvantaged among us, which we ignore at our peril. We have much more to learn about optimal strategies for supporting young children and their families who are confronted by a wide range of difficult circumstances, but we have already accumulated a body of knowledge which can do a great deal of good if it is put to appropriate use. Utilizing this knowledge is, to a large extent, a matter of choice: politicians and other policy makers determine what resources are to be allocated for matters such as early childhood education and infant mental health. Those who are actively involved in these fields have an obligation to provide policy makers with the best possible information and advice with regard not only to existing needs and appropriate options for dealing with them but also to promising avenues of research and practice which deserve to be explored in order to develop new options. Many conditions which have an adverse impact on the development of children could be eliminated, or at the very least ameliorated, if societies decided to commit sufficient resources to the task.

Children and their families, especially those who are grappling with adverse conditions of one sort of another – and those who grapple with adversity often struggle simultaneously with numerous adverse factors – need and can benefit greatly from varied sources of support. These may include mentors who can provide guidance and advice, social resources, and other types of support systems located in the family, the community, and the larger society. There are a number of programs and approaches which have been shown to be effective in improving outcomes for young children and their families, particularly those who are at risk for developing infant mental health problems, and some of the most important ones are described in this book. If sufficient resources were dedicated to this undertaking, programs like these could be expanded to serve larger populations and research could be directed to improve existing approaches and to develop new ones.

Our knowledge about what is best for the development of infants and young children needs to find expression in a variety of ways. One of the most important of these is to infuse mental health principles into existing systems which deal with young children – families, educational systems, community settings, and cultural organizations. Relevant knowledge has to be disseminated to those who are involved in providing services to young children and their families, and these individuals need to be offered ongoing support in the form of consultations provided by mental health professionals with multidisciplinary training. Much can also be accomplished by establishing prevention programs which are aimed at proactively reducing the incidence of mental health problems before they occur. In addition, there will always be children and families who need specialized services provided directly to them by trained professionals. Substantial resources must be invested in providing professionals such as these with the best possible training and with ongoing support throughout the course of their careers. All these topics and others will be covered in this book.

To a significant extent this book is an outgrowth of my work in the Early Childhood Graduate Program of the Hebrew University of Jerusalem, which is dedicated to training professionals to work in various aspects of the field of early childhood. This program offers three tracks. One of these is devoted to the study of community services and policy, including program development, with a view to increasing awareness of early childhood issues and improving community services among policy makers; another provides consultation and support for the staff of child care centers and endeavors to increase understanding of their needs and experiences and support them as they support the children in their care. The latest addition to this program is a track dedicated to training professionals who will provide services directly to children and their families according to the principles of infant and early childhood mental health, as there are always children and families who need direct support in order to achieve optimal outcomes.

The aim of this book is to build a bridge between existing research knowledge and practice in the field of infant and early childhood mental health, and its structure reflects this aim. The emphasis of the first half of the book is on the theoretical and research underpinnings of the field of infant mental health, while its second half emphasizes evidence-based interventions utilized to assess the efficacy of the practical application of these research principles. The first chapter offers a conceptualization of the field of infant and early childhood mental health and a historical survey of its growth as well as an overview of the topics covered in the remainder of the book. The second chapter deals with the developmental context in which infant and early childhood mental health must be understood, and the third chapter treats the necessity of approaching these topics with awareness of and sensitivity to cultural contexts. The fourth chapter discusses the age-old "nature versus nurture" controversy and the contributions of recent research to a more profound and nuanced appreciation of the complementary roles of both. The fifth chapter deals with risk factors which increase the likelihood of mental health problems in infants and young children. The sixth chapter, which may be seen as the pivot on which the book turns, is devoted to the relational context which is crucial to understanding and improving mental health in infants and young children, and integrates research and practice from this perspective. The seventh chapter discusses the crucial concept of resilience, which allows some children and families to function well despite adversity, and ways in which resilience can be strengthened. The eighth chapter is devoted to the theoretical bases of intervention programs in infant and early childhood mental health, while the ninth chapter discusses the notion of evidence-based interventions and presents a number of specific evidence-based programs. The tenth chapter deals with infant and early childhood mental health consultation, which is designed to offer support and expert guidance for the staff of existing frameworks from the mental health perspective. The final chapter addresses imperatives for policy makers and professionals in the field of infant and early childhood mental health.

I would like to conclude this preface by acknowledging some of the individuals and institutions who have shaped my work and contributed, directly or indirectly, to the present book. I owe a debt of gratitude to the students I have taught over the years at David Yellin College and at the Hebrew University of Jerusalem, from whom I have learned a great deal and who have both stimulated and challenged me; and perhaps even more to the many children and families with whom I have had the privilege of working, who have shared their lives, their struggles, and their aspirations with me and provided a never-ending source of inspiration. I would like to express my thanks to my husband, Robert Brody, for his unfailing support and assistance during the writing of this book and always. The Harris Foundation of Chicago deserves my heartfelt thanks, as well as the thanks of many others, for its generous support of the field of infant mental health in general, and specifically for supporting the establishment of the program in Infant and Early Childhood Mental Health at the Hebrew University of Jerusalem which I am privileged to head. Finally, I am grateful to Miranda Dijksman and Hendrikje Tuerlings of Springer Verlag for inviting me to publish this book in the series *Children's Well-being: Indicators and Research*, and to my colleagues Asher Ben-Arieh, Sheila Kamerman, and Shelley Phillips, the editors of this series.

Jerusalem, Israel Cory Shulman

Contents

1 Conceptualization of the Field of Infant and Early Childhood Mental Health 1
Introduction 1
History 2
Beginning Steps 2
Formulation of Core Concepts 3
Attachment Becomes One of the Central Constructs 4
Mindfulness and Reflective Thinking 6
Defining Infant Mental Health 7
Defining Organizations in Europe and the United States 8
The Role of Emotions in Infant and Early Childhood Mental Health 8
Early Mental Health and Later Development 9
Theoretical Models of Infant Mental Health 10
Normative Theories of Development and Infant Mental Health 11
The Effect of the Quality of Early Experiences 11
Development in the Earliest Years 12
Developmental Change 13
Implications of Early Development for Later Development 14
The Developing Sense of Self 15
References 16

2 Social and Emotional Development in Infant and Early Childhood Mental Health 23
Introduction 23
Conceptualizing Early Development 24
Brain and Behavior in Early Development 26
Cognitive Development 26
Developmental Tasks: Reciprocal Connections 28

Developmental Context of Social and Emotional Functioning in the Early Years 29
Bonding 29
Research Paradigms 30
Individual Differences in Emotional Development 31
Temperament 31
Developmental Stages and Social and Emotional Growth 34
The Underpinnings of Theory of Mind 35
Foundation for the Concern for Others 36
Issues of Concern 37
References 38

3 Social and Cultural Contexts in Infant and Early Childhood Mental Health 43
Introduction 43
Understanding Social Behavior in the Early Years 44
Conducting Research into Socialization of Young Children 45
Changes at the End of the First Year in Gaze Behavior 47
Infant Socialization in the Home Culture 48
Implicit and Explicit Socialization 49
Parenting 51
Parental Awareness 51
Parenting Styles 52
Research Methodology in Cross-Cultural Infant and Early Childhood Mental Health 54
Research Strategies and Instruments 54
The Culturally Determined "Ideal Child" 55
Cultural Differences in Childrearing 56
Cultural Differences in Attachment Behavior 58
Risk Factors Perceived Through a Cultural Lens 60
References 61

4 The Nature-Versus-Nurture Controversy and Its Implications for Infant and Early Childhood Mental Health 67
Introduction 67
History of the Nature Versus Nurture Controversy 68
Individual Differences in Infancy and Early Childhood and Behavioral Genetics 69
Research Methods for Studying Behavioral Genetics 70
Findings from Behavioral Genetics Research 71
Intervention Strategies Based on Behavioral Genetics 72
Gene-Environment Interplay 72
General Models of the Nature-Nurture Controversy 75
References 76

5 Risk Factors in Infant and Early Childhood Mental Health 81
Introduction 81
The Conceptualization of Risk 82
Identifying Risk Factors 84
Longitudinal Research 84
Changes in Familiar Situations as a Risk Factor 85
Parental Characteristics and Risk 86
Research Methodologies for Studying Risk 87
Employing Statistical Models to Explain Risk 89
Environmental Risk Factors in Infancy: Poverty 90
Parental Risk Factors: Depression 93
Child Risk Factors: Prematurity 94
Risk Factors for Early Infant and Child Mental Health in Developing Countries 96
References 97

6 The Relational Context of Infant and Early Childhood Mental Health 101
Relationships as a Bridge Between Theory and Intervention 101
The Relational Imperative in Infant Mental Health 102
Zero-to-Three Diagnostic System 103
Emotional Availability 105
Parenting Across Cultures 108
Attachment 111
Interrelational Context 112
Child Characteristics in the Relational Context 112
Jealousy 112
Social Cognition in Infants 114
Attunement 117
References 118

7 Resilience in Children and Families 125
Introduction 125
Resilience Models 126
Risk and Resilience in a Relational Context 128
Family and Community Resilience 129
Research in Resilience 131
Longitudinal Resilience Research Designs 132
Longitudinal Resilience Research Statistics 133
Longitudinal Resilience Research Models 135
Applications of Resilience Research 137
Implications for Intervention 138
References 140

8 Theoretical Bases of Intervention in Infant and Early Childhood Mental Health . . . 145
Introduction . . . 145
Psychodynamic Theory . . . 146
Attachment-Based Theory . . . 148
Developmental Theories of Infant Mental Health . . . 150
Sameroff: Transactional Model . . . 150
Greenspan: Developmental, Individual-Differences, Relationship-Based Model (DIR) . . . 152
Bagnato: Convergent Model . . . 153
Als: Synactive Theory of Development . . . 153
Ayres: Sensory Integration Theory of Development . . . 154
Brazelton: Touchpoints Model . . . 155
Guralnick: Multidisciplinary Collaborative Team Work Model . . . 156
References . . . 156

9 A Survey of Evidence-Based Interventions in Infant and Early Childhood Mental Health . . . 159
Introduction . . . 159
Research Methodology and Designs Which Assess Intervention Effectiveness . . . 161
Evidence-Based Practice . . . 162
Child Parent Psychotherapy . . . 164
Incredible Years® . . . 167
Parent Child Interaction Therapy . . . 170
Interaction Guidance . . . 171
Home Visiting Intervention . . . 174
References . . . 175

10 Early Childhood Mental Health Consultation . . . 181
Introduction . . . 181
Issues to be Considered in Mental Health Consultation in Early Childhood . . . 182
The Consultative Model and Its Principles . . . 184
The Consultation Setting . . . 186
The Adult Client . . . 187
The Consultant . . . 188
The Consultative Relationship . . . 190
Consultative Skills . . . 192
Reflective Practice . . . 192
Problem-Solving . . . 193
Capacity Building . . . 195
Research Findings . . . 196
Challenges in Early Childhood Mental Health Consultation . . . 198
References . . . 199

11 Applications of Infant and Early Childhood Mental Health Research in Policy and Practice 203
Introduction 203
Policy Agenda: Promoting Infant and Early Childhood Mental Health 204
Policy Agenda: Creating Mental Health Informed Systems 205
Support Programs for Families at Risk 207
Incorporating Mental Health Perspectives in Policy Decisions 209
Policy Agenda: Establishing Prevention Programs 210
Policy Agenda: Training Professionals 212
Policy Agenda: Incorporating Diversity-Informed Tenets 213
Conclusions and Recommendations for Policymakers, Researchers and Practitioners 214
References 216

Index 219

Chapter 1
Conceptualization of the Field of Infant and Early Childhood Mental Health

Introduction

Infancy and early childhood are critical developmental periods during which the brain and the body of young children undergo rapid change. Developments in physical, intellectual, social and emotional domains which occur during this time have been found to have a profound effect on subsequent well being (Belsky & Fearon, 2002; Fox, Henderson, Marshall, Nichols, & Ghera, 2005; Schore, 2001; Sroufe, 2000; Sroufe, Carlson, Levy, & Egeland, 1999). The study of these developments has evolved into a separate, integrative field of scientific inquiry called infant and early childhood mental health. This is an evolving interdisciplinary discipline which seeks to elucidate the interplay between aspects of normal and abnormal development in the early years, the relationships among various developmental domains, and the multifaceted factors which affect infant and early childhood mental health. Although this is an emerging field, the myriad of books, research projects and practical interventions which have appeared over the last 30 years gives evidence of the magnitude of interest in this field. This book will review the state of our knowledge, integrating research findings and clinical practices regarding infant mental health in the twenty-first century.

This introductory chapter begins with a history of the field, presenting its evolution through a chronological prism. This historical survey establishes the themes to be discussed throughout the book, including the relationship between research and practice; the tension between intervention strategies and prevention perspectives; and the multidisciplinary approach that is at the foundation of work in the field of infant and early childhood mental health.

After a historical survey, several definitions of infant and early childhood mental health, which reflect the complexity inherent in a field which bridges science and practice in the first years of the child's life, will be presented. Although progress is being made in understanding the seminal processes and identifying important

C. Shulman, *Research and Practice in Infant and Early Childhood Mental Health*, Children's Well-Being: Indicators and Research 13,
DOI 10.1007/978-3-319-31181-4_1

components of mental health in the early years, there is still much to investigate in order to understand the inherent complexity of infant and early childhood mental health. The developmental perspective is crucial to understanding infant and early childhood mental health, as development is the pervasive theme which runs through the significant components of the infant's life. After survival, the infant's physical, emotional and social growth is the first developmental task, and in order for this growth to be successful after survival, growing relationships with primary caregivers are required. The infant develops within the family context in which each family member is the product of his or her own childhood environment, and the cultural context, in which the child is socialized and functions according to certain cultural conventions and circumstances. Sameroff's transactional model (1975, 2009) incorporates development over time, reflecting the multi-layered, relational model which lies at the base of infant and early childhood mental health.

History

Beginning Steps

The field of infant mental health began in the Unites States after the Second World War when Fraiberg, Adelson, and Shapiro (1975) realized the importance of studying both typical and atypical behavior within the mother-child relationship. Selma Fraiberg was working with congenitally blind babies, and as opposed to "mapping" what she saw in these babies onto what was expected from typically developing children, as was the norm at that time, she began to extrapolate knowledge from the differences and deviations she observed in these babies from infants with typical development (Fraiberg, 1977). Her proposed model was based on understanding that the internal world of caregivers influenced their ability to interact with and care for their babies, and became the theoretical foundation for the science of infant mental health. Around the same time as Selma Fraiberg was investigating developmental patterns in blind infants, Martha Harris and Esther Bick (1976) were observing typically developing infants in the United Kingdom. By watching and listening to babies during the first 2 years of their lives, they charted the developmental changes which were occurring. Their focus on the earliest stages of mental development and the interactional patterns between infants and their caregivers formed the underpinning of infant mental health in the UK. Bowlby's (1956) seminal work in attachment incorporated the quality of caregiving as an integral part of the infant's social and emotional development. Attachment theory, which also advanced during the post war years amidst an atmosphere of loss and bereavement, emphasizes that child development is influenced by the manner in which parents and other caregivers treat young children and the ways in which the children experience and understand these interactions.

Continuing to build on this groundwork, Daniel Stern (1974), a psychiatrist and psychoanalytical theorist, and Tronick, Als, and Brazelton (1977) simultaneously began studying mother and infant turn taking, which they described as rhythmical patterns of approach and withdrawal between the mother and infant (Stern, 1974, 1995, 2000, 2009; Tronick & Cohn, 1989). Analysis of videotaped mother-infant interactions revealed a synchronous "dance" comprised of brief periods during which mothers and their children were communicating continually, in an interactive manner. These interactions included subtle, body-based exchanges of looks, vocalizations, eye contact and speech, and reflected a harmonious connection between two individual beings.

When there was a disruption in the interpersonal connection, infants were able to control the interaction by looking away when they needed a break from the input, while mothers who were attuned to their babies were able to engage in this dance by regulating their interaction to meet the baby's needs, thereby repairing disruptions. Mothers who were not able to modulate their interactions according to their children's needs seemed to overwhelm their babies with their intrusiveness or seemed to underwhelm their babies by not responding to them. Some of the less attuned mothers were experiencing depression or dealing with unresolved loss in their own lives (Field, 1994). Infants who experienced extended periods of disruption, rather than attunement, revealed an avoidant style of attachment to the caregiver at ages as early as 3 months. The importance of these findings is evident in view of later research which has found that such early disruptions in mother-child interactions are implicated in a range of longer term adverse child cognitive (Meins, Fernyhough, Russell, & Clark-Carter, 1998; Murray, Fiori-Cowley, Hooper, & Cooper, 1996) and emotional outcomes (Caplan et al., 1989; Coghill, Caplan, Alexandra, Robson, & Kumar, 1986, Dawson, Hessl, & Frey, 1994; Field, Healy, Goldstein, & Guthertz, 1990), including behavioral problems (Murray & Cooper, 1997).

Formulation of Core Concepts

Colwyn Trevarthen (1979), trained as a biologist, began studying infants and posited that even newborns can initiate interactions with adults. He focused on movement and action as reflecting emotional states and postulated that communication, human intersubjectivity and others' emotions are all part of the chronobiology of human development beginning in infancy, manifested in the ability of the infant and young child to regulate their own emotions. Emotion regulation is perceived as adaptive and functional in that it is helpful to the child in attaining goals (Bretherton, Fritz, Zahn-Waxler, & Ridgeway, 1986; Campos & Barrett, 1984). Emotions are important regulators of interpersonal relationships (Charlesworth, 1982; Shiota, Campos, Keltner, & Hertenstein, 2004), thus maintaining contact with the attachment figure (Cassidy, 1994; Trevarthen, 1984) through eye contact, smiling, and other fundamental body movements.

Emotion regulation has been described as serving the function of maintaining the relationship, and the ability to regulate emotion contributes to the infant's more generalized regulation in response to experiences with the caregiver. An example of this synchronization of interactional patterns of infants and their caregivers was documented in infants who experienced rejection. It was suggested as a possible explanation that by avoiding eye contact the infants were trying to minimize negative affect in order to avoid the risk of further rejection (Isabella, Belsky, & von Eye, 1989), whereas infants whose mothers have been relatively unavailable or inconsistently available are thought to maximize negative affect in order to increase the likelihood of gaining the attention of a frequently unavailable caregiver (Isabella & Belsky, 1991). Although seemingly not adaptive behavior, both these patterns of emotion regulation help ensure that the child remains close to the parent and thereby be protected. In addition, emotional regulation helps maintain the dyadic relationship when infants signal to their parents that they will cooperate in maintaining the parent's own state of mind and regulation. This approach to emotion regulation is congruent with work examining the socialization of emotions (Lewis & Saarni, 1985; Thompson, 1994).

Thus, these early theorists facilitated a new way of perceiving infancy by drawing attention to the importance of babies' emotional well being, particularly their capacity for emotional regulation, and to the interrelatedness of influence of the infant and the primary caregiver on this process. Beebe, Lachmann and Jaffe (1997) recognized that this regulation process is bi-directional and dynamic, with considerable co-regulation occurring between the mother and her baby. Fonagy, Steele, Steele, Moran, and Higgitt (1991) emphasized the importance of primary caregivers being able to be mindful of the baby's state. This model of co-regulation has become one of the cornerstones of the infant mental health movement, supported by the recognition of the fact that even very young children are sensitive to the quality of their interactions with other people (Feldman, 2007; Murray & Cooper, 1997; Slade, 2002, 2005). Bowlby's (1969) continuing work, emphasizing the importance of parent-child interactions as critical to the child's development, was reflected in his changing the name of the children's department at Travistock Clinic which he directed to the department for children and parents. He challenged the prevailing notion that humans develop as individual monads, struggling against their own aggressive impulses toward civilization and proposed that people develop as members of interacting systems. He believed that the source of psychopathology was to be found not in internalized Oedipal conflicts but in failed or unavailable infant and early childhood attachments (Wylie & Turner, 2011).

Attachment Becomes One of the Central Constructs

While Bowlby (1969) described how attachment increases the likelihood of infants' survival, researchers have more recently begun to recognize that attachment also has far-reaching functions in terms of the manner in which the proximity of the mother helps infants to modulate or regulate an aroused emotional state until they are able to do so for themselves (Beebe et al., 2010; Leerkes, Blankson, & O'Brien,

2009). Securely attached infants seek comfort when distressed and recover from an aroused, disorganized state when comforted. Insecurely attached infants, however, are unable to use the caregiver to modulate their aroused state and they may over-regulate, under-regulate or even show evidence of both, reflecting conflicting emotions. Consequently, attachment is important both because it provides the infant with a secure base from which to begin to explore the world and because it acts as a prototype for later relations.

Infants' early attachment interactions become internalized as an "internal working model" that enables them to know what to expect from their interactions with other people (Bowlby, 1989). This representational model provides children with a very early set of expectations in relation to "self" and "self with others" that continues to influence them throughout their lives (Prior & Glaser, 2006). While internal models may be modified through experience, they function mainly outside of awareness and therefore are resistant to change (Crittenden, 1990).

Insecurely attached children's expectations range from assuming others will be unresponsive, unavailable, and/or unwilling to meet their needs, to their being threatening, abusive, and/or endangering, and these beliefs follow them throughout their lives (van IJzendoorn & Bakermans-Kranenburg, 1997; Van IJzendoorn, Juffer, & Duyvesteyn, 1995) and may even be passed on to the next generation. Researchers have recently begun to disentangle intergenerational continuities in attachment patterns and have identified significant associations between a parent's style of attachment and his or her child's attachment type (Fonagy, Steele, & Steele, 1991; Kretchmar & Jacobvitz, 2002; Van IJzendoorn, 1992).

From the beginning, infants seek interaction with others and continually influence and respond to their environments. Based on the work of these early theoreticians, it is now acknowledged that the earliest years of life are a critical period during which children make emotional attachments and form the first relationships that may be the foundation for future mental health (Bowlby, 1969, 1989; Fonagy, Gergely, & Jurist, 2004; Sroufe, 2005; Steele, Steele, & Fonagy, 1996; Stern, 1995). Infants need opportunities to attune to others, to learn to regulate or manage their emotions, and to attach to primary caregivers who in turn can reflect and respond to them as individuals. While research linking infants' attachment styles to psychopathology or physical illness in adulthood is limited to a few longitudinal studies (Greenberg, 1999; Kerns & Brumariu, 2014; Main, 1996; Puig, Englund, Simpson, & Collins, 2013), the investigation of the nature of relationships between behavior in the early years and future mental health as adults has focused on assessing associations between relevant attachment events in infancy and early childhood and later psychopathology.

Such links have been investigated using two operationalizations of the attachment constructs, "attachment style" (Hazan & Shaver, 1987, 1994) and "attachment states of mind" (Dozier, Stovall-McClough, & Albus, 2008; Main, Kaplan, & Cassidy, 1985; Miga, Hare, Allen, & Manning, 2010). While these constructs share a conceptual framework, there are key differences between them that lead to different behavioral definitions. The system used by Main and her colleagues assesses states of mind with respect to attachment as a function of discourse coherence and defensive strategy. By contrast, attachment style assesses the individual's self-reported style of forming adolescent and adult attachments. As expected, given these different operationalizations, these variables are not strongly related to each other, but correlations between precursors to later anti-social behavior and anxiety-related pathology have been found among constellations of temperamental and generic vulnerability, dysfunctional parenting, and stressful or disorganized early environments in the preschool years.

Sensitive attunement, warmth, synchrony, and the successful repair of ruptures by caregivers in very early interactions with the baby are associated with later secure attachment of the child (Van Van IJzendoorn, 1992). Providing the child with emotional warmth means ensuring that the child feels valued for his or her uniqueness and thus develops a feeling of self-worth. Emotional warmth includes the child's recognition of his or her own racial and cultural identity and involves helping the child to value these aspects of a sense of self, facilitating the child's formation of secure, stable and affectionate relationships with significant adults who are appropriately responsive to the child's needs. Displaying emotional warmth usually involves appropriate physical contact such as cuddling in order to demonstrate warm regard, praise and encouragement for the child (Owen, Slep, & Heyman, 2012).

Mindfulness and Reflective Thinking

Recent research has also highlighted the importance of the parents' capacity for "mind-mindedness" (Arnott & Meins, 2007; Cohen & Semple, 2010; Ordway, Webb, Sadler, & Slade, 2015). Meins (1999) studied a group of 200 mothers with infant children, half of whom had left school by age sixteen, and the single most important factor in predicting the child's development was how well the mother was able to interpret the baby's feelings. The findings from this study showed that the mothers' ability to interpret their babies' internal states was a better predictor of the children's language and play skills at 8, 14, and 24 months of age than background variables such as income or socioeconomic status. The better the mother was at interpreting the child's mood and intentions, the faster the child developed the ability to represent thoughts and feelings through play, which is an acquired representational system. This research builds on Fonagy's work which describes such mindfulness as "mentalization" (Fonagy et al., 2004) and refers to the capacity of parents to experience babies as intentional beings rather than simply responding to physical characteristics or behaviors. Fonagy suggests that it is the child's experience of being treated as an intentional being that helps children to develop an understanding of mental states in other people and to regulate their own internal experiences.

The importance of attunement in these early interactions has been researched using advanced methodologies involving technologies and computational techniques (Feldman, 2012; Perry, 2009; Ruttle, Serbin, Stack, Schwartzman, &

Shirtcliff, 2011), and the field of neurodevelopmental science has cultivated new research methodologies which emphasize the importance of considering the quality of the early caregiving environment on the developing brain. The quality of interactions with primary caregivers in the baby's environment has been implicated in the way in which babies build their life-long internal sense of self (for an overview, see Gerhardt, 2006; Schore, 2001; Siegel, 2012). The scientific evidence on the significant developmental impacts of early experiences, caregiving relationships and environmental threats, from fields ranging from behavioral genetics and neuroscience to policy analysis and intervention research, is incontrovertible. Virtually every aspect of early human development, from the brain's evolving circuitry to the child's capacity for empathy, is affected by the environments and experiences that are encountered in a cumulative fashion, beginning early in the prenatal period and extending throughout the early childhood years and beyond.

The science of early development is also clear about the specific importance of parenting and of regular caregiving relationships more generally. The centrality of early bonding experiences and the importance of the quality of the caregiver-child relationship for future development is complemented by other influences including inborn temperament, individuation needs, family dynamics and culture, which all lie outside the caregiver-child dyad. The question today is not whether early experience matters but rather how early experiences shape individual development and contribute to children's continued movement along positive pathways.

Defining Infant Mental Health

Linking the adjective "infant" to the state of being implied in "mental health" may seem counterintuitive. Infants are dependent on others who respond to them by providing physical needs such as food, clothing and shelter, as well as emotional needs such as living within a loving, warm, and supportive relationship. To ascribe "mental health" to young, developing, helpless entities, particularly when it brings to mind adult psychiatric issues such as psychopathology and mental disorders resulting in diagnoses, is in tension with the vision of a promising future for the developing child. Stigma, conceptualized as a set of prejudicial attitudes, stereotypes, and discriminatory behaviors towards a subgroup (Corrigan, 2000), has been associated with people who have mental health problems (Link & Phelan, 2006; Link, Struening, Rahav, Phelan, & Nuttbrock, 1997; Phelan, Bromet, & Link, 1998), making the concept of infant mental health problematic. The name makes it sound as if infants' issues and problems are analogous to those of older children, adolescents and adults, whereas infant mental health focuses more on risk and wellbeing than is typically found in the field of adolescent and adult mental health.

Defining Organizations in Europe and the United States

Despite this heuristic argument against the construct of infant mental health, today there are over 3500 books available which address this burgeoning field and over 15,000 articles have been published in professional journals. Although infant mental health has been conceptualized differently by different theoreticians, each definition encompasses a view of the developing child within family and cultural contexts. The World Association of Infant Mental Health (Osofsky, 2000) defines infant mental health as the ability to develop physically, cognitively, and socially in a manner which allows infants and young children to master the primary emotional tasks of early childhood without serious disruption caused by harmful life events. Because infants develop in an environmental context which is responsible for nurturing them, infant mental health involves the psychological balance of the infant-family system. WAIMH's mission is to promote education, research, and study of the effects of mental, emotional and social development during infancy on later normal and abnormal development through international and interdisciplinary cooperation, research collaborations and professional meetings devoted to scientific, educational, and clinical work with infants and their caregivers.

Whereas WAIMH is an international organization, Zero to Three is a nonprofit organization based in the United States that provides parents, professionals and policymakers with the knowledge and the wherewithal to nurture early development, based on empirical and clinical information which has demonstrated that health and development are directly influenced by the quality of care and experiences a child has with his or her parents and other adults early in life. Similarly to WAIMH, Zero to Three (2001) specifies as critical components of infant mental health the developing capacity of the child from birth to 3 year old to experience, regulate and express emotions; to form close and secure interpersonal relationships; to explore the environment and to learn. The development of these abilities occurs in the context of family, community and cultural expectations for young children, rendering infant mental health synonymous with healthy social-emotional development (Zeanah, Berlin & Boris, 2011), which is more fully discussed in Chap. 2.

The Role of Emotions in Infant and Early Childhood Mental Health

Babies learn to experience, regulate and express emotions in the context of supportive relationships with adults who are able to read and respond to their cues. Babies who are having difficulty coping with external stimulation (as manifested in crying, fussiness, gaze aversion, and distressed facial expressions) need adults who notice their discomfort and who are able to support them by making the adjustments that help them regain their calm. Furthermore, when adults provide sensitive and responsive care, babies form trusting relationships, which in turn foster their ability to explore their environment and to engage with others. Regardless of whether care is provided at home, in child care or with relatives and/or friends, babies need adults who understand and are in tune with their needs and know how to respond to those needs by creating a warm, responsive and nurturing environment (Honig, 2002; Juffer, Bakermans-Kranenburg, & van IJzendoorn, 2012; Sroufe, 2000).

Freud (1955) was the father of psychoanalytical theory and therefore was among the first to define mental health, although he was referring to mental health in adults. He perceived a person's mental health to be at the base of the capacity to work well and to love well. In an attempt to extrapolate from Freud's adulthood conceptualization to one appropriate for young children, Lieberman and Van Horn (2011) define mental health for infants and young children as the capacity to grow well and love well, while concomitantly recognizing that growing well is different from working well and that a dependent young child loves those who afford the protection, care and security which they cannot provide for themselves. Thus, when examining mental health in the first years of life, it is imperative to realize the dynamic nature of development and relationships which is at the base of infant and early childhood mental health.

Early Mental Health and Later Development

As more and more infants survive and develop into adolescence and adulthood, the fields of infant mental health and child development complement one another, with research focusing on the long-term effects of early development. One of the most pressing research needs is to identify variables in infancy which are predictive of positive developmental outcomes in childhood, adolescence and adulthood. In this manner, the connection between early experience and infant characteristics on the one hand, and later developmental, behavioral and adaptive outcomes on the other hand, can be isolated and possibly be targeted for intervention programs. The significance of infant and early childhood mental health is accentuated, as it is linked to emotional well being and affects children's abilities to cope with the challenges of life at all stages of development.

In the 1960s, the awareness that poor development in early life had deleterious consequences, including the need for supplementary or special education services and potentially a lifetime on welfare or in prison, led to the establishment of early intervention programs in kindergartens, such as Head Start, as preventative measures (Love et al., 2005; Webster-Stratton, 1998; Zigler & Muenchow, 1992). Research into these initial early intervention programs revealed positive results in the area of learning and a decrease in dropping out of school or the repetition of bad behavior patterns, resulting in expulsion from school (Farrington, 1994; Vimpani, 2004), but emphasized the need for even earlier interventions beginning in preschool or even before (Love et al., 2002), which might possibly prevent some of the later downward spiral seen in children at risk for mental health problems as they develop. This continual interface between mental health and child development highlights the fact that additional research into infant development can help shed light on the developmental processes which stimulate mental health and which may lead to the development of more effective interventions (Bakermans-Kranenburg, Van IJzendoorn, & Juffer, 2003; Guralnick, 1997; Sameroff & Fiese, 2000).

Changes in laws regarding gender discrimination, children's rights and quality of day care services have also contributed to the surge in research in infant development. Social service agencies are faced with overwhelming numbers of cases of children with difficulties not being addressed in child care frameworks, and research can provide the knowledge base which is needed in order to determine when early development is proceeding well and when it is not. In addition to legal and social changes over the last 50 years, there has been an increase in cultural awareness and the realization that there is no such thing as "the right way" to raise a child (Brooks & Goldstein, 2001) but that infant care practices are culturally determined (Contreras, Narang, Ikhlas, & Teichman, 2002; Rubin & Chung, 2013). For example, Western societies foster independence and individuality in infants, while in many African societies family solidarity and being part of the collective are central to child rearing practices (Keller et al., 2006; Keller, Völker, & Yovsi, 2005). These cross-cultural differences will be discussed more comprehensively in Chap. 3.

Theoretical Models of Infant Mental Health

The various theoretical models upon which infant mental health has been based and through which it has been empirically evaluated offer different theoretical perspectives on the process of human development. Among the most prominent of these are the ecological model articulated by Bronfenbrenner (1979) and subsequently expanded to a bio-ecological model by Bronfenbrenner and Ceci (1994); the transactional model first formulated by Sameroff and Chandler (1975); the concepts of vulnerability and resilience applied to a wide variety of biological and environmental conditions by Werner (1985), Rutter (2012) and Rutter and Sroufe (2000); the process of parenting model developed by Belsky (1984); the social support model for families of children with disabilities proposed by Dunst (2000) and operationalized by Foley and Hochman (2006); the developmental context perspective proposed by Lerner and Busch-Rossnagel (2013); the biosocial model for high risk populations by Rutter (2005); the principles of developmental psychopathology posited by Cicchetti (2013); and the social context model constructed by the MacArthur Foundation research network on Psychopathology and Development (Boyce, Sokolowski, & Robinson, 2012). Various models highlight different elements, but all focus on the interrelatedness of the genetic and environmental aspects, developmental and interactional components and normality and pathology.

Bronfenbrenner (1979, 1986) originally suggested that environment shapes development through a model in which the child is at the center, surrounded by parents and family, all of whom are functioning within a particular social milieu that provides social services which are determined, among other things, by the cultural, political, and economic macrocosm. This model has been used to posit and assess the interaction between the various layers of the model, and as a system for establishing interventions. Currently known as the bioecological model (Bronfenbrenner & Ceci, 1994; Bronfenbrenner & Morris, 2006), this model provides a theoretical framework for incorporating the multi-layered, interactional, dynamic nature of the study of infant mental health. Likewise, Sameroff's (1975, 2000, 2009, 2013) transactional model deals with the reciprocal nature of infant and early childhood mental health, focusing on the interactions between the child and his or her experiences over time. Resilience models focus on strengths and weaknesses in adaptive functioning in high risk populations. All these models provide theoretical frameworks from which operational variables can be defined and can serve as outcome measures in research paradigms. Similarly, some psychopathology models focus on development while others focus on the social milieu in which the child is developing, serving as a reminder that young children's environments are both physical and social.

Normative Theories of Development and Infant Mental Health

All these models examine desired outcomes derived from normative theories while taking variability into account, and relate to unfolding domains of development under the interactive influences of genetic predisposition and individual experience. Development which results from interaction with the environment has been formulated as either environment-expectant or environment-dependent learning. Experience-expectant learning refers to the brain being primed for exposure to a particular environmental experience which results in the rewiring of the brain and the establishment of a new neural pathway, while experience-dependent learning denotes the acquisition of additional skills which develop over the lifespan and for which there are no optimal periods. The developmental trajectories of experience-expectant skills are relatively less susceptible to intervention, while those of experience-dependent skills are affected more significantly, but no area of human competence is completely predetermined by intrinsic factors (Andersen 2003; Johnson & de Haan, 2015). Young children's relationships with their primary caregivers and other environmental experiences significantly impact their cognitive, linguistic, emotional, social, and moral development.

The Effect of the Quality of Early Experiences

These relationships promote growth most significantly when they are nurturing, individualized, and responsive in a contingent and reciprocal manner, and characterized by a high level of "goodness of fit" (Winnicott, 1984). Their impact on development is mediated through the nature and the quality of the experiences that they offer. Early childhood development can be seriously compromised by impairments in regulation. The causes of such impairments are multiple and often revolve around disturbances in what should be close relationships between the children and their primary caregivers.

The mental health of young children has been theorized in a number of ways, each of which produces different domains of scientific inquiry and implications for early childhood intervention. Most problems incorporated in the field of infant mental health are matters of multiple risks, where physical, mental and emotional difficulties need to be addressed simultaneously. Infant mental health does not deal with individual factors, but with the alteration of a dynamic system whose reorganization can lead to better, more optimal developmental outcomes for an infant (Cicchetti & Toth, 1997; Tronick & Beeghly, 2011).

Development in the Earliest Years

In order to understand infant development and its interplay with infant mental health, researchers have focused on the earliest years of life. The assumptions upon which the empirical study of development is based have changed and will continue to change. Today such research is based on the central assumption that infants grow and develop within the family context, not in isolation. Most aspects of infant development are best understood when perceived in terms of the relationships between infants and the adults around them. Parents and their infants have mutual and constantly changing effects on one another. In addition, infants come into the world with inborn characteristics, formulated as temperament (Thomas & Chess, 1977). The caregiver-child interaction and experience are not the only causes of individual differences; rather, genetic and prenatal factors determine some individual differences even before postnatal experience begins, with some infants seemingly born more vulnerable than others, and therefore more adversely affected by unfavorable environments.

Although it is difficult to cope with poor environmental conditions, beginning in the 1990s, researchers focused on resilience, even in very young children, which somehow seems to enable resilient children to function in less than optimal conditions without necessarily having serious adverse long-term effects, as opposed to others who are less resilient and who respond deleteriously to the same conditions. In addition, infants are born with the ability to learn (Gopnik, Meltzoff, & Kuhl, 1999), and within the first days and weeks of life, infants have an ability to change their behavior according to responses from those in their environment. Even the very young infant is a complex person with many characteristics and abilities which cannot be separated from one another.

Today, it is accepted that research cannot investigate abilities in isolation, but must rather investigate an interwoven pattern of abilities and the manner in which different abilities affect the child's functioning and progress. For example, language development can best be understood as a method for interacting with others (social development) and expressing needs and desires (emotional development) and not as an isolated skill. Similarly, emotional development is recognized as being the foundation for learning, supporting the premise that developmental trajectories of young children are determined by multiple factors, and that each factor affects more than one infant characteristic. Research has also operationalized the fact that these developmental capabilities and individual attributes are to be found on a continuum, not simply present or absent, or good or bad, and needs to be specified and characterized. This is particularly important to remember when assessing difficulties, issues and problems which do not appear in isolation. Each problem needs to be considered in its full complexity, not as an artificially simplified characteristic, while remembering that the infant's early experiences have an effect on later development.

Developmental Change

Underlying almost all research in infant mental health is a concern with the rules that govern the nature of development and subsequent developmental change. Development is defined as the changes which occur through the process of natural growth, and is the result of learning from the environment and maturation, with learning being the change which results from experience, and maturation referring to the changes that occur as a result of biological factors. These two simultaneously occurring processes interact and the combined effect is greater than either would have had if it had occurred in isolation. Since "interaction" describes the shared effect at a given moment in time, Sameroff (1983) proposed the term "transaction" to describe changes in the nature of an interaction that occur over time as a result of continuing interaction. In other words, not only do maturation and learning interact, but also the nature of their interaction changes over time. The concept of transactions in development is an extraordinarily salient abstraction, as it takes into account changes in infants which affect the manner in which they experience the world and the manner in which the world experiences them.

In addition to the transactional approach to development, the study of infant development can be based on a dynamic systems perspective, which stresses the importance of interrelations between and among factors (Endsley, 1995). As infant mental health researchers have realized the complexity of relevant factors and the reciprocal impact they have on one another, they have adopted the systems approach to development. A dynamic-action system is a group of factors that influence each other and that are in a constant process of change, with the components of the system working together according to its own rules. Thus the system is self-organizing. Since no two systems have the same rules, each system is unique, and so even if all the components are the same, the outcome may be different. This variability in outcomes is limited by the possible configurations of the components of the system. Because the components are constantly interacting and as a result dynamically reconfiguring themselves, they can actually change into new components, which might result in the system beginning to function according to an entirely new set of rules.

Furthermore, infant mental health researchers are interested in patterns of developmental change. Different aspects of development show different patterns of change. Many are not linear, such as changes in size or the acquisition of a new ability that is based on an existing skill. In infant mental health, researchers are less concerned with specific stages of development and more concerned with the internal changes that involve a readiness to be affected by experience. The term "critical period" or "sensitive period" refers to a stage of special predisposition during development when events in the environment have an effect on development that they would not have had earlier and will not have to the same degree at a later stage. Critical periods have been demonstrated in a number of studies of animals, most famously the ducklings that imprinted on Konrad Lorenz (1937). Although the notion of critical periods is different for animals and humans, it remains a useful concept when assessing social and emotional development.

Implications of Early Development for Later Development

Infant mental health is based on the assumption that there are critical periods in early development and that early experience affects later development and behavior (Bornstein, 1989). Although a direct connection has not been unequivocally determined, most researchers agree that attempts to treat problems which began in infancy later in life are not always successful. Thus, it is important to understand the domains of infant mental health in order to address them in a timely and appropriate manner.

The central areas which define early mental health bridge different developmental domains including emotional, social and adaptive development. They include the young child's capacity to experience, tolerate and express a range of emotions without being overwhelmed (Berardi, Pizzorusso, & Maffei, 2000). Like other aspects of development, emotional growth depends on a combination of internal and external factors (Winnicott, 1965), and differentiation between them is not always easy. Infants differ one from another from birth in their individual responsiveness to the world around them, their sensitivities to stimulation and their reactions to that stimulation. Therefore one aspect of mental health in infancy revolves around infants' and young children's ability to regulate their emotional state (Gross & Muñoz, 1995; Schore, 2001).

Infant mental health extends beyond the internal world of infants to the interaction with people surrounding them and deals with the young child's ability to form and maintain mostly trusting intimate relationships with caregivers. Through secure attachment with the primary caregiver, young children learn about the world around them and gain the ability to explore the unknown and return to the safe haven provided by the caregiver when they feel the need. Finally, along with optimal conditions for emotional growth and a secure and supportive relationship with caregivers, the third developmental task to be included in the field of infant mental health is the young child's capability to learn age-appropriate culturally expected skills, in order to affiliate with the social context in which he or she will have to function. Socialization occurs within these complex, ever-changing dynamic systems. Not only do individual traits and family values affect the ability to function successfully, but cultural values, economic and political concerns also influence the process of socialization. Thus, throughout infancy and toddlerhood developmental changes occur in the child. These changes are stagelike in nature and follow a predictable sequence, usually with specific timing (Fischer, 1980; Flavell, 1982; Kagan, 1980). There are qualitative differences at different points in time and there are developmental tasks (Havighurst, 1972) which need to be mastered at a particular point in development in order for development to continue successfully. Facilitating the successful development of infants and young children is one of the primary purposes of the field of infant mental health.

In addition to attaining developmental motor, cognitive and language milestones, one of the most important developmental tasks for infants during the first year of life is to learn to manage their emotions and to increase their ability to maintain a balanced state. Zeanah (2012) posits that an issue of sensory, behavioral or emotional regulation can be identified for every challenge or problem in infancy. Infants' needs are immediate, and since even the most sensitive and responsive parent cannot always respond immediately, the ability to contain the child's intense and difficult feelings while waiting can be as important as the actual resolution. Bion (1984) described containment as the way in which one person could encompass the powerful feelings of another and could make them more manageable through touch, gesture and speech, while Winnicott (1960) described how parents continue to consciously include the needs of their baby in their minds, and consequently the infant experiences a sense of security because the caregiver conveys understanding of his or her needs, responds to distress signals and contains the infant's difficult feelings. As this pattern is consistently repeated the infant learns what to expect and that caregivers can be trusted. Babies who learn to co-regulate their emotions with their caregivers also gradually learn how to self-regulate their own emotions, which is a necessary developmental skill.

The Developing Sense of Self

The final topic in early development to be addressed in this introductory chapter is the child's "sense of self", which is based on the assumption that each child is unique and each child experiences the world in a unique manner. The manner in which the world assumes meaning is unique for each child, and by the same token each child affects the world uniquely. The continuing interchange of the child and his or her unique meaning of the world is the basis of the child's sense of self. Thus, the field of infant mental health focuses on each unique individual, emphasizing individual differences as expressed in temperament, parental characteristics which affect parenting styles, and transactional changes in the caregiver-child relationship over time (Sameroff, 2010). The field of infant mental health is fundamentally interested in the multiple levels at which the child develops, ranging from the cellular and genetic to cultural and societal levels. There is a complex interaction among these levels throughout the lifespan, but because so many of these changes occur during infancy, they affect the young child's developing sense of self and must be addressed when studying infant mental health. The infant comes into the world with certain inborn capacities, vulnerabilities and proclivities. These parameters and traits come into contact with the caregivers whose responses to the child begin the process of formulating a sense of self (Rochat, 2014).

Research in the field of infant mental health consists of characterizing variables which interact to determine the emotional state of the very young child and which are involved in the child's developing sense of self. Consolidating a sense of self and making sense of the world by actively exploring and organizing the world occurs within the context of human relationships and results from the transactions between the active self and a responsive environment. Infants' earliest experiences with others and the intense relationship which is built between the parents and the child during the first 6 months of life are the foundation of the emerging self. As intentional communication and turn-taking emerge, infants begin to experience more self-knowledge as their interactional repertoire increases along with their control over their own and others' behavior. By the end of the first year of the baby's life, there is a broad sense of self and the beginnings of empathy (Davidov, Zahn-Waxler, Roth-Hanania, & Knafo, 2013), and with expanding symbolic knowledge of the world, including pretend play and language, the child begins to refer to self and others, can identify self in the mirror (Bischof-Köhler, 2012) and begins limit testing (Winnicott, 1965). Thus, the developing sense of self is both influenced by and influences the young child, the parents, the whole family system, other factors in the environment, and the quality of interaction among these variables. The interface between the infant's biological and genetic potentials, the nature and the quality of the young child's most significant relationships and the social and cultural context in which the child is being raised is one of the central aspects of the study of infant mental health.

References

Andersen, S. L. (2003). Trajectories of brain development: Point of vulnerability or window of opportunity? *Neuroscience & Biobehavioral Reviews, 27*(1), 3–18.

Arnott, B., & Meins, E. (2007). Links among antenatal attachment representations, postnatal mind-mindedness, and infant attachment security: A preliminary study of mothers and fathers. *Bulletin of the Menninger Clinic, 71*(2), 132–149.

Bakermans-Kranenburg, M. J., Van IJzendoorn, M. H., & Juffer, F. (2003). Less is more: Meta-analyses of sensitivity and attachment interventions in early childhood. *Psychological Bulletin, 129*(2), 195–215.

Beebe, B., Lachmann, F., & Jaffe, J. (1997). Mother—Infant interaction structures and presymbolic self-and object representations. *Psychoanalytic Dialogues, 7*(2), 133–182.

Beebe, B., Jaffe, J., Markese, S., Buck, K., Chen, H., Cohen, P., . . . & Feldstein, S. (2010). The origins of 12-month attachment: A microanalysis of 4-month mother–infant interaction. *Attachment & Human Development, 12*(1–2), 3–141.

Belsky, J. (1984). The determinants of parenting: A process model. *Child Development, 55*(1), 83–96.

Belsky, J., & Fearon, R. M. P. (2002). Infant–Mother attachment security, contextual risk, and early development: A moderational analysis. *Development and Psychopathology, 14*, 293–310.

Berardi, N., Pizzorusso, T., & Maffei, L. (2000). Critical periods during sensory development. *Current Opinion in Neurobiology, 10*(1), 138–145.

Bion, W. R. (1984). *Learning from experience* (Vol. 22). Sterling, VA: Stylus Publishing, LLC.

Bischof-Köhler, D. (2012). Empathy and self-recognition in phylogenetic and ontogenetic perspective. *Emotion Review, 4*(1), 40–48.

Bornstein, M. H. (1989). Sensitive periods in development: Structural characteristics and causal interpretations. *Psychological Bulletin, 105*(2), 179–197.

Bowlby, J. (1956). *The growth of independence in the young child.* Publisher not identified.

Bowlby, J. (1969). *Attachment and loss: Vol. 1. Attachment.* New York, NY: Basic Books.

Bowlby, J. (1989). *Attachments and loss.* Los Angeles, CA: Continuing Education Seminars.

Boyce, W. T., Sokolowski, M. B., & Robinson, G. E. (2012). Toward a new biology of social adversity. *Proceedings of the National Academy of Sciences, 109*(Suppl 2), 17143–17148.

Bretherton, I., Fritz, J., Zahn-Waxler, C., & Ridgeway, D. (1986). Learning to talk about emotions: A functionalist perspective. *Child Development, 56*, 529–548.

Bronfenbrenner, U. (1979). Contexts of child rearing: Problems and prospects. *American Psychologist, 34*(10), 844–850.

Bronfenbrenner, U. (1986). Ecology of the family as a context for human development: Research perspectives. *Developmental Psychology, 22*(6), 723–742.

Bronfenbrenner, U., & Ceci, S. J. (1994). Nature-nurture reconceptualized in developmental perspective: A bioecological model. *Psychological Review, 101*(4), 568–586.

Bronfenbrenner, U., & Morris, P. A. (2006). The bioecological model of human development. In R. M. Lerner (Ed.), *Handbook of child psychology: Vol. 1. Theoretical models of human development* (6th ed., pp. 793–828). New York, NY: Wiley.

Brooks, R., & Goldstein, S. (2001). *Raising resilient children: Fostering strength, hope, and optimism in your child.* New York, NY: MacGraw Hill.

Campos, J. J., & Barrett, K. C. (1984). Toward a new understanding of emotions and their development. In C. E. Izard, J. Kagan, & R. B. Zajonc (Eds.), *Emotions, cognition, and behavior* (pp. 229–263). Cambridge, UK: Cambridge University Press.

Caplan, H. L., Cogill, S. R., Alexandra, H., Robson, K. M., Katz, R., & Kumar, R. (1989). Maternal depression and the emotional development of the child. *The British Journal of Psychiatry, 154*(6), 818–822.

Cassidy, J. (1994). Emotion regulation: Influences of attachment relationships. *Monographs of the Society for Research in Child Development, 59*(2-3), 228–249.

Charlesworth, W. R. (1982). An ethological approach to research on facial expressions. In C. E. Izard (Ed.), *Measuring emotions in infants and children* (pp. 317–334). Cambridge, UK: Cambridge University Press.

Cicchetti, D. (2013). An overview of developmental psychopathology. In *The Oxford handbook of developmental psychology* (Vol. 2, pp. 455–480). Oxford: Oxford University Press.

Cicchetti, D., & Toth, S. L. (1997). Transactional ecological systems in developmental psychopathology. In S. S. Luthar, J. Burack, D. Cicchetti, & J. Weisz (Eds.), *Developmental psychopathology: Perspectives on adjustment, risk, and disorder* (pp. 317–349). New York: Cambridge University Press.

Coghill, S. R., Caplan, H. L., Alexandra, H., Robson, K., & Kumar, R. (1986). Impact of maternal postnatal depression on cognitive development of young children. *British Medical Journal, 292*, 1165–1167.

Cohen, J. A. S., & Semple, R. J. (2010). Mindful parenting: A call for research. *Journal of Child and Family Studies, 19*, 145–151.

Contreras, J. M., Narang, D., Ikhlas, M., & Teichman, J. (2002). A conceptual model of the determinants of parenting among Latina adolescent mothers. In J. M. Contreras, K. Kerns, & A. Neal-Barnett (Eds.), *Latino children and families in the United States: Current research and future directions* (pp. 155–177). Westport, CT: Praeger Publishers/Greenwood Publishing Group.

Corrigan, P. W. (2000). Mental health stigma as social attribution: Implications for research methods and attitude change. *Clinical Psychology: Science and Practice, 7*(1), 48–67.

Crittenden, P. M. (1990). Internal representational models of attachment relationships. *Infant Mental Health Journal, 11*(3), 259–277.

Davidov, M., Zahn-Waxler, C., Roth-Hanania, R., & Knafo, A. (2013). Concern for others in the first year of life: Theory, evidence, and avenues for research. *Child Development Perspectives, 7*(2), 126–131.

Dawson, G., Hessl, D., & Frey, K. (1994). Social influences on early developing biological and behavioral symptoms related to risk for affective disorder. *Development and Psychopathology, 6*, 759–779.

Dozier, M., Stovall-McClough, K. C., & Albus, K. E. (2008). Attachment and psychopathology in adulthood. In J. Cassidy & P. R. Shaver (Eds.), *Handbook of attachment: Theory, research, and clinical applications* (2nd ed., pp. 718–744). New York, NY: Guilford Press.

Dunst, C. J. (2000). Revisiting" rethinking early intervention". *Topics in Early Childhood Special Education, 20*(2), 95–104.

Endsley, M. R. (1995). Toward a theory of situation awareness in dynamic systems. *Human Factors: The Journal of the Human Factors and Ergonomics Society, 37*(1), 32–64.

Farrington, D. (1994). Early developmental prevention of juvenile delinquency. *RSA Journal, 142*(5454), 22–34.

Feldman, R. (2007). Parent–Infant synchrony: Biological foundations and developmental outcomes. *Current Directions in Psychological Science, 16*(6), 340–345.

Feldman, R. (2012). Oxytocin and social affiliation in humans. *Hormones and Behavior, 61*(3), 380–391.

Field, T. (1994). The effects of mother's physical and emotional unavailability on emotion regulation. *Monographs of the Society for Research in Child Development, 59*(2–3), 208–227.

Field, T., Healy, B., Goldstein, S., & Guthertz, M. (1990). Behavior-state matching and synchrony in mother-infant interactions of nondepressed versus depressed dyads. *Developmental Psychology, 26*, 7–14.

Fischer, K. W. (1980). A theory of cognitive development: The control and construction of hierarchies of skills. *Psychological Review, 87*(6), 477–531.

Flavell, J. H. (1982). On cognitive development. *Child Development, 53*, 1–10.

Foley, G. M., & Hochman, J. D. (Eds.). (2006). *Mental health in early intervention: Achieving unity in principles and practice*. Baltimore, MD: Brookes Publishers.

Fonagy, P., Gergely, G., & Jurist, E. L. (Eds.). (2004). *Affect regulation, mentalization and the development of the self.* London, UK: Karnac Books.

Fonagy, P., Steele, M., & Steele, H. (1991). Intergenerational patterns of attachment: Maternal representations during pregnancy and subsequent infant-mother attachments. *Child Development, 62*, 891–905.

Fonagy, P., Steele, M., Steele, H., Moran, G. S., & Higgitt, A. C. (1991). The capacity for understanding mental states: The reflective self in parent and child and its significance for security of attachment. *Infant Mental Health Journal, 12*(3), 201–218.

Fox, N. A., Henderson, H. A., Marshall, P. J., Nichols, K. E., & Ghera, M. M. (2005). Behavioral inhibition: Linking biology and behavior within a developmental framework. *Annual Reviews of Psychology, 56*, 235–262.

Fraiberg, S. (1977). *Insights from the blind: Comparative studies of blind and sighted infants.* New York, NY: Basic Books.

Fraiberg, S., Adelson, E., & Shapiro, V. (1975). Ghosts in the nursery: A psychoanalytic approach to the problems of impaired infant-mother relationships. *Journal of the American Academy of Child Psychiatry, 14*(3), 387–421.

Freud, S. (1955). From the history of an infantile neurosis. In *The standard edition of the complete psychological works of Sigmund Freud, Volume XVII (1917–1919): An infantile neurosis and other works* (pp. 1–124). New York, NY: Random House.

Gerhardt, S. (2006). Why love matters: How affection shapes a baby's brain. *Infant Observation, 9* (3), 305–309.

Gopnik, A., Meltzoff, A. N., & Kuhl, P. K. (1999). *The scientist in the crib: Minds, brains, and how children learn*. New York, NY: William Morrow & Co.

Greenberg, M. T. (1999). Attachment and psychopathology in childhood. In J. Cassidy & P. R. Shaver (Eds.), *Handbook of attachment: Theory, research, and clinical applications* (pp. 469–496). New York, NY: Guildford Publications.

Gross, J. J., & Muñoz, R. F. (1995). Emotion regulation and mental health. *Clinical Psychology: Science and Practice, 2*(2), 151–164.

Guralnick, M. J. (1997). Effectiveness of early intervention for vulnerable children: A developmental perspective. *American Journal on Mental Retardation, 102*(4), 319–345.

Harris, M., & Bick, E. (1976). The contribution of observation of mother-infant interaction and development to the equipment of a psychoanalyst or psychoanalytic psychotherapist. *Collected Papers of Martha Harris and Esther Bick*, 225–239.

Havighurst, R. J. (1972). *Developmental tasks and education*. New York, NY: McKay Company.

Hazan, C., & Shaver, P. (1987). Romantic love conceptualized as an attachment process. *Journal of Personality and Social Psychology, 52*(3), 511–524.

Hazan, C., & Shaver, P. R. (1994). Attachment as an organizational framework for research on close relationships. *Psychological Inquiry, 5*(1), 1–22.

Honig, A. S. (2002). *Secure relationships: Nurturing infant/toddler attachment in early care settings*. National Association for the Education of Young Children, 1509 16th Street, NW, Washington, DC 20036.

Isabella, R. A., & Belsky, J. (1991). Interactional synchrony and the origins of infant-mother attachment: A replication study. *Child Development, 62*(2), 373–384.

Isabella, R. A., Belsky, J., & von Eye, A. (1989). Origins of infant-mother attachment: An examination of interactional synchrony during the infant's first year. *Developmental Psychology, 25*(1), 12–21.

Johnson, M. H. & de Haan, M. (2015). *Developmental cognitive neuroscience (4th edition)*. New York, NY: Wiley.

Juffer, F., Bakermans-Kranenburg, M. J., & van IJzendoorn, M. H. (Eds.). (2012). *Promoting positive parenting: an attachment-based intervention*. London, UK: Routledge.

Kagan, J. (1980). *Infancy: Its place in human development*. Cambridge, MA: Harvard University Press.

Keller, H., Lamm, B., Abels, M., Yovsi, R., Borke, J., Jensen, H., ... & Chaudhary, N. (2006). Cultural models, socialization goals, and parenting ethnotheories: A multicultural analysis. *Journal of Cross-Cultural Psychology, 37*(2), 155–172.

Keller, H., Völker, S., & Yovsi, R. D. (2005). Conceptions of parenting in different cultural communities: The case of West African Nso and Northern German women. *Social Development, 14*(1), 158–180.

Kerns, K. A., & Brumariu, L. E. (2014). Is insecure parent–child attachment a risk factor for the development of anxiety in childhood or adolescence? *Child Development Perspectives, 8*(1), 12–17.

Kretchmar, M. D., & Jacobvitz, D. B. (2002). Observing mother-child relationships across generations: Boundary patterns, attachment, and the transmission of caregiving. *Family Process, 41*(3), 351–374.

Leerkes, E. M., Blankson, A. N., & O'Brien, M. (2009). Differential effects of maternal sensitivity to infant distress and nondistress on social-emotional functioning. *Child Development, 80*(3), 762–775.

Lerner, R. M., & Busch-Rossnagel, N. A. (Eds.). (2013). *Individuals as producers of their development: A life-span perspective*. Amsterdam, The Netherlands: Elsevier.

Lewis, M., & Saarni, C. (Eds.). (1985). *The socialization of emotions* (Vol. 5). New York, NY: Springer.

Lieberman, A. F., & Van Horn, P. (2011). *Psychotherapy with infants and young children: Repairing the effects of stress and trauma on early attachment*. New York, NY: Guilford Press.

Link, B. G., & Phelan, J. C. (2006). Stigma and its public health implications. *The Lancet, 367* (9509), 528–529.

Link, B. G., Struening, E. L., Rahav, M., Phelan, J. C., & Nuttbrock, L. (1997). On stigma and its consequences: Evidence from a longitudinal study of men with dual diagnoses of mental illness and substance abuse. *Journal of Health and Social Behavior, 38*, 177–190.

Lorenz, K. Z. (1937). The companion in the bird's world. *The Auk, 54*, 245–273.

Love, J. M., Kisker, E. E., Ross, C. M., Schochet, P. Z., Brooks-Gunn, J., Paulsell, D., . . . & Brady-Smith, C. (2002). *Making a difference in the lives of infants and toddlers and their families: The impacts of early Head Start* (Volumes I-III: Final technical report [and] appendixes [and] local contributions to understanding the programs and their impacts).

Love, J. M., Kisker, E. E., Ross, C., Raikes, H., Constantine, J., Boller, K., . . . & Fuligni, A. S. (2005). The effectiveness of early head start for 3-yearold children and their parents: Lessons for policy and programs. *Developmental Psychology, 41*(6), 885–901.

Main, M., Kaplan, N., & Cassidy, J. (1985). Security in infancy, childhood and adulthood: A move to the level of representation, growing points of attachment theory and research. *Monographs of the Society for Research in Child Development, 50*, 66–104.

Main, M. (1996). Introduction to the special section on attachment and psychopathology: 2. Overview of the field of attachment. *Journal of Consulting and Clinical Psychology, 64*(2), 237–243.

Meins, E. (1999). Sensitivity, security and internal working models: Bridging the transmission gap. *Attachment and Human Development, 1*, 325–342.

Meins, E., Fernyhough, C., Russell, J., & Clark-Carter, D. (1998). Security of attachment as a predictor of symbolic and mentalising abilities: A longitudinal study. *Social Development, 7*, 1–24.

Miga, E. M., Hare, A., Allen, J. P., & Manning, N. (2010). The relation of insecure attachment states of mind and romantic attachment styles to adolescent aggression in romantic relationships. *Attachment & Human Development, 12*, 463–481.

Murray, L., & Cooper, P. J. (1997). Effects of postnatal depression on infant development. *Archives of Disease in Childhood, 77*(2), 99–101.

Murray, L., Fiori-Cowley, A., Hooper, R., & Cooper, P. (1996). The impact of postnatal depression and associated adversity on early mother-infant interactions and later infant outcome. *Child Development, 67*(5), 2512–2526.

Ordway, M. R., Webb, D., Sadler, L. S., & Slade, A. (2015). Parental reflective functioning: An approach to enhancing parent-child relationships in pediatric primary care. *Journal of Pediatric Health Care, 29*(4), 325–334.

Osofsky, J. D., & Fitzgerald, H. E. (2000). *WAIMH handbook of infant mental health (volume 1): Perspectives on infant mental health*. Chichester, UK: Wiley.

Owen, D. J., Slep, A. M., & Heyman, R. E. (2012). The effect of praise, positive nonverbal response, reprimand, and negative nonverbal response on child compliance: A systematic review. *Clinical Child and Family Psychology Review, 15*(4), 364–385.

Perry, B. D. (2009). Examining child maltreatment through a neurodevelopmental lens: Clinical applications of the neurosequential model of therapeutics. *Journal of Loss and Trauma, 14*(4), 240–255.

Phelan, J. C., Bromet, E. J., & Link, B. G. (1998). Psychiatric illness and family stigma. *Schizophrenia Bulletin, 24*(1), 115–126.

Prior, V., & Glaser, D. (2006). *Understanding attachment and attachment disorders: Theory, evidence and practice*. London, UK: Jessica Kingsley Publishers.

Puig, J., Englund, M. M., Simpson, J. A., & Collins, W. A. (2013). Predicting adult physical illness from infant attachment: A prospective longitudinal study. *Health Psychology, 32*(4), 409–417.

Rochat, P. (Ed.). (2014). *Early social cognition: Understanding others in the first months of life*. New York, NY: Psychology Press.

Rubin, K. H., & Chung, O. B. (Eds.). (2013). *Parenting beliefs, behaviors, and parent-child relations: A cross-cultural perspective*. New York, NY: Psychology Press.

Rutter, M. (2005). Environmentally mediated risks for psychopathology: Research strategies and findings. *Journal of the American Academy of Child & Adolescent Psychiatry, 44*(1), 3–18.

Rutter, M. (2012). Resilience as a dynamic concept. *Development and Psychopathology, 24*(02), 335–344.

Rutter, M., & Sroufe, L. A. (2000). Developmental psychopathology: Concepts and challenges. *Development and Psychopathology, 12*, 265–296.

Ruttle, P. L., Serbin, L. A., Stack, D. M., Schwartzman, A. E., & Shirtcliff, E. A. (2011). Adrenocortical attunement in mother–child dyads: Importance of situational and behavioral characteristics. *Biological Psychology, 88*(1), 104–111.

Sameroff, A. J. (1983). Developmental systems: contexts and evolution. In W. Kessen (Series Ed.) & P. H. Mussen (Vol. Ed.), *Handbook of child psychology: Vol. 4. History, theories, and method* (pp. 238–294). New York, NY: Wiley.

Sameroff, A. (1975). Transactional models in early social relations. *Human Development, 18*(1-2), 65–79.

Sameroff, A. (2000). Ecological perspectives on developmental risk. In J. D. Osofsky & H. E. Fitzgerald (Eds.), *WAIMH handbook of infant mental health* (Infant mental health in groups at high risk, Vol. 4, pp. 1–33). New York, NY: Wiley.

Sameroff, A. (2009). *The transactional model*. Washington, DC: American Psychological Association.

Sameroff, A. J. (2010). A unified theory of development: A dialectic integration of nature and nurture. *Child Development, 81*, 6–22.

Sameroff, A. J., & Chandler, M. J. (1975). Reproductive risk and the continuum of caretaking casualty. *Review of Child Development Research, 4*, 187–244.

Sameroff, A. J., & Fiese, B. H. (2000). Transactional regulation: The developmental ecology of early intervention. In J. P. Shonkoff & S. J. Meisels (Eds.), *Handbook of early childhood intervention* (pp. 135–159). Cambridge, UK: Cambridge University Press.

Schore, A. N. (2001). Effects of a secure attachment relationship on right brain development, affect regulation, and infant mental health. *Infant Mental Health Journal, 22*(1–2), 7–66.

Shiota, M. N., Campos, B., Keltner, D., & Hertenstein, M. J. (2004). Positive emotion and the regulation of interpersonal relationships. In P. Philippot & R. Feldman (Eds.), *The regulation of emotion* (pp. 127–155). New York, NY: Psychology Press.

Siegel, D. J. (2012). *The developing mind: How relationships and the brain interact to shape who we are*. New York, NY: Guilford Press.

Slade, A. (2002). Keeping the baby in mind: A critical factor in perinatal mental health. *Zero to Three, 22*(6), 10–16.

Slade, A. (2005). Parental reflective functioning: An introduction. *Attachment & Human Development, 7*(3), 269–281.

Sroufe, L. A. (2000). Early relationships and the development of children. *Infant Mental Health Journal, 21*(1–2), 67–74.

Sroufe, L. A. (2005). Attachment and development: A prospective, longitudinal study from birth to adulthood. *Attachment & Human Development, 7*(4), 349–367.

Sroufe, L., Carlson, E. A., Levy, A. K., & Egeland, B. (1999). Implications of attachment theory for developmental psychopathology. *Development and Psychopathology, 11*(01), 1–13.

Steele, H., Steele, M., & Fonagy, P. (1996). Associations among attachment classifications of mothers, fathers, and their infants. *Child Development, 67*(2), 541–555.

Stern, D. N. (1974). The goal and structure of mother-infant play. *Journal of the American Academy of Child Psychiatry, 13*(3), 402–421.
Stern, D. N. (1995). *Motherhood constellation*. London, UK: Karnac Books.
Stern, D. N. (2000). *The interpersonal world of the infant: A view from psychoanalysis and developmental psychology*. New York, NY: Basic Books.
Stern, D. N. (2009). *The first relationship: Infant and mother*. Cambridge, MA: Harvard University Press.
Thomas, A., & Chess, S. (1977). *Temperament and development*. New York, NY: Brunner/Mazel.
Thompson, R. A. (1994). Emotion regulation: A theme in search of definition. *Monographs of the Society for Research in Child Development, 59*(2-3), 25–52.
Trevarthen, C. (1979). Communication and cooperation in early infancy: A description of primary intersubjectivity. In M. Bullowa (Ed.), *Before speech: The beginnings of interpersonal communication* (pp. 321–348). Cambridge, UK: Cambridge University Press.
Trevarthen, C. (1984). Emotions in infancy: Regulators of contact and relationships with persons. In K. Scherer & P. Eckman (Eds.), *Approaches to emotion* (pp. 129–157). Hillsdale, NJ: Lawrence Erlbaum Associates.
Tronick, E., Als, H., & Brazelton, T. B. (1977). Mutuality in mother-infant interaction. *Journal of Communication, 27*(2), 74–79.
Tronick, E., & Beeghly, M. (2011). Infants' meaning-making and the development of mental health problems. *American Psychologist, 66*(2), 107–119.
Tronick, E., & Cohn, J. F. (1989). Infant-mother face-to-face interaction: Age and gender differences in coordination and the occurrence of miscoordination. *Child Development, 60*, 85–92.
Van IJzendoorn, M. H. (1992). Intergenerational transmission of parenting: A review of studies in nonclinical populations. *Developmental Review, 12*(1), 76–99.
Van IJzendoorn, M. H., & Bakermans-Kranenburg, M. J. (1997). Intergenerational transmission of attachment: A move to the contextual level. In L. Atkinson & K.J. Zucker (Eds.), *Attachment and Psychopathology* (pp. 135–170) New York, NY: Guilford Press.
Van IJzendoorn, M. H., Juffer, F., & Duyvesteyn, M. G. (1995). Breaking the intergenerational cycle of insecure attachment: A review of the effects of attachment-based interventions on maternal sensitivity and infant security. *Journal of Child Psychology and Psychiatry, and Allied Disciplines, 36*, 225–225.
Vimpani, A. (2004). Challenges for professionals working with children placed in kinship care and their families: A clinical study and literature review. *Developing Practice: The Child, Youth and Family Work Journal, 10*, 24–35.
Webster-Stratton, C. (1998). Preventing conduct problems in Head Start children: strengthening parent competencies. *Journal of Consulting and Clinical Psychology, 66*(5), 715–730.
Werner, E. E. (1985). Stress and protective factors in children's lives. In A.R. Nicol (Ed.), *Longitudinal Studies in Child Psychology and Psychiatry* (pp. 335–355). Chichester, England: Wiley.
Winnicott, D. W. (1960). The theory of the parent-infant relationship. *International Journal of Psychoanalysis, 41*(6), 585–595.
Winnicott, D. W. (1965). The maturational processes and the facilitating environment: Studies in the theory of emotional development. In *The international psycho-analytical library* (pp. 37–55). London, UK: The Hogarth Press and the Institute of Psycho-Analysis.
Winnicott, D. W. (1984). *Delinquency and deprivation*. London, UK: Routledge.
Wylie, M. S., & Turner, L. (2011). The attuned therapist. *Psychotherapy Networker, 35*, 19–27.
Zeanah, C. H. (2012). *Proposal to include child and adolescent age related manifestations and age related subtypes for PTSD in DSM-V*. Arlington, VA: American Psychiatric Association.
Zeanah, C. H., Berlin, L. J., & Boris, N. W. (2011). Practitioner review: Clinical applications of attachment theory and research for infants and young children. *Journal of Child Psychology and Psychiatry, 52*(8), 819–833.
Zigler, E., & Muenchow, S. (1992). *Head start*. New York, NY: Basic Books.

Chapter 2
Social and Emotional Development in Infant and Early Childhood Mental Health

Introduction

Infancy and early childhood are periods of extraordinary developmental changes, as the child begins to walk independently and thus gain more independence in the physical and social world. Through these new interactions with the world around them, children develop a sense of self and self-other relations, as well as an awareness of the cultural milieu and its practices. These practices are the foundation of beginning moral evaluations of one's own and others' behavior, and the acceptance of adults' rules for behavior. Evolving regulatory strategies allow young children to align their behavior with parental and societal expectations. As children move from infancy to toddlerhood and through early childhood, attaining language, motor and cognitive developmental skills, their social and emotional competence changes profoundly and forms the underpinnings of their mental health. This is the period in which self-concept, self-regulation, emotional control, empathy, and altruism develop, alongside a deeper understanding of interpersonal interactions and communication.

By examining these abilities through a developmental lens, it is possible to gain a more comprehensive understanding of the mechanisms underlying infant and early childhood mental health, the interrelatedness among the developing systems and the distinctiveness of social emotional development. A focus on infant and early childhood mental health through a developmental lens serves as the basis of this chapter which will include a discussion of research in the biology of social emotional development, its behavioral manifestations, and the importance of social relationships for development. Developmental trajectories will be presented across multiple systems including social, emotional, cognitive and linguistic development, and across processes such as regulatory, reflective, and representational, in an attempt to conceptualize infant and early childhood mental health on the basis of

C. Shulman, *Research and Practice in Infant and Early Childhood Mental Health*,
Children's Well-Being: Indicators and Research 13,
DOI 10.1007/978-3-319-31181-4_2

empirical findings in developmental research, while emphasizing the intrapersonal and interactional variables involved in development through early childhood.

Conceptualizing Early Development

Immediately after birth, the child is called an infant, which comes from the Latin word, infans, which means without speech. As the child begins to walk, the word toddler is often applied, describing the unsteady walk of the young child at this age, when cognitive, linguistic, emotional, social and motor abilities are rapidly changing. Children growing out of the period of toddlerhood are referred to as preschoolers, reflecting the sociological framework and the time at which young children begin to spend more time in an educational framework. Not all cultures have the same division of early childhood. For example, in Arabic and Italian there is only one inclusive term for all young children until they enter school. The selective manner in which young children are labelled, and consequently viewed, in a particular culture or social group is both reflected and dictated by linguistic groupings.

It appears that the word "toddler" first appeared as a grouping for economic reasons, when a group of retailers wanted to market a new line of clothing for young children between infancy and the preschool years (Cook, 2004). By using a new label, toddler, a new niche was created and a specialty line was generated. Interestingly, developmentalists do not typically define these periods in terms of exact ages, but rather by the acquisition of skills which operationalize each period (Brownell & Kopp, 2010). For example, some define toddlerhood as beginning at 18 months, whereas others consider 18 month olds as babies and begin using the label toddler at 24 months. The flexibility in determining beginning and endpoint demarcations of each developmental period reflects the recognition that development is not a simple, linear process and does not necessarily occur in a set sequence, and yet it is possible to specify and characterize typical and atypical developmental trajectories.

By researching the skills and competencies that emerge over the first 3 years of life from a developmental stance, it may be possible to relate to questions regarding the nature and course of change, the mechanisms underlying it, and its implications for infant and early childhood mental health. The development of social emotional competence is most clearly characterized by its changes over time, rather than by examining a skill at a particular point in time under circumscribed conditions. The developmental prism may offer a way of understanding the supports and resources necessary for social emotional competence which lies at the heart of infant mental health. Similarly it is possible to investigate the degree to which presumed competencies are robust at different ages under similar circumstances and under different circumstances at similar ages.

It is important to understand how these competencies are measured and defined in order to decide if findings from different methodologies are comparable. For example, when studying empathy, it is possible to find empirical support for the claim that 18 month olds have empathy, but it is not clear if this is only towards the child's mother, or in a particular emotional valence (Svetlova, Nichols, &

Brownell, 2010), or when other cognitive, social and attentional demands are not being placed on the young child. Likewise it is important to understand whether these findings emerged in natural settings or in the laboratory and whether the responses were spontaneous or elicited (Brownell, Svetlova, & Nichols, 2009; Spinrad & Stifter, 2006). Only by taking into consideration questions regarding how children's social emotional competencies change over time and how they vary as a function of setting will it be possible to investigate the complexities of social emotional development in the first years of life and their implications for infant and early childhood mental health.

In addition to recognizing the need for understanding the implications of the various ways in which empirical findings regarding the development of social emotional skills can be interpreted, it is important to appreciate that theoretical disagreements exist about the nature of change in social emotional development. Some theorists posit that children are born with innate, discrete domains of functioning (e.g., Onishi & Baillargeon, 2005), which develop according to a set timetable (e.g., Fletcher et al., 1995; Leslie, 1987), while others claim that developmental change can be conceptualized as a series of self-related processes maturing from bodily experiences, as the infant links his or her own body and actions and others' bodies and actions (Meltzoff, 2007; Meltzoff & Moore, 1998; Trevarthen, 1979). Tomasello (1999) conceptualizes early social and emotional development as the outcome of an early ability to mentally simulate others' internal psychological states, extrapolating downward to younger ages from adult developmental models. Middle ground can be found in the argument that social and emotional development in the first years of life can be conceptualized as the gradual emergence of social emotional abilities through continuous interactions between social and cognitive processes, increasing in complexity over time and with experience and the appearance of qualitatively new capacities. Thus development can be conceptualized as the result of the interaction between the developmental processes and the growing differentiation and specialization of brain functioning and physiological structures from earlier and simpler levels (e.g., Nelson & Fivush, 2004).

An interesting example of this differentiation appears along gender lines by the end of the first year, when infants seem to associate men's voices with pictures of men and women's voices with women's pictures (Green, Kuhl, Meltzoff, & Stevens, 1991), providing support for the claim that they are already able to discriminate cross-modally and associate auditory stimuli with visual ones as a result of the attention they pay to the social world around them. Infants tend to look more at mothers (as opposed to fathers) when no particular emotional valence in facial expression is exhibited, whereas when discerning between happy and fearful expressions, infants will look more at the fearful expression regardless of gender (Hirshberg & Svejda, 1990). One possible explanation for this is that children differentiate by gender because they experience mothers and fathers differently as a consequence of their divergent parenting styles. It has been shown that mothers' interactions with children characteristically include more soothing behavior, whereas more physical and exciting playful interactions are associated with fathers. These divergent parenting styles become even more pronounced at the toddler stage, when mothers tend to make more attempts to control and socialize the toddlers' behavior than fathers do. Although mothers are more intrusive than fathers at this age, they tend to be less directive than fathers, using cajoling or questioning techniques, such as "Would you like to have lunch now?" or "Everyone is going out". Fathers' style has been characterized as more directly assertive, exerting direct pressure on the toddler to comply. On the other hand, mothers have been shown to be more likely to carry a screaming child upstairs and place him in a crib than fathers (McKinney & Renk, 2008).

Brain and Behavior in Early Development

Cognitive Development

Regardless of the theoretical orientation, it is clear that the first years of life for the growing child are grounded in interacting systems and processes. As technology improves it becomes possible to trace physiological changes in the developing brain and look for concomitant behavioral manifestations, in order to understand some of the correlations between brain and behavior during this period of pervasive developmental change. Evolutionary adaptations have led to unique and specialized developments in the human brain of particular attributes, traits and functioning (Decety & Jackson, 2004; Donald, 1991; Finlay, Darlington, & Nicastro, 2001). By studying certain developmental milestones, such as object permanence, which is the ability to understand that objects and people continue to exist even when they are out of sight, a skill which requires stable and permanent mental representations through variations in time and space, it is possible to understand the cognitive experience of developing children in greater depth. Object permanence is one of the many skills at the base of infant and early childhood mental health, as children need to grasp that those who provide for them and emotionally nurture them continue to exist and are available even when unseen and that, although surface characteristics can change, the fundamental existence and identity of the caregivers remain constant in the child's life.

By extending original Piagetian tasks of object permanence (Piaget, 1952) to nonhuman primates (Call, 2001; Collier-Baker & Suddendorf, 2006) and toddlers (Collier-Baker & Suddendorf, 2006; Kopp, Sigman, & Parmelee, 1974) and by realizing the emotional and social aspects inherent in achieving object permanence above and beyond the cognitive elements, the study of object permanence has become seminal in providing support for the hypothesis that young children acquire an elemental understanding of their animate (social) and inanimate (object) worlds within an environment that provides numerous possibilities for developing secure attachmentswith caregivers as they appear, disappear and reappear. Significantly, it is this fundamental ability to represent permanence in the physical and social world that provides the foundation for the formation of multiple, complex interpersonal relationships and the ability to communicate about the world with others, foundational skills of infant and early childhood mental health.

In addition to the young child's growing cognitive abilities which serve as the foundation for social learning, it is the infant's ability to inhibit his or her behavior appropriately which supports social and emotional development in the first years of life. The study of young children's aggressive behavior leads to an understanding of developmentally adaptive and non-adaptive behavior. It is possible to observe physical aggression as early as 12 months and normatively it peaks in the second year of life, declining in the early preschool years (Tremblay et al., 2005). Normative decline in aggressive behavior may result from increased inhibitory control, self-regulatory strategies, understanding of others' feelings and intentions and the ability to use language to negotiate interpersonal challenges. Differential patterns of aggression can be partially explained by parenting style and by parents' responses to aggression (Khoury-Kassabri, 2010), and are mediated by the child's gender, temperament, and neurodevelopmental functioning, as well as by family values and resources (Calkins & Johnson, 1998; Fagot & Hagan, 1991; Hay, Heron, & Ness, 2005; Martin & Ross, 2005; Shaw, Keenan, & Vondra, 1994).

Some risk factors for negative outcomes in infant and early childhood mental health have been identified and include adverse child, parent, family and environmental variables, which contribute to persistent aggression lasting longer than would be expected from typical developmental stages. This association between risk factors and adverse outcomes seems to operate additively and interactively (NICHD Early Child Care Research Network, 2004). However, it is inappropriate to discuss risk factors without noting that a variety of social and emotional developmental capabilities, including the ability to empathize, prosocial behaviors, ability to read others' intentions, interest in social play, acquiring self-regulatory mechanisms, and understanding self in relation to others, may be correlated with other more positive outcomes and have been conceptualized as protective factors. Outcomes for any particular child are the result of the dynamic interplay between that child's risk and protective factors interacting within a developmental context (Rutter & Sroufe, 2000).

The study of behaviors associated with positive and adverse outcomes in infant mental health has also guided research into the connection between brain and behavior. Specifically, researchers (e.g., Dawson, Klinger, Panagiotides, Hill, & Spieker, 1992; Happe & Frith, 2014) have focused on the frontal lobe and the prefrontal cortex which lies at the top of the frontal lobe and has been linked to developing executive functioning in the human brain. These areas have been associated with abilities to differentiate among conflicting thoughts, to determine the consequences of activities, to work toward a defined goal, to predict outcomes, to choose how to act based on experience, and to connect emotions to memories. The developing child uses the frontal lobe in the search for understanding similarities and differences between things and events, as well as in learning about socially acceptable behavior. Along with crucial learning experiences, the frontal lobe is involved in attaining personal and cooperative goals, intellectual generativity and initiating and maintaining social relationships.

Developmental Tasks: Reciprocal Connections

The earliest developmental task necessary in order to attain these fundamental capabilities lies in sensory, emotional, and behavioral regulatory functions, which have become a major focus in the field of infant and early childhood mental health. There is some disagreement among researchers regarding the relative influence of the frontal lobe in social emotional functioning in the earlier years, with Amodio and Frith (2006) claiming the ventro-medial and the dorso-lateral are the primary brain areas involved in the development of executive functioning and LeBar and Cabeza (2006), while Wood and Grafman (2003) focused on the orbitofrontal region of the brain. Although they may not agree regarding the exact location in the brain responsible for social development, they do agree that this is the area of brain in which reciprocal connections between the frontal lobe and other areas of the brain such as the amygdala and parietal cortex are found (Raz & Buhle, 2006). The prefrontal cortex, which rests at the nexus of cognitive, motor and language abilities, is pivotal in human social and emotional functioning (Sabbagh, Xu, Carlson, Moses, & Lee, 2006), but without basic regulatory processes, which develop in infancy and early childhood, it would be very difficult to achieve the ability to understand and empathize with others and to consciously reflect on one's and others' behavior and internal states, including beliefs, desires, and intentions, known as theory of mind (Frith & Frith, 2003; Wellman, Cross, & Watson, 2001).

As the brain develops and matures, at the end of the first year, frontal lobe activation increases, particularly in the prefrontal cortex (Casey, Tottenham, Liston, & Durston, 2005). Social and emotional development related to frontal lobe maturation is manifest in cognitive, emotional and regulatory systems. These interrelated systems scaffold across developmental domains to support and complement development and subsequent mental health in the very young child. Behavior inhibition, controlled attention, modulation of emotion and the understanding of cultural mores and norms relate to the regulatory systems (Calkins & Fox, 2002), whereas the developing child's sense of self, which includes personal identity and awareness of familial roles and social status, is part of an ability to evaluate one's actions and goals (Eisenberg, Vaughan, & Hofer, 2011; Seth, Baars, & Edelman, 2005).

These skills advance within the context of cognitive and linguistic development as the young child gains information about the social world, including the knowledge that others have minds and thoughts which might differ from the child's and the growing ability to understand and appraise emotions (Zelazo, Craik, & Booth, 2004). Thus, development is not only sequential, with more advanced skills building on prerequisite abilities, but also structural, with similarly timed, mutually constrained systems sustaining parallel growth in different developmental domains (Johnson & Munakata, 2005). For example, as children persist in a difficult task, turning to a parent for help instead of tantrumming, there is evidence that emotional regulation has progressed (Kochanska, Murray, & Coy, 1997), and similarly as children learn to evaluate their own and other's actions, their monitoring of themselves increases and supports their sense of self (Zelazo et al., 2004). Finally, as toddlers begin to use language to label feelings, their emotional regulation improves (Havighurst, Wilson, Harley, Prior, & Kehoe, 2010; Kopp, 1989). These developmental processes have mostly been studied in cross-sectional methodologies related to individual differences (Calkins & Fox, 2002), but they merit longitudinal investigation in order to identify how and when each process changes within and across domains of development (Kochanska, Aksan, & Joy, 2007).

Developmental Context of Social and Emotional Functioning in the Early Years

The developmental context for social and emotional growth, like other aspects of development, depends on internal and external variables, both of which have been extensively studied, emphasizing the importance of distinguishing between those factors which are associated with the child and those which are the result of experiences with others. The fundamentals of emotional development occur within a social context, which will be covered more fully in the next chapter. This chapter will focus on the development of the emotional and social skills which the infant acquires during the first years of life.

Bonding

The critical emotional events of the young child's world involve the development of a deep emotional connection with parents and caregivers. The earliest developmental change in the emotional domain occurs at birth. Considerable interest in maternal-infant bonding following birth has resulted in research literature, much of which is based on personal narratives not on empirical findings. It is important to carefully address this initial bonding in order to avoid misunderstanding and exaggeration. It is not clear that animal models are particularly helpful in understanding human bonding, as parenting factors are more complex than the results obtained from animal models, such as mice (Newport, Stowe, & Nemeroff, 2002), chimpanzees (Tomonaga et al., 2004; Warneken & Tomasello, 2009) and rats (Wynne-Edwards & Timonin, 2007).

The basic assumption in bonding is that parents are particularly primed to develop positive feelings about their newborn, who is particularly attractive to the parents immediately after birth, when the neonate is more awake, alert and responsive than he or she will be the following day. This is important as the parents experience a change in attitude and are more ready to respond to their baby's needs (Slade, 2003). Bonding makes it easier to care for the infant well, and satisfying the infant's needs becomes so important that the parent actually experiences pain when the child is hungry or cries for another reason (Granju & Kennedy, 1999). Bonding also decreases the likelihood that the child will experience physical abuse. Bonding must not be oversimplified. It is not simply a matter of contact with the baby, rather emotional bonding results from a complex dynamic system in which many factors interact to produce the desired outcome.

The factors which influence bonding lie within the parent and within the child, and investigation of these factors over the last 20 years has helped to identify early risk factors for positive outcomes in infant mental health. Parental risk factors can include parental grief from losing a parent or someone else with whom the parent had a close relationship. This is particularly true when the lost person is a child – a miscarriage or stillbirth within the previous year, or the death of a twin while the other twin survives – because fears that this child will also die can interfere with the bonding process (Boyle, Vance, Najman, & Thearle, 1996; Hutti, Armstrong, Myers, & Hall, 2015). Parental depression and/or other mental health conditions have also been found to interfere with this important initial bonding process.

Characteristics of the baby which may affect bonding include the baby's health, alertness and responsiveness. Parental attention is less drawn to a drowsy or uninterested baby (Thoman, 1975). The quantity of eye contact and facial expressions which the baby exhibits will also affect parental responsiveness, as these are two fundamental interactional pathways. Situational risk factors may include delayed opportunities to establish contact with the baby, which may arise with a pre-term birth or the need for intensive care (Goldberg, 1979). Further discussion of the roles which parenting and risk factors play in infant mental health can be found in later chapters.

Research Paradigms

Research into emotional and social development in infancy concentrates on experimental approaches, on carefully controlled observations in the laboratory and in the home, and, on clinical work, which collects information about infants, toddlers and preschoolers and their families when there is a problem and the families turn to professionals for help. The relationship between empirical research and clinical practice, including child care procedures, is not always clear. Therefore it is necessary to analyze and integrate information obtained from studies of behavior in the laboratory and from examining spontaneous behavior in naturalistic settings. Behavioral studies of emotional development in infancy focus on behavior and its ramifications. Research goals include looking for causal connections, testing specific hypotheses, and/or assessing service provision. In infant mental health, research often occurs while directly working with infants and their families, wherein the goals are to assess the outcomes of intervention programs and to strengthen emotional and social development in order to support children and families who are at risk for developing or are already experiencing mental health problems. When a young child shows emotional difficulties it also affects the family and therefore intervention techniques support the child and the caregiver-infant relationship, as well as the parents and the familial system.

In research paradigms with young children it is imperative to gather information from parents and caregivers who spend many hours with the infant as well as from questionnaires, reports and observational studies. Observations of behavior done by trained observers focusing on operational definitions of the variables being investigated are perceived as valid and reliable, as the observers have been trained systematically and typically inter-observer reliability is calculated, in which observations from two or more observers are correlated. In addition, specific experimental tasks based on measurements of responses to a controlled stimulus may be used in order to understand changes with age and maturation. An example of this type of research paradigm is the "still-face procedure" which assesses a child's reaction to an expressionless, unresponsive adult face (Tronick, Als, Adamson, Wise, & Brazelton, 1979), which is discussed more fully in chapter 6. The development of pro-social behavior and empathy in very young children is also investigated using such paradigms (Davidov, Zahn-Waxler, Roth-Hanania, & Knafo, 2013).

Individual Differences in Emotional Development

Temperament

Children are different from birth in theirindividual responsiveness to the world. One of the important emphases in infant mental health research is to understand, specify and quantify these differences, especially in the early months, remembering that it is very difficult to distinguish between individual differences resulting from the child's biological nature and those resulting from early experience. The term used to designate individuality in young children is temperament (Thomas, Chess, & Birch, 1970), which refers to the biological factors which help determine the child's personality later in life. Temperamental factors are constitutional characteristics which determine behavioral responses of the infant to the environment. When a characteristic is genuinely temperamental it will change less as a result of experience, but it may be expressed differently at different ages (Rothbart, Ahadi, & Evans, 2000). To be considered temperamental, a characteristic must be present at birth and remain with the individual throughout life, although this refers to the underlying biological characteristic and not necessarily to the specific manner in which it is manifested behaviorally. Newborns, 2 year olds and preschoolers have different behavioral profiles, but display behavioral stability and continuity in their basic temperamental characteristics.

The study of continuity and stability in temperament is complicated by the rapidity of developmental change in infancy. A temperamental characteristic like activity level can be expressed in restlessness in a 2 month old and in jumping in an 18 month old. The measurement of continuity of temperament focuses on different behaviors at various ages but all are assumed to be an expression of the same underlying temperamental characteristic. A second approach to the study of continuity in temperament centers on comparing the behavior of an individual relative to other infants of the same age group. For example, 2 month old babies cry more than 6 month olds do, and by comparing the crying baby at two and at 6 months of age, it is possible to see if the amount of crying of one child in relation to other infants remains the same or differs with maturation (McCall, 1986). If the child cried more than most other children at 2 months of age and also at 6 months, this would support the continuity of temperament of that characteristic.

In addition it is possible to assess continuity of temperamental factors it is necessary to perform longitudinal research which shows similarities over time. Not all characteristics are equally stable and it may be that there is more continuity in a characteristic after 6 months of age than earlier (Pettit & Bates, 1984; Rothbart et al., 2000). Vaughn et al. (1992) suggest that, given that individual differences occur within a social context, it is important to also examine temperament within the social interactions the infant experiences, in order to identify those characteristics which are more and those which are less affected by environmental factors and the quality of interactions with parents and caregivers.

Questionnaires and detailed structured interviews with parents and caregivers who know the infant well are frequently used as a measure of temperamental styles, because they have had many experiences with the infant's reactions and can assess his or her usual response pattern to everyday situations. It would not be efficient or even appropriate for a researcher to spend the amount of time that would be necessary to describe typical patterns of behavior of an individual infant. Nevertheless, it is essential to remember that parents have their own biases and characteristics which affect their reporting, as was evidenced by the fact that mothers who were more anxious during their pregnancies reported their children's behavior as more fussy and difficult (Mebert, 1991). The questionnaires used are generally based on the nine temperament characteristics outlined originally by Thomas et al. (1970), and are coded on a continuum between highest and lowest levels of the factor being rated. By not simply noting if a particular trait exists or not ("0" is not present or "1" is present), Likert scoring reflects a spectrum of expression. Although few infants are rated in the extreme areas of the continuum, it is still crucial to remember that this is not a measure of pathology but rather of individuality. The nine factors can be found in Table 2.1.

Rothbart (1981, 2007) proposed an additional framework for organizing temperamental traits, in which temperament is viewed as the individual personality differences in infants and young children that are present prior to the development of higher cognitive and social aspects of personality. For Rothbart, temperament is defined as individual differences in reactivity and self-regulation that manifest in the domains of emotion, activity and attention. Moving away from classifying infants into categories, Rothbart suggested that temperament should be conceptualized dimensionally and identified three core dimensions of temperament. Three broad factors, surgency (extraversion), negative affect, and effortful control, emerged after a factor analysis methodology was applied to data from 3, 6, and

Table 2.1 Nine temperamental factors based on Thomas et al. (1970)

Trait	Description
Activity level	A measure of the level of movement and activity which characterizes the child
Rhythmicity	A measure of the predictability of the child's physiological functioning including sleeping, eating and eliminating
Distractibility	A measure of the child's ability to concentrate
Approach and withdrawal	A measure of the child's reaction to unfamiliar situations
Adaptability	A measure of the child's capacity to learn to tolerate routines and rules
Attention span and persistence	A measure of the child's ability to remain on task
Intensity of reaction	A measure of the degree of intensity of the child's overall reactions
Threshold of responsiveness	A measure of the intensity of stimulation required in order to capture the child's attention
Quality of mood	A measure of the positive or negative valence of the child's mood

12 month old infants. Extraversion as a dimension of temperament is characterized by positive anticipation, impulsivity, increased levels of activity and a desire for sensation, and reflects the degree to which a child is generally happy and active and enjoys vocalizing and seeking stimulation, which is why it has been labeled as surgency. The dimension of negative affect includes fear, frustration, sadness, anger, and discomfort, and represents the degree to which a child is shy and not easily calmed. Finally, effortful control delineates the child's ability to focus and shift attention, inhibitory control, and perceptual sensitivity. An example of behaviors associated with this profile would be the child who is not easily distracted, is able to inhibit one response in order to depend on a more effective strategy in problem solving and is able to focus on a goal and plan to achieve it.

Questionnaires (Rothbart, Ahadi, Hershey, & Fisher, 2001) have been developed to study these three dimensions of temperament and longitudinal studies have revealed predictable, stable correlations with later behavior. For example, 10 month olds with higher levels of surgency/extraversion were more likely to develop externalizing problems like acting out and less likely to develop internalizing problems such as shyness or low self-esteem (Eisenberg et al., 2009). Anger is related to later externalizing problems, while fear is associated with internalizing difficulties, whereas fear which is expressed as behavioral inhibition as early as 8–10 months predicts later levels of fear (Rueda & Rothbart, 2009). Similarly, higher levels of effortful control at age seven also predicted lower externalizing problems in middle childhood (Kochanska, Koenig, Barry, Kim, & Yoon, 2010). These three dimensions also revealed an interaction effect, with children with high negative affect showing decreased internalizing and externalizing problems when they were also high on effortful control (Posner & Rothbart, 2009). Effortful control shows stability from infancy into the school years and also predicts moral development (Augustine & Stifter, 2015; Kochanska, Barry, Jimenez, Hollatz, & Woodard, 2009).

These conceptualizations of temperamental traits do not judge them as better or worse, or the baby as good or bad; rather, the issues concerning temperament revolve around goodness of fit, or the extent to which the temperament of the infant and the caregiver work well together. Differences and similarities in temperament styles can either help a parent and child feel close and comfortable or make things difficult between them. Infants who are irritable or fussy, however, seem to negatively affect their mothers' ability to respond positively to them very early in development (van den Boom & Hoeksma, 1994). Sadly, even for the babies who became less irritable by age 5–6 months, the mothers' attitudes toward the children did not improve, and they soothed their babies less and were less responsive to the babies' positive signals. Thus, temperamental characteristics are not good or bad in and of themselves, but rather must be assessed within the context of the fit between the caregiver and the infant. In addition to the goodness of fit between infant and adult temperaments, it is likewise critical to assess parental attitudes and expectations, cultural values, and even aspects of the physical environment, which can all influence the long-term effects of a particular temperament. Rather than investigating a certain temperamental pattern on its own, it should be assessed according to how well it fits into the environment in which the child is developing.

Developmental Stages and Social and Emotional Growth

Throughout infancy and toddlerhood, developmental changes occur in the young child's social and emotional behavior. Not only do these changes follow predictable stages, they also support one another and develop structurally (Havighurst, 1972; Zigler, 2012). Instead of delineating particular skills sequentially, researchers have begun to assume that it is important to investigate which tasks are being mastered concomitantly, providing scaffolding for the next level of developmental tasks. As previously mentioned, initially it is important for the infant to achieve the ability to calm down when distressed, excited or emotionally aroused. This ability to self-regulate allows the infant to watch, learn, explore and be interested in the world (Greenspan & Wieder, 2007). Self-regulation has been described as the ability to learn how to modulate, tolerate, and endure experiences of negative affect (Kopp, 1989).

Newborns' emotions seem to be in control of them, rather than the infant controlling his or her emotions. For example, once the baby begins to cry, unless comfort is offered the infant will continue to cry until exhausted, when he or she falls into a deep sleep because the infant hasn't yet acquired strategies for calming down without adult help. In the course of only a short few months, the infant who is well cared for will begin to develop self-regulation techniques. Part of this learning is by chance, as the infant finds his or her thumb and begins to suck, which is comforting, and some of it comes about as a result of an attentive and available parent, who, for example, is always looking for the most comforting position in which to hold her irritable baby. As the mother learns what is best for the baby, the baby learns it too and will then try to find that comfortable spot again, knowing it can be attained. Other early self-regulating practices include gaze aversion, closing eyes when not sleeping, looking at hands, and rubbing or tugging hair, clothes, or ears. Some babies do these activities while nursing, another regulatory activity although not in the infant's control. By the end of 3 months, the infant has only partially gained self-regulation, but is already quite different in his or her ability to self-regulate from the totally unregulated newborn.

The Underpinnings of Theory of Mind

As mentioned previously, mental representationof objects and people becomes more mature by the end of the first year. The developing capacity for mental representation makes it possible for the infant to think not only of another person but also of what that person might think or know. At this stage, young children are beginning to develop a theory of mind and the ability to empathize with others who may feel differently than they. This still unsophisticated theory of mind is the assumption that people have minds and that they are aware of experiences and intentions. Trevarthen's (1979) hypothesis of intersubjectivity assumes that, from the time of birth, infants have the ability to recognize human beings as people and to predict some of their actions, and also to share some control over their actions, thus understanding in a very basic way others' feelings. Hobson (1993) elaborated on this primitive intersubjectivity and suggested that each early emotion is associated with a universal experience and with facial and vocal expression, and that the infant can therefore know that a particular expression on a parent's face, combined with other signals, indicates the same feeling that the baby experiences and expresses similarly.

Cognitive and affective abilities work together as the infant uses social referencing of the parents' expressions and behaviors to understand what parents think about the world around them. Theory of mind develops as the growing child's feelings match those of her parents and when there is evidence that different people have different minds with different feelings and thoughts. Meltzoff and Gopnik (1993) posit that the earliest development of theory of mind in young children is cultivated by an early awareness of body movements which are accompanied by specific sensations, in other people and in themselves. Theory of mind in infancy would then be advanced by the many reciprocal social imitation games played during the first year of life. Some support for this premise is provided by the fact that young children do seem to be fascinated by adults who imitate them (Meltzoff, 2002).

One aspect of even a developing theory of mind is that it is not only an awareness of self and subjectivity, but also an awareness of others and how they feel. Until a sense of self is present, social emotions cannot develop. Some aspects of self-recognition are in place by the end of the first year, when the baby can point to body parts when they are labelled, even when they are not visible, reflecting some sense of permanence in his body awareness (Lewis & Brooks, 1978). When the infant can recognize himself or herself in the mirror, a picture or a video, it is clear that he or she can now imagine how he or she looks to other people (Asendorpf, Warkentin, & Baudonnière, 1996). The ability for self-recognition in a mirror emerges between 15 and 18 months, when the toddler appears to be embarrassed when seeing his or her reflection in the mirror. An experimental task developed to assess achievement of this developmental task is called the rouge technique: a red dot is put on the child's forehead or nose and when he or she sees it in the mirror, the toddler immediately puts his hand on the spot if he recognizes himself or herself (Anderson, 1984; Bertenthal & Fischer, 1978).

Foundation for the Concern for Others

In recent years, empirical research has raised questions regarding some of our preconceptions about infants' emotional and social developmental capabilities. Specifically, concern for others has been thought to emerge during the second year of life (Hoffman, 2010), based on the assumption that in order to be empathic to others, a child must have a sense of self and the other, because otherwise they would interpret others' distress as their own. Davidov et al. (2013) presented empirical evidence contradicting these assumptions and proposed an alternative theory of the early development of empathy, which does not depend on self-reflective abilities and exists already in the first year of life. Their findings point to the fact that infants can show empathic concern for others earlier in life than previously thought. Although Hoffman (2008) viewed empathy as an innate capability, he posited that it only emerged in the second year of life after self-recognition was attained. However, it now appears that concern for others, an emotional response consisting of tender feelings on behalf of a distressed other, may be present in the first year of life.

Previously it was accepted that the young infant cannot remain focused on the other in distress nor feel for the other, as infants became overly aroused from the other's distress, leading to self-distress (Eisenberg, Fabes, & Spinrad, 2006; Eisenberg et al., 2009). Davidov et al. (2013) argue that the processes underlying infants' emphatic self-distress may not stem from confusion between the distress of others and that of the self, but rather that the infant is likely having difficulties regulating the emotional arousal induced by others' distress. An optimal level of emotional arousal is necessary for empathic concern. The ability to regulate the arousal created by the other's distress is not yet sufficiently developed in the first year of life. When infants were exposed to only mild and brief distress they were able to regulate their arousal more effectively than when they experienced more prolonged and intense distress of others (Hay et al., 2005; Roth-Hanania, Davidov, & Zahn-Waxler, 2011). In addition, since they found no significant correlations between self-recognition and empathic concern, Zahn-Waxler, Radke-Yarrow, Wagner, and Chapman (1992) proposed that self-knowledge was not necessary in order to experience concern for others. Instead they suggest that a simpler, implicit form of self-recognition (rather than self-knowledge) is sufficient for experiencing concern for others, which is based on the infant's subjective experience of his or her own sensory experience and self-generated actions (Gallagher & Meltzoff, 1996). Thus infants can differentiate between self-generated movements and being moved by someone else (Rochat & Hespos, 1997), and between crying and hearing someone else's crying, because it feels different to them (Dondi, Simion, & Caltran, 1999).

By positing that the capacity for empathic concern exists in the first year and does not depend on self-reflective abilities, Davidov et al. (2013) have changed the way reciprocal emotional development in the first year is understood and studied. Infants' cognitive, emotional and social competencies are often underestimated, and focusing on concern for others during the first year may lead to knowledge regarding the social brain and the neural, hormonal and autonomic substrates of early empathy (Light & Zahn-Waxler, 2011), and to more developmentally appropriate assessment procedures in which the distress is not overwhelming for the young infant. Through the use of appropriate empirical research designs, it may be possible to identify parameters that facilitate infants' development of concern for others.

The vast majority of infants attain the emotional developmental milestones successfully as a result of their biological endowment and a good enough caregiving environment which supports their mental health. These emotionally healthy young children may experience some emotional upheaval, just as emotionally healthy adults do. Unfortunately, a small number of infants experience major difficulties in their emotional development, and a focus on infant mental health can be effective in helping these children. Sadly, although some of these problems can be ameliorated, some are not only not curable, they may not even be preventable.

Issues of Concern

Many of the emotional manifestations that concern parents of infants and toddlers are a matter of temperament. Some issues like thumb sucking may be a result of temperament. Children who are not distractible and who are intense in their reactions seem to be more likely to persist in sucking past year one (Newson, Newson, & Mahalski, 1982). Tantrums and negativism are a normal part of toddlerhood and should be seen as a struggle of the child to attain independence. Although these individual behaviors are developmentally appropriate during the toddler period, they should diminish as the child matures and develops other behavioral strategies for expressing independence.

Sleeping and eating difficulties are usually manifestations of normal developmental variability in infants and toddlers. Changes in sleeping patterns and appetite are oftentimes signs of developmental transitions from one stage to another.

Although these are not pathological problems in and of themselves, they can be made into pathological problems by less than optimal responding by the adults in the infants' life. Fear of strangers and anxiety about separation are normal parts of attachment, as is distress following longer periods of separation.

When these problems are more than just issues of development in their intensity, frequency and severity they may need more specific interventions. The field of developmental psychopathology deals with understanding normal pathways of development in order to follow significant deviations from the norm and to identify factors which are involved in those deviations (Sroufe, 2000; Stern, 1985, 1995). Developmental psychopathologists are also interested in the factors that enable some infants to resist stress and continue to develop in a normative way despite the difficulties they encounter. These issues will be covered more comprehensively in Chaps. 5 and 7.

References

Amodio, D. M., & Frith, C. D. (2006). Meeting of minds: The medial prefrontal cortex and social cognition. *Nature Neuroscience Reviews, 7*, 268–277.

Anderson, J. R. (1984). The development of self-recognition: A review. *Developmental Psychobiology, 17*(1), 35–49.

Asendorpf, J. B., Warkentin, V., & Baudonnière, P. M. (1996). Self-awareness and other-awareness. II: Mirror self-recognition, social contingency awareness, and synchronic imitation. *Developmental Psychology, 32*(2), 313–321. http://dx.doi.org/10.1037/0012-1649.32.2.313.

Augustine, M. E., & Stifter, C. A. (2015). Temperament, parenting, and moral development: Specificity of behavior and context. *Social Development, 24*(2), 285–303.

Bertenthal, B. I., & Fischer, K. W. (1978). Development of self-recognition in the infant. *Developmental Psychology, 14*(1), 44–50.

Boyle, F. M., Vance, J. C., Najman, J. M., & Thearle, M. J. (1996). The mental health impact of stillbirth, neonatal death or SIDS: Prevalence and patterns of distress among mothers. *Social Science & Medicine, 43*(8), 1273–1282.

Brownell, C. A., & Kopp, C. B. (Eds.). (2010). *Socioemotional development in the toddler years: Transitions and transformations*. New York, NY: Guilford Press.

Brownell, C. A., Svetlova, M., & Nichols, S. (2009). To share or not to share: When do toddlers respond to another's needs? *Infancy, 14*(1), 117–130.

Calkins, S. D., & Fox, N. A. (2002). Self-regulatory processes in early personality development: A multilevel approach to the study of childhood social withdrawal and aggression. *Development and Psychopathology, 14*, 477–498.

Calkins, S. D., & Johnson, M. C. (1998). Toddler regulation of distress to frustrating events: Temperamental and maternal correlates. *Infant Behavior and Development, 21*, 379–395.

Call, J. (2001). Object permanence in orangutans (Pongo pygmaeus), chimpanzees (Pan troglodytes), and children (Homo sapiens). *Journal of Comparative Psychology, 115*(2), 159–171.

Casey, B. J., Tottenham, N., Liston, C., & Durston, S. (2005). Imaging the developing brain: What have we learned about cognitive development? *Trends in Ccognitive Sciences, 9*(3), 104–110.

Collier-Baker, E., & Suddendorf, T. (2006). Do chimpanzees (Pan troglodytes) and 2-year-old children (Homo sapiens) understand double invisible displacement? *Journal of Comparative Psychology, 120*(2), 89–97.

Cook, D. T. (2004). *The commodification of childhood: The children's clothing industry and the rise of the child consumer*. Durham, NC: Duke University Press.

Davidov, M., Zahn-Waxler, C., Roth-Hanania, R., & Knafo, A. (2013). Concern for others in the first year of life: Theory, evidence, and avenues for research. *Child Development Perspectives, 7*(2), 126–131.

Dawson, G., Klinger, L. G., Panagiotides, H., Hill, D., & Spieker, S. (1992). Frontal lobe activity and affective behavior of infants of mothers with depressive symptoms. *Child Development, 63*, 725–37.

Decety, J., & Jackson, P. L. (2004). The functional architecture of human empathy. *Behavioral and Cognitive Neuroscience Reviews, 3*(2), 71–100.

Donald, M. (1991). *Origins of the modern mind: Three stages in the evolution of culture and cognition.* Cambridge, MA: Harvard University Press.

Dondi, M., Simion, F., & Caltran, G. (1999). Can newborns discriminate between their own cry and the cry of another newborn infant? *Developmental Psychology, 35*(2), 418–426.

Eisenberg, N., Fabes, R. A., & Spinrad, T. L. (2006). Prosocial behaviour. *Handbook of Child Psychology, 3*, 646–718.

Eisenberg, N., Valiente, C., Spinrad, T. L., Cumberland, A., Liew, J., Reiser, M., & Losoya, S. H. (2009). Longitudinal relations of children's effortful control, impulsivity, and negative emotionality to their externalizing, internalizing, and co-occurring behavior problems. *Developmental Psychology, 45*(4), 988–1008.

Eisenberg, N., Vaughan, J., & Hofer, C. (2011). Temperament, self-regulation, and peer social competence. In *Handbook of peer interactions, relationships, and groups* (pp. 473–489). New York, NY: Guilford Press.

Fagot, B. I., & Hagan, R. (1991). Observations of parent reactions to sex-stereotyped behaviors: Age and sex effects. *Child Development, 62*, 617–628.

Finlay, B. L., Darlington, R. B., & Nicastro, N. (2001). Developmental structure in brain evolution. *Behavioral and Brain Sciences, 24*(2), 263–278.

Fletcher, P. C., Happe, F., Frith, U., Baker, S. C., Dolan, R. J., Frackowiak, R. S., & Frith, C. D. (1995). Other minds in the brain: a functional imaging study of "theory of mind" in story comprehension. *Cognition, 57*(2), 109–128.

Frith, U., & Frith, C. D. (2003). Development and neurophysiology of mentalizing. *Philosophical Transactions of the Royal Society of London. Series B, Biological Sciences, 358*(1431), 459–473.

Gallagher, S., & Meltzoff, A. N. (1996). The earliest sense of self and others: Merleau-Ponty and recent developmental studies. *Philosophical Psychology, 9*(2), 211–233.

Goldberg, D. (1979). *Manual of the general health questionnaire.* Windsor, Canada: NFER Publishing Company.

Granju, K. A., & Kennedy, B. (1999). *Attachment parenting: Instinctive care for your baby and young child.* New York, NY: Simon and Schuster.

Green, K. P., Kuhl, P. K., Meltzoff, A. N., & Stevens, E. B. (1991). Integrating speech information across talkers, gender, and sensory modality: Female faces and male voices in the McGurk effect. *Perception & Psychophysics, 50*(6), 524–536.

Greenspan, S. I., & Wieder, S. (2007). *Infant and early childhood mental health: A comprehensive developmental approach to assessment and intervention.* Washington, DC: American Psychiatric Publications.

Happé, F., & Frith, U. (2014). Annual research review: Towards a developmental neuroscience of atypical social cognition. *Journal of Child Psychology and Psychiatry, 55*(6), 553–577.

Havighurst, R. J. (1972). *Developmental tasks and education.* New York, NY: McKay Company.

Havighurst, S. S., Wilson, K. R., Harley, A. E., Prior, M. R., & Kehoe, C. (2010). Tuning in to kids: Improving emotion socialization practices in parents of preschool children–findings from a community trial. *Journal of Child Psychology and Psychiatry, 51*(12), 1342–1350.

Hay, A. D., Heron, J., & Ness, A. (2005). The prevalence of symptoms and consultations in pre-school children in the Avon longitudinal study of parents and children (ALSPAC): A prospective cohort study. *Family Practice, 22*(4), 367–374.

Hirshberg, L. M., & Svejda, M. (1990). When infants look to their parents: I. Infants' social referencing of mothers compared to fathers. *Child Development, 61*(4), 1175–1186.
Hobson, R. P. (1993). The intersubjective domain: Approaches from developmental psychopathology. *Journal of the American Psychoanalytic Association, 41*, 167–192.
Hoffman, M. L. (2010). Empathy and prosocial behavior. In M. Lewis, J. M. Haviland-Jones, & L. F. Barrett (Eds.), *Handbook of emotions-third edition* (pp. 440–455). New York, NY: Guilford Press.
Hutti, M. H., Armstrong, D. S., Myers, J. A., & Hall, L. A. (2015). Grief intensity, psychological well-being, and the intimate partner relationship in the subsequent pregnancy after a perinatal loss. *Journal of Obstetric, Gynecologic, & Neonatal Nursing, 44*(1), 42–50.
Johnson, M. H., & Munakata, Y. (2005). Processes of change in brain and cognitive development. *Trends in Cognitive Sciences, 9*(3), 152–158.
Khoury-Kassabri, M. (2010). Attitudes of Arab and Jewish mothers towards punitive and non-punitive discipline methods. *Child & Family Social Work, 15*(2), 135–144.
Kochanska, G., Aksan, N., & Joy, M. E. (2007). Children's fearfulness as a moderator of parenting in early socialization: Two longitudinal studies. *Developmental Psychology, 43*(1), 222–237.
Kochanska, G., Barry, R. A., Jimenez, N. B., Hollatz, A. L., & Woodard, J. (2009). Guilt and effortful control: Two mechanisms that prevent disruptive developmental trajectories. *Journal of Personality and Social Psychology, 97*(2), 322–333.
Kochanska, G., Koenig, J. L., Barry, R. A., Kim, S., & Yoon, J. E. (2010). Children's conscience during toddler and preschool years, moral self, and a competent, adaptive developmental trajectory. *Developmental Psychology, 46*(5), 1320–1332.
Kochanska, G., Murray, K., & Coy, K. C. (1997). Inhibitory control as a contributor to conscience in childhood: From toddler to early school age. *Child Development, 68*(2), 263–277.
Kopp, C. B. (1989). Regulation of distress and negative emotions: A developmental view. *Developmental Psychology, 25*(3), 343–354.
Kopp, C. B., Sigman, M., & Parmelee, A. H. (1974). Longitudinal study of sensorimotor development. *Developmental Psychology, 10*(5), 687–695.
LeBar, K. S., & Cabeza, R. (2006). Cognitive neuroscience of emotional memory. *Nature Reviews Neurosciences, 7*, 297–314.
Leslie, A. M. (1987). Pretense and representation: The origins of "theory of mind". *Psychological Review, 94*(4), 412–426.
Lewis, M., & Brooks, J. (1978). Self-knowledge and emotional development. In M. Lewis & L. A. Rosenblum (Eds.), *The development of affect* (pp. 205–226). New York, NY: Springer.
Light, S., & Zahn-Waxler, C. (2011). The nature and forms of empathy in the first years of life. In J. Decety (Ed.), *Empathy: From bench to bedside* (pp. 109–130). Cambridge, MA: MIT Press.
Martin, J. L., & Ross, H. S. (2005). Sibling aggression: Sex differences and parents' reactions. *International Journal of Behavioral Development, 29*, 129–138.
McCall, R. B. (1986). Issues of stability and continuity in temperament research. In R. Plomin & J. Dunn (Eds.), *The study of temperament: Changes, continuities and challenges* (pp. 13–25). Hillsdale, NJ: Erlbaum.
McKinney, C., & Renk, K. (2008). Differential parenting between mothers and fathers: Implications for late adolescents. *Journal of Family Issues, 29*(6), 806–827.
Mebert, C. J. (1991). Dimensions of subjectivity in parents' ratings of infant temperament. *Child Development, 62*(2), 352–361.
Meltzoff, A. N. (2002). Imitation as a mechanism of social cognition: Origins of empathy, theory of mind, and the representation of action. In U. Goswami (Ed.), *Blackwell handbook of childhood cognitive development* (pp. 6–25). Oxford, UK: Blackwell Publishers.
Meltzoff, A. N. (2007). 'Like me': A foundation for social cognition. *Developmental Science, 10* (1), 126–134.
Meltzoff, A. N., & Gopnik, A. (1993). The role of imitation in understanding persons and developing a theory of mind. In S. Baron-Cohen, H. Tager-Flusberg, & D. J. Cohen (Eds.),

Understanding other minds: Perspectives from autism (pp. 335–366). Oxford, UK: Oxford University Press.

Meltzoff, A. N., & Moore, M. K. (1998). Infant intersubjectivity: Broadening the dialogue to include imitation, identity and intention. In S. Bråten (Ed.), *Intersubjective communication and emotion in early ontogeny* (pp. 47–62). Cambridge: Cambridge University Press.

Nelson, K., & Fivush, R. (2004). The emergence of autobiographical memory: A social cultural developmental theory. *Psychological Review, 111*(2), 486–511.

Newport, D. J., Stowe, Z. N., & Nemeroff, C. B. (2002). Parental depression: Animal models of an adverse life event. *American Journal of Psychiatry, 159*(8), 1265–1283.

Newson, J., Newson, E., & Mahalski, P. A. (1982). Persistent infant comfort habits and their sequelae at 11 and 16 years. *Journal of Child Psychology and Psychiatry, 23*, 421–436.

NICHD Early Child Care Research Network. (2004). Trajectories of physical aggression from toddlerhood to middle childhood: Predictors, correlates, and outcomes. *Monographs of the Society for Research in Child Development, 69*(4), vii–1.

Onishi, K. H., & Baillargeon, R. (2005). Do 15-month-old infants understand false beliefs? *Science, 308*(5719), 255–258.

Pettit, G. S., & Bates, J. E. (1984). Continuity of individual differences in the mother-infant relationship from six to thirteen months. *Child Development, 55*, 729–739.

Piaget, J. (1952). *The origins of intelligence in children* (Vol. 8, No. 5, p. 18). New York, NY: International Universities Press.

Posner, M. I., & Rothbart, M. K. (2009). Toward a physical basis of attention and self-regulation. *Physics of Life Reviews, 6*(2), 103–120.

Raz, A., & Buhle, J. (2006). Typologies of attentional networks. *Nature Reviews Neuroscience, 7*, 367–379.

Rochat, P., & Hespos, S. J. (1997). Differential rooting response by neonates: Evidence for an early sense of self. *Early Development and Parenting, 6*(34), 105–112.

Rothbart, M. K. (1981). Measurement of temperament in infancy. *Child Development, 52*, 569–578.

Rothbart, M. K. (2007). Temperament, development and personality. *Current Directions in Psychological Science, 16*(4), 207–212.

Rothbart, M. K., Ahadi, S. A., & Evans, D. E. (2000). Temperament and personality: Origins and outcomes. *Journal of Personality and Social Psychology, 78*(1), 122–135.

Rothbart, M. K., Ahadi, S. A., Hershey, K. L., & Fisher, P. (2001). Investigations of temperament at three to seven years: The children's behavior questionnaire. *Child Development, 72*(5), 1394–1408.

Roth-Hanania, R., Davidov, M., & Zahn-Waxler, C. (2011). Empathy development from 8 to 16 months: Early signs of concern for others. *Infant Behavior and Development, 34*(3), 447–458.

Rueda, M. R., & Rothbart, M. K. (2009). The influence of temperament on the development of coping: The role of maturation and experience. *New Directions for Child and Adolescent Development, 124*, 19–31.

Rutter, M., & Sroufe, L. A. (2000). Developmental psychopathology: Concepts and challenges. *Development and Psychopathology, 12*, 265–296.

Sabbagh, M. A., Xu, F., Carlson, S. M., Moses, L. J., & Lee, K. (2006). The development of executive functioning and theory of mind: A comparison of U.S. and Chinese preschoolers. *Psychological Science, 17*, 74–81.

Seth, A. K., Baars, B. J., & Edelman, D. B. (2005). Criteria for consciousness in humans and other mammals. *Consciousness and Cognition, 14*(1), 119–139.

Shaw, D. S., Keenan, K., & Vondra, J. I. (1994). Developmental precursors of externalizing behavior: Ages 1 to 3. *Developmental Psychology, 30*(3), 355–364.

Slade, A. (2003). Holding the baby in mind: Discussion of Joseph Lichtenberg's "communication in infancy". *Psychoanalytic Inquiry, 23*(3), 521–529.

Spinrad, T. L., & Stifter, C. A. (2006). Toddlers' empathy-related responding to distress: Predictions from negative emotionality and maternal behavior in infancy. *Infancy, 10*(2), 97–121.
Sroufe, L. A. (2000). Early relationships and the development of children. *Infant Mental Health Journal, 21*(1–2), 67–74.
Stern, D. (1985). *The interpersonal world of the infant*. New York, NY: Basic Books.
Stern, D. N. (1995). *Motherhood constellation*. London, UK: Karnac Books.
Svetlova, M., Nichols, S. R., & Brownell, C. A. (2010). Toddlers' prosocial behavior: From instrumental to empathic to altruistic helping. *Child Development, 81*(6), 1814–1827.
Thoman, E. B. (1975). How a rejecting baby affects mother-infant synchrony. In Ciba Foundation Symposium 33, *Parent-infant Interaction* (pp. 185–186). Amsterdam, The Netherlands: Elsevier.
Thomas, A., Chess, S., & Birch, H. G. (1970). The origin of personality. *Scientific American, 223*, 102–109.
Tomasello, M. (1999). *The cultural origins of human cognition*. Cambridge, MA: Harvard University Press.
Tomonaga, M., Tanaka, M., Matsuzawa, T., ... & Bard, K. A. (2004). Development of social cognition in infant chimpanzees (Pan troglodytes): Face recognition, smiling, gaze, and the lack of triadic interactions. *Japanese Psychological Research, 46*(3), 227–235
Tremblay, R. E., Nagin, D. S., Séguin, J. R., Zoccolillo, M., Zelazo, P. D., Boivin, M., ... & Japel, C. (2005). Physical aggression during early childhood: Trajectories and predictors. *The Canadian Child and Adolescent Psychiatry Review, 14*(1), 3–9.
Trevarthen, C. (1979). Communication and cooperation in early infancy: A description of primary intersubjectivity. In M. Bullowa (Ed.), *Before speech: The beginnings of interpersonal communication*. Cambridge, UK: Cambridge University Press.
Tronick, E., Als, H., Adamson, L., Wise, S., & Brazelton, T. B. (1979). The infant's response to entrapment between contradictory messages in face-to-face interaction. *Journal of the American Academy of Child Psychiatry, 17*(1), 1–13.
van den Boom, D. C., & Hoeksma, J. B. (1994). The effect of infant irritability on mother-infant interaction: A growth curve analysis. *Developmental Psychology, 31*, 581–590.
Vaughn, B. E., Stevenson-Hinde, J., Waters, E., Kotsaftis, A., Lefever, G. B., Shouldice, A., ... & Belsky, J. (1992). Attachment security and temperament in infancy and early childhood: Some conceptual clarifications. *Developmental Psychology, 28*(3), 463–473.
Warneken, F., & Tomasello, M. (2009). Varieties of altruism in children and chimpanzees. *Trends in Cognitive Sciences, 13*(9), 397–402.
Wellman, H. M., Cross, D., & Watson, J. (2001). Meta-analysis of theory-of-mind development: the truth about false belief. *Child Development, 72*(3), 655–684.
Wood, J. N., & Grafman, J. (2003). Human prefrontal cortex: Processing and representational perspectives. *Nature Reviews Neuroscience, 4*, 139–147.
Wynne-Edwards, K. E., & Timonin, M. E. (2007). Paternal care in rodents: Weakening support for hormonal regulation of the transition to behavioral fatherhood in rodent animal models of biparental care. *Hormones and Behavior, 52*(1), 114–121.
Zahn-Waxler, C., Radke-Yarrow, M., Wagner, E., & Chapman, M. (1992). Development of concern for others. *Developmental Psychology, 28*(1), 126–136.
Zelazo, P. D., Craik, F. I., & Booth, L. (2004). Executive function across the life span. *Acta Psychologica, 115*(2), 167–183.
Zigler, E. F. (2012). The motivational perspective. In S. Kreitler (Ed.), *Cognition and motivation: Forging an interdisciplinary perspective* (pp. 433–449). Cambridge, UK: Cambridge University Press.

Chapter 3
Social and Cultural Contexts in Infant and Early Childhood Mental Health

Introduction

Child development and culture are inseparable. The development of social emotional behavior, in particular, has cultural overtones. Humans develop through social interactions which occur within a cultural framework through which appropriate social norms and customs are to be passed on to the developing child. Children are surrounded by their culture and acquire cultural knowledge through their experience of their parents' expectations, attitudes, and child-rearing practices (Greenfield, Keller, Fuligni, & Maynard, 2003; Harkness & Super, 1996).

In multi-cultural societies the cultural milieu can be divided into the home culture and the societal culture. Home culture refers to the attitudes, routines and cultural background of the immediate family (Greenfield, Suzuki, & Rothstein-Fisch, 2006). Because children interact with the individuals in their home culture on a daily basis, they learn from the implicit values transmitted through their relationships with family members. Children are likewise exposed to the culture of the larger society, through interactions with outside sources such as schools, peers, and the media, thereby absorbing the general cultural values inherent in the society within which they are being socialized. In many cases the cultural system within the home mirrors the values of the general cultural climate, whereas in other situations the cultural climate of the home may differ significantly from the cultural climate of the society at large. Immigrant families often find themselves in difficult situations when their children receive conflicting messages from home and from the outside world. In assessing the behaviors of parents and children from diverse backgrounds, mental health professionals must be aware of these intercultural dynamics.

Socialization is the process through which the infant learns about social rules and attitudes. It comes about through experiencing the world with other people and includes social conventions, such as toilet training, and moral universals, such as

C. Shulman, *Research and Practice in Infant and Early Childhood Mental Health*,
Children's Well-Being: Indicators and Research 13,
DOI 10.1007/978-3-319-31181-4_3

attitudes toward aggression (Phillips, 2013). Some of this rule-governed behavior occurs through imitation (Buttelmann, Zmyj, Daum, & Carpenter, 2013), some through social referencing of adults (Over & Carpenter, 2012), and other behaviors through direct instruction of the child (Dean, Kendal, Schapiro, Thierry, & Laland, 2012; Keller, 2013). Through socialization the infant becomes a toddler and preschooler who behaves in ways that are similar to others in his or her cultural group. The well-socialized person's behavior is similar to that of others in his or her culture in terms of aggressiveness, compliance, friendliness to strangers, autonomy and other behaviors considered appropriate in a particular cultural context.

Socialization occurs within the context of a complex, ever-changing, dynamic system. Differently from emotional development, which focuses on the individual child and at most on the parent-child dyad, including the parent's attentiveness to the child's signaling, the study of socialization investigates family systems and groups defined by similar cultural norms of behavior. Socialization is the process of working toward achieving the goals which define the family or cultural grouping, so that infants and young children grow up into adaptive and productive adults.

The present chapter deals with infant socialization, emphasizing parent-child relations as a socializing agent, as well as transferring cultural expectations, and the implications of these expectations for infant and early childhood mental health. We will focus first on family influences and on the complex ways in which caregivers and infants interact, reciprocally influencing one another, with an emphasis on the impact that the home culture has on the socialization process, and then proceed to address the manner in which societal culture influences the developing infant and young child, while recognizing that the appropriateness of particular caregiving techniques is specific to a given culture. For example, in western societies leaving an infant under the care of an "older" sibling who is six would be seen as negligent, whereas in African tribes it is perfectly acceptable. Thus, the information presented in this chapter is predicated on the premise that there is no one way to socialize an infant but rather socialization occurs within a cultural context, which must be taken into consideration when assessing socialization and its outcomes.

Understanding Social Behavior in the Early Years

The themes of social synchrony, the coordination of nonverbal behaviors between social partners during interpersonal exchange (Atzil, Hendler, & Feldman, 2011) and social reciprocity were presented as part of the context of emotional development in the previous chapter and will be covered in the current chapter from the perspective of interpersonal interactions in which socialization takes place. Social reciprocity occurs when the acts of two or more persons support each other in a relationship and their actions become similar to one another (Feldman, Gordon, Influs, Gutbir, & Ebstein, 2013). The earliest social reciprocities become established between parents and their very young children, supporting the premise that there is an interpersonal bias in behavioral responding.

In typical development, the social acts of others are seen as playing a role in the behavioral organization of socialization, because they are readily enmeshed in the ongoing behaviors of the child and because they are more compelling than nonsocial events (Bowlby, 1956). The supposition that social stimuli are more salient than nonsocial events presupposes the synchronous development of sensory and attentional abilities between infants and adults. Through this synchrony behavior, patterns of the adult and the child can organize internal states, in addition to internal states organizing behavior patterns. In this regard social behavior is seen as the leading edge of highly flexible adaptive functions which are responsive to changing internal and external circumstances. Thus social relationships, ranging from each distinctive dyadic relationship to the culture within which a child is developing form the basis on which socialization is built.

Requisite adaptations within dyadic relationships also affect all levels of the social interactional interplay, including incorporating the social rules which reinforce behavior norms in a particular cultural setting. Given the developmental and behavioral changes in members of family systems, the necessity to continuously modify familial relationships makes the family system a dynamic one which undergoes change, and those changes have an impact on the family members as well. The bias of family systems to maintain continuity within familial relationships and to preserve the integrity of the system itself establishes the family as a central socializing agent in the life of the very young child.

One of the major emphases of the socialization process is to promote social competence in the developing child, which revolves around the importance of reciprocity in relationships. Social skills are situation specific, with few if any interpersonal behaviors appropriate in all settings, for social norms vary and are determined by both situational and cultural factors. Thus a major purpose of socialization is to help the young child understand the social and behavioral demands of different circumstances and adapt skills effectively according to the requirements of the social context (Berns, 2012). The definition of social competence differs from one study to another and there are inherent difficulties in comparing results from different empirical research investigations. Nevertheless, there is overall agreement that the essence of social behavior consists of the ability to relate to others in a mutually reinforcing and reciprocal manner and to adapt social skills to the varying demands of different interpersonal contexts.

Conducting Research into Socialization of Young Children

After defining the components of social behavior being studied, it is essential to understand the research methodologies used to define and evaluate social interactional parameters in research paradigms. Research makes use of interviews, questionnaires, developmentally appropriate social/cognitive tasks and observational measures in order to examine the appropriateness of social behavior to the social milieu in which it is manifest. Direct observations of children's social interactions have been used in order to identify at which ages particular behaviors emerge, to specify differences between adult-child social interactional patterns and peer interactional patterns, to compare different cultures and their expected social behaviors, and finally to evaluate the effectiveness of intervention programs.

The data collected and subsequently analyzed is typically quantitative in nature, expressing the rate, frequency or percentage of interactive behaviors, and the coding systems range from simply counting the presence or absence of target behaviors to highly sophisticated rating systems. Despite the popularity of observational techniques it is important to remember that the effects of observer presence, the expectations of the observers and the participants, be they infants or adults, differences in sampling procedures, observer drift, and other variables may influence results, making it imperative to exercise caution in interpreting observational findings (Elwick, Bradley, & Sumsion, 2014). Perhaps the most salient problem in observational techniques is determining which aspects of social competence to observe. Simply defining and observing specific facets of social behavior does not necessarily guarantee that such behaviors are critical for socialization and adaptive social functioning. Given the lack of construct validity (the ability of the chosen instruments to measure the constructs being investigated) in most observational studies, it is impossible to know whether the behavioral constructs evaluated are in fact related to social competence, or, as stated above, whether the behaviors rated can be compared across studies. In addition the generalizability of findings from observational studies remains questionable and the differential role of specific behaviors in a variety of settings must always be considered. Finally, the validity of cross-sectional sampling procedures also requires reexamination, since there are indications that cross-sectional findings may be only weakly correlated with the results of longitudinal studies (Carmona, Buunk, Peiró, Rodríguez, & Bravo, 2006; Egeland, 1991).

In addition to naturalistic observation of children's behavior, many studies assess social behavior through simulating real-life situations in the laboratory. This may be done by role playing or by establishing a relationship and then manipulating aspects of the social interaction, but the external validity of these paradigms has been questioned (Whiten, 1991) and therefore the interpretation of the findings of such studies must also be treated with caution. Depending on the type of behavior being assessed and the age of the child, interviews, questionnaires and other social experimental tasks can be used to validate findings. Although each of these techniques has its own limitations, they can serve as useful adjuncts to other methods of assessment. In general, despite the aforementioned drawbacks, direct observational methods, particularly with infants, remain the most accepted research methodology in assessing behavior within a social context.

Research into social competence is based on delineating the young child's competencies at particular ages and how the infant transitions from one developmental stage to the next. Consider for example the development of joint attention (Akhtar & Gernsbacher, 2007; Moore & Dunham, 2014; Mundy et al., 2007), which involves attending together with another person to a common event or object external to both participants. In order to be considered joint attention, there must be three mutual points of shared attention, one to the other person, one to the event or object and one back to the other person. Alternatively, the three points can begin with the event or object, and one of the participants looks at the object, then to the other observer and back to the object (Meltzoff & Moore, 1998). The ability to follow others' looks and points to objects and events in the world and to draw others' attention to the things in the world which interest us is often considered an ultimate social achievement of late infancy along with the consolidation of primary attachments, which together constitute the foundational skills for learning about the world from others. However, the mechanisms involved in these skills and their relationship with other social skills remain unclear.

Changes at the End of the First Year in Gaze Behavior

One possible explanation for the changes observed in social behavior at the end of the first year is that by the end of the first year of life, the infant seems to understand that gaze can be intentional (Tomasello, 1999; Woodward, 2005), which means that the very young child has already acquired initial comprehension of others' mental states. The infant's knowledge regarding gaze and other social signals is predicated on his or her understanding that people are influenced by their experiences in the world and that their behavior is governed by the context in which it occurs. This set of abilities opens the infant up to direct socialization, as he or she can begin to interpret others' motives and intentions. Because of this, caregivers should be able to teach a wide variety of novel behaviors, as the 12 month old is able to understand the caregiver's mind more flexibly than a younger infant. Infants at this age also contribute more directly to learning in the social context by sharing information, emotions, and preferences, as well as by observing others and appropriating relevant behavior into their own repertoire.

Another explanation could be that infants by the end of their first year have learned general tenets regarding rule-governed behavior, including spatial and temporal relationships between one's own and others' movements and behavior, and about the objects in the world to which these behaviors (gazing, pointing, smiling, and frowning) are directed. Likewise they learn that adults' language refers to something in the physical world that they are referencing (Ruffman & Perner, 2005). This explanation does not yet incorporate a young child having a more developed theory of mind (Moore, 2007), which will continue to mature during toddlerhood. This interpretation has the young child understanding less of the social world and therefore requires parents and adults to accommodate the limited social understanding of the young child in their socializing attempts.

In this view, both socializing and social learning processes change significantly during the years of toddlerhood. For example, Lillard et al. (2013) perceive pretend play as an important context for social learning. Pretend play begins around 12–-14 months of age and the ability to represent something which is not present is dependent on the skillfulness of the adult or older child who is playing with the one year old. Parents provide toddlers who are not yet skilled pretenders with specific reliable behavioral cues which signify the playful aspect of pretending as something different from the real world. The earliest instances of pretending occur in the context of social play, during which the infant receives clear behavioral cues from the interaction with a partner who demonstrates how to participate in and interpret play actions. Development of pretending constitutes a gradual shift from the child's conceptualization of the world as immediate and concrete to pretense, which is the foundation of underlying abstract mental states. This shift is partially driven by explicit socialization, with parents adapting the amount and nature of their support for their child's understanding of pretense as the child's skills and capabilities change.

The toddler's early word learning facilitates parental socialization as the child participates in functional socializing contexts of social life until he or she begins to understand the words associated with familiar routines. Homer and Nelson (2009) view children as continuously scaffolded by adults as they become more involved in everyday activities and begin to communicate more socially. Children are motivated to learn language as a tool for more complete participation in shared activities (Akhtar & Martinez-Sussman, 2007). As parents expand their young child's world they increase the meanings which are shared between them. This means that the earliest language emerges from caregivers' socialization of their children, in keeping with an emphasis on general social and emotional competence (Harris, Donnelly, Guz, & Pitt-Watson, 1986; Hay & Cook, 2007). Nelson (2009) posits that the language that a child first learns is idiosyncratic, learned mimetically and not appropriate outside the familiar routines in which it was acquired. This suggests that the 12 month old's words and gestures are learned differently and serve different purposes for the child and the adults than those of the 24 or 36 month old child. Thus it can be argued that language is also acquired contextually and it is important to consider the context when assessing infant mental health issues, questions and problems.

Infant Socialization in the Home Culture

Understanding how children absorb and learn about the social world around them is crucial, particularly when studying the impact of early experience on social outcomes. Whatever formulations of development are employed, they must be complex and must take into account the quality of early interactions and experience (Sameroff, 2010, Sroufe, 2000). Research in the twenty-first century also focuses on genetic factors involved in development, and evidence from temperament studies, such as the fact that anxious adults give birth to inhibited children (Fox, Henderson, Marshall, Nichols, & Ghera, 2005), seems to imply that it is less crucial to study the effects of early experience. However, by investigating how genetic factors and experience interact to produce individual characteristics, it may be possible to understand how to optimize the socialization of young children. We may hypothesize that genetically transmitted characteristics of the infant, including temperament, influence the way that infant is treated by the adults who care for him or her.

Implicit and Explicit Socialization

Recognizing the mutual interactional impact that young children and adults have on one another is crucial for understanding infant and early childhood mental health, which is based on relationship building, the foundation upon which social emotional competence develops. During the first three years of life, socialization moves from indirect or implicit to direct or explicit socialization. In the first year, children are socialized through touch and soothing or comforting behavior. This includes sleeping arrangements, carrying the child, feeding and eating routines, social play and toilet training. For example, interaction around feeding, which occurs many times throughout the day, every day, is a socializing experience. It involves learning socially and culturally acceptable foods and beginning to understand when and where people eat.

If the parent is sensitive to the baby's cues and appropriately understands the baby's signal that he or she is hungry, the baby begins to expect that people care about his or her wellbeing, but if the caregiver is unavailable or insensitive to those signals, the child does not expect to be cared for or understood. Communication during feeding, even as the child begins to self-feed, is part of the socialization process regarding relationships between people. As purposeful communication is related to empathy and sense of self, it is a basic component to be addressed when evaluating infant mental health status.

In general, it is important to view all child rearing tasks as somehow related to socialization (Mercer, 1981). Infants learn from their caregivers what is culturally appropriate and how things are done in their affiliatory group. This socialization process occurs in all developmental domains, as the infant learns the rhythm and style of motoric activity, such as internalizing the postures and gestures which characterize a particular group and are unfamiliar to another. Similarly, at the emotional level, it involves learning attitudes and fears; at the physical level, learning what food is acceptable to eat and when and where it is appropriate to sleep; and cognitively it involves language as the communicative tool through which these messages are made explicit. For example, as the infant develops from the unconscious imitation of other family members to the messages transmitted initially through touch (implicitly) to the more explicit messages conveyed, socialization occurs. As previously mentioned, a tired or fussy infant self-calms by employing techniques that were initially provided by a concerned and sensitive caregiver.

Parents and caregivers begin to use overt instruction, correction of inappropriate or undesirable behaviors and explanations to communicate specific expectations, standards and rules for socially acceptable behavior (Forman & Kochanska, 2001;

Perez & Gauvain, 2007; Thompson & Goodvin, 2007). Parents also begin to communicate how pleased or displeased they are with their children's behavior. These evaluations reflect cultural mores and transmit messages regarding normative or norm-violating behavior to the children themselves. Explicit socialization emerges along with children's emerging abilities to reflect on their own and others' behavior and goals, to regulate their behavior consciously and strategically, and to begin to understand others' expectations with regard to their behavior. They are more attentive to verbally communicated messages and instructions, which are a main source of explicit socialization. Praise, encouragement, prohibitions and punishment require shared meaning and shared motivations (Owen, Slep, & Heyman, 2012; Perez & Gauvain, 2007).

It is possible to assume that conflict between the child and parents and other caregivers is another expression of explicit socialization. Social conflicts arise during this period as young children challenge restrictions and expectations which are not the same as the child's own goals and preferences. These conflicts reveal that children understand their parents' goals and desires, compare them to their own and recognize that they are not the same. In addition, at this age children realize that they can control their own behavior, which then affects their parents' behavior. Thus, parent-child conflicts are normative, a vital component of explicit socialization emerging out of the child's growing autonomy and the parent's efforts to encourage the child's adherence to culturally appropriate behavior. If either the child or the parent does not understand the importance of this developmental socialization pathway or responds in a maladaptive manner, problems in infant mental health can occur (Frick & Morris, 2004).

Explicit socialization is the sequel to the bonding and attachment which occur between the parent and the child during the first year of life, and it involves learning a broad set of rules which govern accepted socially and culturally normative behavior. One of the most important roles that parents play in the socialization of their young children is to guide their children to comply with rules which govern acceptable behavior. Successful socialization regarding rules provides the foundation for interaction with other children, caregivers, adults, neighbors and others in their social group. In early childhood, rules are simple and often revolve around safety and prohibitions. In addition, this is the time that children are instructed about expectations regarding respect for others, like not taking things without permission, and respect for property, like not coloring on the walls, and the young child is expected to comply and behave appropriately. This period of explicit socialization in the home by the parents is a time for teaching the child to be able to wait for attention, to organize and attain goals, and to internalize behavioral conventions and expectations (Greenspan & Wieder, 2007; Shonkoff & Philips, 2000). Internalization of rules depends on the young child's ability to understand and accept the parent's message. To achieve this, the parent must get the child's attention, give clear and consistent messages, and signal how important compliance with the rule is to the parent. Socialization of prosocial behavior is also accomplished by modeling the desired behaviors. The parent's demonstration of sympathy when the child is hurt or needs help, rather than mocking behavior, is one of the most powerful tools of instruction.

Parenting

Parental Awareness

The role of socializing the young child is one of the most important aspects of parenting. Although most parents are able to cope with the complexities of parenting, they do so by instinct and motivated by love. But good parents must also be able to reason about how to care for their infant and be mindful of their parenting (Duncan, Coatsworth, & Greenberg, 2009). A sense of love and connection is critical but it does not necessarily provide the knowledge that parents need in order to fulfill their role and to cope with the never-ending job of raising a young child successfully into adulthood.

This parental awareness of the parenting role has been conceptualized as parental or maternal reflective functioning (Fonagy, Steele, & Steele, 1991; Ordway, Sadler, Dixon, & Slade, 2014), which was defined as the capacity to understand that one's own and another's behaviors are linked in meaningful ways to underlying mental states, to feelings, wishes, thoughts, and desires. Reflective functioning suggests an awareness that an individual's behavior is a reflection of internal therefore unobservable, changing, dynamic, intentions and emotions. As such reflective functioning enables the parent to reflect on his or her own feelings and mental states, as well as having an interpersonal component that provides the parent the opportunity to distinguish between inner and outer reality, and pretend play and personal, mental and emotional processes which occur as a result of the infant-parent communication (Fonagy, Target, Steele, & Steele, 1998).

Essential to maternal reflective functioning is the capacity to recognize that the child, no matter how young, has mental states, which leads to the essence of reflective functioning which is the ability to link the awareness of the child's and/or the parent's own internal state to behavior or to other internal states. Here is an example of maternal reflective functioning about her toddler's behavior and her frustration. "Sometimes he seems so upset (child's mental state) and I don't really understand why (link to mother's mental state). It seems like he is trying to tell me what he wants and I respond but it turns out that he wanted something else (child's mental state). I get confused (mother's mental state) when I try the wrong thing because I don't know what he wants or what he is feeling (link to child's mental state). That's so hard for me, particularly when he starts to tantrum (child's behavior). Sometimes I try to calm him down, pick him up but he isn't ready to calm down because he still is angry (appreciation of the child's mental state). When that happens, I realize that it's me who wants to hold him, but he doesn't want that, so I try to give him more time (distinction between her feelings and those of the child)" (adapted from Slade, 2005).

Reflective functioning allows the caregiver to reflect on complex and often uncomfortable mental states without feeling overwhelmed. This ability allows the adult to fully appreciate the intersubjective nature of the parent-child relationship and to recognize not only the influence that she has on her child, but that specifically what she does and thinks profoundly affects the relationship she has with her child. The higher the level of parental awareness in general and of reflective functioning specifically, the more capable the parent is of dealing with the challenges of child rearing. Optimal outcomes in young children are associated with higher levels of parental awareness (Brophy-Herb et al., 2011; Feldman, Eidelman, & Rotenberg, 2004) and of maternal insightfulness (Koren-Karie, Oppenheim, Dolev, Sher, & Etzion-Carasso, 2002). Insightfulness refers to the parent's capacity to invoke motives that underlie the child's behavior (Oppenheim & Koren-Karie, 2002).

Parenting Styles

Parents can be quite different from one another, and even fathers and mothers of the same child, living in the same households can have different childrearing philosophies and practices. It is important to remember that there is no such thing as a perfect parent and that no one style is better than another, but specific behavioral correlates have been found to be associated with different parenting styles. The concept of parenting style reflects systematic and sometimes subtle differences in approaches to raising children and is an attempt to link parenting to children's behavioral outcome. Unfortunately most of the research in this area is correlational, making it difficult to understand the causal relationships between parenting styles and later outcomes. The seminal research in this area was conducted by Diana Baumrind (1966, 1967), who studied 100 preschool aged children, and using naturalistic observation and parental interviews identified four dimensions of parenting which include disciplinary strategies, warmth and nurturance, communication styles and expectations of maturity and control. Using factor analysis statistics, Baumrind (1966) identified three parenting style categories with differing profiles regarding the four dimensions of parenting, and further research by Maccoby and Martin (1983) added a fourth parenting style category.

The four parenting styles are defined as authoritarian, authoritative, permissive and uninvolved. The authoritarian parent attempts to shape, control, and evaluate the behavior and attitudes of the child in accordance with a set standard of conduct, usually an absolute standard, often theologically motivated and/or formulated by a higher authority. If a parent belongs in this category, he or she values obedience as a virtue and favors punitive measures to curb the child's will whenever the child's actions or beliefs conflict with the actions and beliefs of the parent. The child is to be kept in his or her place, with restricted autonomy, and is assigned household responsibilities in order to inculcate respect for work. The preservation of order and traditional structure is a highly valued goal and therefore verbal give and take is not encouraged.

The authoritative parent seems similar to the authoritarian parent in that there are attempts to direct the child's activities and there is a strong sense of right and wrong; however, when the parent is authoritarian, he or she decides what is right, whereas an authoritative parent presents the issues in a rational, issue-oriented manner, employing verbal negotiations, sharing with the child the reasoning behind the policy, and soliciting objections when the child refuses to conform. Both autonomous self-will and disciplined conformity are valued, so that the parent exerts firm control when the child and parent disagree but does not limit the child with unexplained restrictions. While recognizing and enforcing the adult perspective, the authoritative parent also appreciates the child's individual interests. The authoritative parent affirms the child's present behavior and qualities, but also sets standards for future conduct and uses reason to shape and reinforce behavior to achieve stated objectives, without basing decisions simply on group consensus or the individual child's desires.

Differently from both the authoritarian and authoritative parent, the permissive parent typically behaves in a non-punitive, accepting and affirmative manner towards the child's impulses, desires, and actions. The parent consults with the child about policy decisions and gives full explanations for family rules. Few demands for household responsibility and orderly behavior are placed on the child. The parent is seen as a resource for the child to use as necessary or desired, not as an ideal to be emulated or as an active agent responsible for shaping or altering the child's ongoing or future behavior. The child is allowed to regulate his or her own activities as much as possible, while the parent avoids exercising control and does not encourage the child to obey externally defined standards. An uninvolved parenting style is characterized by few demands, low responsiveness and little communication. While these parents fulfill the child's basic needs, they are generally detached from their child's life. In extreme cases, these parents may even reject or neglect the needs of their children.

Parenting styles in early childhood have been associated with various child developmental outcomes, with authoritarian parenting styles generally leading to children who are obedient and proficient but who rank lower in happiness, social competence and self-esteem. Authoritative parenting styles, on the other hand, tend to result in children who are happy, capable and successful (Maccoby, 1992). Children of permissive parents often rank lowest in happiness and in self-regulation, and are more likely to experience difficulty with authority, which typically expresses itself in poor school performance. Uninvolved parenting styles result in children who tend to lack self-control, have low-self-esteem and are less socially competent. Despite these findings which seem to support authoritative parenting, not all parents adopt that style. Some potential reasons that parents are not all authoritative in their parenting stem from personality, family size, parental background, culture, educational and socioeconomic levels and religious beliefs.

Empirical findings reveal that parental use of corporal punishment has adverse effects on children's social and behavioral adjustment (Davidov & Khoury-Kassabri, 2013; Taylor, Lee, Guterman, & Rice, 2010), but despite its negative effects, corporal punishment remains a common disciplinary technique among parents (Khoury-Kassabri, 2010). In an attempt to understand this behavior within the family and cultural systems in which the child is developing, Khoury-Kassabri, Attar-Schwartz, and Zur (2014) analyzed the effects of corporal punishment within the family system on multiple levels in an attempt to understand the influence of cultural and family contexts on young children's behavior and adjustment difficulties. Two thousand four hundred and forty-seven Arab mothers reported in anonymous questionnaires that they strongly supported the use of corporal punishment. The use of corporal punishment mediated the association between mothers' lower perceived self-efficacy in disciplining their children, parental disagreement with regard to disciplinary methods and maternal stress in predicting children's mental health problems. These results emphasize the need to understand children's social and emotional development within the context of the family system and culture within the family when interpreting children's adaptive behavior.

It is also important to remember that when two parents are raising a child together there may be differences in their styles and if the mother has, for example, an authoritative style while the father has more of a punitive approach, the child may not experience a cohesive parenting style. In order to create a consistent approach to parenting, parents should learn to cooperate and combine the different elements of their unique parenting styles. Prevention and intervention programs should address parents' awareness of the influence of their disciplinary styles on their children's behavioral outcomes. Understanding diverse cultural values and associated child rearing practices reveals the strengths of socialization and should be appreciated with regard to diverse cultural groups in the field of infant and early childhood mental health. Knowledge can be acquired through training, education, or experience with a culture in various contexts.

Research Methodology in Cross-Cultural Infant and Early Childhood Mental Health

Research Strategies and Instruments

Research on cross-cultural socialization processes utilizes a variety of approaches, including naturalistic observational techniques as well as experimental designs. Because socialization is the result of a combination of biological and environmental factors, research designs often focus on interactions (Zahn-Waxler, 1995, 2002). Tronick (2013) surveyed different research strategies employed to study early emotional and social development in a unique integrative methodology. Firstly, mothers were trained to make systematic observations of emotional events in their children's lives; secondly, responses to mild emotional events, such as bumping an elbow, were experimentally tested in the laboratory; and finally, an apartment was set up in the laboratory as a home environment in which mothers and their children could be observed interacting in a naturalistic setting.

Another useful strategy in researching cultural contextual effects on infant and early childhood developmental and behavioral outcomes is the use of checklists. Two behavioral checklists specifically adapted for use with very young children are frequently used as mental health outcome measures. The Child Behavior Checklist

(CBCL: Achenbach, Edelbrock, & Howell, 1987) is a 100-item measure that asks parents to rate the degree to which their children's behavior is described in a statement (not true, somewhat true, very true). Behaviors such as non-compliance, defiance, inability to wait and uncooperativeness, and other clusters of behaviors have all been associated with negative mental health outcomes. Designed to assess even younger children's behavior, the Infant Toddler Social and Emotional Assessment (ITSEA: Briggs-Gowan & Carter, 2006) is a 165-item questionnaire which parents complete in a similar manner to the CBCL.

Because the adult's role in socialization is a powerful one, techniques for assessing the general environment and particular adult characteristics are also relevant for assessing the context in which the infant or toddler is developing. The use of reliable and valid measures for interpreting observations in the home environment allows for comparisons across investigations as well as providing a useful way to focus on salient variables in the observation. The Home Measurement of Environment (HOME: Caldwell & Bradley, 1984) has been used in the homes of infants and toddlers, from birth to three years of age. It focuses on maternal responsivity and acceptance as well as the physical organization of the home environment, including the appropriateness of play materials and opportunities for stimulation. Some research tools focus on emotional characteristics of parents, including the Beck Depression Inventory (BDI-II: Beck, Steer, & Brown, 1996), which is a 21-question multiple choice self-report inventory, and the Adult Attachment Interview (AAI: Fonagy et al., 1991), which includes twenty questions which focus on adults' reminiscences about their childhood.

An additional technique is ethnography, which involves the qualitative description of events in a group's everyday life. Originally ethnography was a strategy used exclusively by anthropologists, but it is now a favored technique in infant research. Ethnography is the observation, often through videotaping, of people within their own cultural context, going about their lives in their own homes. Its goal is to understand how life is seen by those living it and being studied (Freel, 1996). Ethnography is a qualitative research technique and is therefore affected by the researcher's subjective view and is most helpful in generating rather than testing theories.

The Culturally Determined "Ideal Child"

Differences in behavioral expectations and in values between cultures are reflected in the preferred endpoints of child development and in how parenting is involved in achieving those goals. Two alternative cultural frameworks have been formulated, both of which are a bit simplistic. In one model, parents want their children to be independent, self-fulfilled and autonomous individuals who enter social relationships and responsibilities by personal choice (Miller, Feldman, & Pasta, 2002). This is typically associated with Western societies, and is part of a greater social model called individualism (Triandis, 1989), where self-realization and the attainment of happiness have been conceptualized as indicators of positive mental health. The other model places greater significance on interdependence (Greenfield, 1994), and is part of a broader social model called collectivism (Triandis, 1989), in which the primary goal of development is interdependence, such that the mature individual sees himself or herself embedded in a network of relationships and responsibilities to others, with personal achievements measured by service to the collective, most often the family and family members. This model has been associated with more traditional, nonwestern societies, such as those in Africa or the Far East.

These models not only generate preferred development and socialization goals, they also function as interpretive frameworks, guiding evaluation of others' behaviors, thoughts, and feelings. As interpretive frameworks the models clarify reasons for cultural differences and the values underlying cross-cultural variability in actions and internal states. As cultural models, individualism and collectivism integrate group differences across developmental domains and different periods of development and provide theoretical, cultural and developmental coherence to what appear prima facie to be unconnected group differences.

Children are first fully exposed during infancy to the cultural beliefs, practices and meanings that surround them and are characteristic of the members of the developing child's community, which are among the most meaningful influences on the child's future (Weisner, 2002). During this developmental period, culture determines the pathway for future choices; it is crucial to be aware of cultural assumptions, as a lack of understanding of cultural foundations can cause problems in communicating with and advising parents. Knowledge of cultural aspects of infancy is essential for all early childhood practitioners including pediatricians, nurses, educators and infant mental health professionals. An understanding of the diverse developmental trajectories set in infancy may provide insight into different observed behavioral patterns, even at a later stage in life. Because it is not possible in the scope of this chapter to address discrete behaviors, the focus will be on paying attention to ethnic diversity and on providing meaning to cultural differences. It is important to note that in this chapter cultural models are not limited to national or ethnic groups, but include any way of grouping people which has an effect on the socialization process and developmental goals of young children. Cultural models and developmental goals operate in a context of economic, social, psychological and physical factors, which can include influences of socioeconomic level, rural/urban locality, level of education and other social markers.

Cultural Differences in Childrearing

Cultural views and goals seem to demand a particular way to parent, making it difficult for people to realize that there are many ways to raise a child. For example, in the field of infant mental health, sleeping and eating disturbances are typically the reason for referral during the first year in Western countries (Craig & Boardman, 1997). Although sleep disturbances are reported as a major concern of parents of young children in the United States (Brazelton, 1999), they are rarely reported in Japan (Kawasaki, Nugent, Miyashita, Miyahara, & Brazelton, 1994) and nonexistent in Kenya (Super & Harkness, 1982). In order to understand these differences it may be helpful to learn from other cultures. In tribal families where co-sleeping is the accepted norm, night waking is not seen as problematic because of the convenience of the sleeping arrangements. Yet it is important to note that in the absence of cultural pressure on babies to sleep through the night or have regular bedtimes, Super and Harkness found that Kenyan babies slept an average of three hours a night until 8 months of age. Sleeping arrangements are an integral part of whole systems of cultural meaning and ecological constraints, and as we look cross-culturally, new options for change appear. On the other hand, it is important not to try to insert different cultural norms, such as co-sleeping, in Western societies, without recognizing that there may be a mismatch between the child's socialized dependence and the parents' own culturally shaped need for independence.

Different cultural models are translated into what is perceived as appropriate parenting behavior, based on cultural beliefs. For example, Kenyan mothers think that western mothers are too slow to respond to their infants' crying, which is the child's communicative system. Likewise they see toddlers as unruly and think that mothers excessively praise their children instead of teaching them to act respectfully. Western mothers are appalled that Kenyan mothers leave their infants with five or six year old children watching them. Since Kenyan mothers do not look at their babies while they are breastfeeding, and do not praise their toddlers' often unsuccessful attempts at a new skill, Western mothers see them as authoritarian and punitive with their children (Dixon, Tronick, Keefer, & Brazelton, 2014). Thus, the importance of understanding parenting as reflecting socialization practices cannot be overestimated, as parents embody and represent the broader cultural context and accompany their children as they become members of that culture. Parents and their children establish their own family culture with specific norms, customs and values which reflect the cultural and ethnic norms of the larger group.

One of the goals of the socialization process is for parents to pass on strategies which will promote the survival of their children and foster their social and cultural competence (Keller et al., 2004). Socialization strategies embody the accumulated knowledge of individuals in a given environment and they are hierarchically organized, with the most abstract level consisting of socialization goals which express the developmental achievements which parents want to impart to their children. Socialization goals are translated into a system of parental ideas (Goodnow, 1988; Lancy, 2014), beliefs (Cheah & Chirkov, 2008) and ethnotheories (Carra, Lavelli, & Keller, 2014; Harkness & Super, 1996). These ideas are expressed in behavioral strategies, interactions and communication within particular contexts.

Cultural Differences in Attachment Behavior

Cross-cultural differences can be observed in parental goals as they are manifest in attachment behaviors. The manner in which attachment style is assessed in Western society is through the use of the strange situation paradigm (Ainsworth, Blehar, Waters, & Wall, 1978). The strange situation paradigm is based on engineering a situation in which the child is meant to feel stress. Children, beginning at the age of one year, are brought into a room in a laboratory where they play with the mother in the presence of an unfamiliar adult. The children's responses are observed and coded when playing with the mother, when the mother leaves and they are left with an unfamiliar adult, and when they are left totally alone. In addition their responses upon reunification with their mothers are observed and analyzed by reliable trained coders.

The behaviors displayed by the children in the strange situation paradigm are supposed to reflect patterns of emotional expressiveness and attachment. From observing the infant's behavior in these situations, the attachment of infants can be categorized as secure, avoidant, resistant, or disorganized. During the strange situation paradigm, securely attached infants are typically relaxed when they play with their mother, whereas insecure-avoidant infants tend to prefer to play with the stranger and may possibly ignore their mothers. Insecure-ambivalent infants typically play with their mothers and with the stranger but do not seem to be relaxed. When separated from their mothers and left with the stranger, securely attached infants become distressed but calm down when they are reunited with their mothers. At separation from their mothers, some insecure-avoidant infants become stressed but many do not, and they do not seem to regain their emotional balance when their mother returns, whereas insecure-ambivalent infants are stressed when they are alone with the stranger and they are clingy when reunited with their mothers but seem to remain stressed. Finally, disorganized infants are unable to cope with the whole situation and they either respond by exhibiting stereotypical behaviors or become completely unresponsive emotionally. They seem not to be at ease with either the stranger or their mothers. Emotional stress in this situation has also been measured by physiological stress markers including levels of cortisol (Engert, Plessow, Miller, Kirschbaum, & Singer, 2014; Hertsgaard, Gunnar, Erickson, & Nachmias, 1995).

Because the strange situation paradigm seemed inappropriate for the Cameroonian setting, where infants are used to being separated from their mothers but are never without adult company, Otto (2009) explored emotional expression when meeting a stranger in an adapted paradigm which involved a female stranger visiting the family, meeting the family and picking the infant up. The approach of the stranger presented the observers with the opportunity to see how the infant responded to strangers, and picking up the infant presented an opportunity to see how he or she responded to physical contact with a stranger and the response when returned to the mother. In addition to looking for behavioral markers, salivary cortisol was taken from the children's mouths before and after the stranger's visit.

Most of the infants showed no emotional response to meeting the stranger or being touched by the stranger and no elevation in cortisol levels, while a smaller group was calm upon meeting the stranger but became distressed when touched, with a concomitant rise in cortisol levels. Finally, a third group of infants showed negative response from the beginning, and they had elevated cortisol levels just from proximal closeness with a stranger. These results reinforce the claim that although attachment is a universal construct, it maintains a culture-specific manifestation (Otto & Keller, 2014). These findings reveal that in Cameroon, securely attached children are characterized by calmness and minimal emotional expression, whereas Western infants reveal stress when with a stranger and are really at ease only with their own mothers. The socialization goal of calmness is central to Cameroonian mothers, as the children adapt to multiple and changing caregivers (Johow & Voland, 2014).

In addition to emotional expressiveness, maternal sensitivity has been postulated as one of the main components which mothers bring to the mother-child dyad and it is perceived as indispensable for secureattachment (Van IJzendoorn, Juffer, & Duyvesteyn, 1995). This generalization, however, does not take into account the cultural reasons for an infant's behavior or for a mother's interpretation of that behavior. Because mothers transmit the culture to their children, it is important to consider the cultural reasons at the base of their interactions as well. For example, in Japan, babies who are categorized as insecurely attached are usually of the resistant type, whereas in the United States, the insecurely attached children are more often avoidant, with avoidant attachment types almost nonexistent in Japan (Takahashi, 2005; Van IJzendoorn & Kroonenberg, 1988).

Cultural differences in parenting may provide a possible interpretation for the variation in attachment styles. Japanese mothers rarely leave their children in the care of strangers or babysitters, as they see being one with their infant as an important developmental goal (Kawakami, Takai-Kawakami, & Kanaya, 1994). Thus, the separations which occur in the strange situation are particularly stressful for the child (and for the mother). Lamb and Sternberg (1990) confirmed that unaccustomed separations from the mother can cause anxiety which is expressed in the strange situation paradigm. This was measured when babies were introduced to day care, where despite the increase in anxiety, habituation to day care helped the behavioral manifestations abate. Further evidence for this hypothesis emerged in a study which focused on working Japanese mothers who were living in the United States (Durrett, Otaki, & Richards, 1984), in which researchers found the archetypal resistant pattern (from the Japanese cultural goal of becoming one with their baby) as well as the avoidant type, as these babies were probably more familiar with being left with babysitters than their compatriots in Japan. Of course, there were also securely attached children in each cultural group.

It appears that the separation history of the infant affects the infant's responses to the strange situation paradigm (Lubiewska, 2013) and that separation history is in part determined by cross-cultural variability in values and culture-specific factors such as being in day care. It is possible that the higher proportion of resistant infants in Japan is due to the differences in daily separation patterns experienced by

Japanese mothers and their infants and by mothers and their infants in the United States. The results of another study which examined attachment types of German mothers and their infants could be attributed to cultural and socialization factors as well. German infants were more avoidant than both the Japanese and the Unites States samples. In Germany, parents desire their children to be non-clingy and independent, and therefore the greater proportion of avoidant children may be viewed as a culturally desirable trait (Campos & Barrett, 1984; Grossmann & Grossmann, 1991). Since securely attached children were the predominant type in all three cultures, it is possible that the secure pattern of attachment is the norm for the mother-infant interaction pattern, with the alternatives (e.g., avoidant, resistant and/or disorganized) reflecting cultural variations.

Risk Factors Perceived Through a Cultural Lens

After presenting the processes involved in socialization and acculturation of the young child, which is accomplished through parenting practices and social interaction, it is imperative to address risk factors in socialization as a focus in infant mental health. Risk factors are those characteristics of the infant, the caregiver or the context that have the potential to harm development (Cicchetti, 2013). An accumulation of risk factors can negatively influence socialization. Rarely will a single risk factor be identified in an infant's life, because typically risk factors occur in clusters. Because they generally occur in multiples, it is difficult to discover the nature of the effect of any single factor on infant development. Certain factors tend to occur with certain others, reflecting co-morbidity. Contextual or environmental risk factors seem to affect different children in different ways (Rutter, 2005) and function as a dynamic system. The outcome for a particular infant results from the combined impact of all the risk factors present in his or her life circumstances.

Risk factors in the infant include the physical health status of the child, temperament and poor social competence. Infant vulnerability is a poorly defined construct but is a real risk factor, as some infants appear to be unusually strongly affected by events that would not affect more resilient children (Crittenden, 1985). Some risk factors involve experiences over which there is no control. This can include changes in the infant's life which are too rapid or too frequent and events such as the death of a parent, a new sibling, family travel or internal or external changes in living accommodations (Braungart-Rieker & Stifter, 1996). Parental characteristics can also put the socialization of the infant at risk. These can include physical or emotional problems or substance abuse, all of which can have deleterious effects on infant development. Living with ongoing exposure to violence and/or trauma and/or with poverty are environmental stressors for infants. These and other risks factors are more fuly discussed in Chap. 5.

References

Achenbach, T. M., Edelbrock, C., & Howell, C. (1987). Empirically-based assessment of the behavioral/emotional problems of 2- and 3-year old children. *Journal of Abnormal Child Psychology, 15*, 629–650.

Ainsworth, M. D., Blehar, M. C., Waters, E., & Wall, S. (1978). *Patterns of attachment: Assessed in the strange situation and at home*. Hillsdale, NJ: Erlbaum.

Akhtar, N., & Gernsbacher, M. A. (2007). Joint attention and vocabulary development: A critical look. *Language and Linguistics Compass, 1*(3), 195–207.

Akhtar, N., & Martinez-Sussman, C. (2007). Intentional communication. In C. Brownell & C. Kopp (Eds.), *Socioemotional development in the toddler years: Transitions and transformations* (pp. 201–220). New York, NY: Guilford Press.

Atzil, S., Hendler, T., & Feldman, R. (2011). Specifying the neurobiological basis of human attachment: Brain, hormones, and behavior in synchronous and intrusive mothers. *Neuropsychopharmacology, 36*(13), 2603–2615.

Baumrind, D. (1966). Effects of authoritative parental control on child behavior. *Child Development, 37*(4), 887–907.

Baumrind, D. (1967). Child care practices anteceding three patterns of preschool behavior. *Genetic Psychology Monographs, 75*, 43–88.

Beck, A. T., Steer, R. A., & Brown, G. (1996). *BDI-II, Beck depression inventory: Manual*. San Antonio, TX: Psychological Corp.

Berns, R. (2012). *Child, family, school, community: Socialization and support*. Stamford, CT: Cengage Learning.

Bowlby, J. (1956). *The growth of independence in the young child*. Publisher not identified.

Braungart-Rieker, J. M., & Stifter, C. A. (1996). Infants' responses to frustrating situations: Continuity and change in reactivity and regulation. *Child Development, 67*(4), 1767–1779.

Brazelton, T. B. (1999). How to help parents of young children: The touchpoints model. *Journal of Perinatology, 19*(6), S6–S7.

Briggs-Gowan, M. J., & Carter, A. (2006). *Manual for the infant–toddler social and emotional assessment (ITSEA)–version 2*. San Antonio, TX: Psychological Corp.

Brophy-Herb, H. E., Schiffman, R. F., Bocknek, E. L., Dupuis, S. B., Fitzgerald, H. E., Horodynski, M., … & Hillaker, B. (2011). Toddlers' social-emotional competence in the contexts of maternal emotion socialization and contingent responsiveness in a low-income sample. *Social Development, 20*(1), 73–92.

Buttelmann, D., Zmyj, N., Daum, M., & Carpenter, M. (2013). Selective imitation of in-group over out-group members in 14-month-old infants. *Child Development, 84*(2), 422–428.

Caldwell, B. M., & Bradley, R. H. (1984). *Home observation for measurement of the environment*. Little Rock, AR: University of Arkansas at Little Rock.

Campos, J. J., & Barrett, K. C. (1984). Toward a new understanding of emotions and their development. In C. E. Izard, R. Kagan, & R. B. Zajonc (Eds.), *Emotions, cognition, and behavior* (pp. 229–263). Cambridge, UK: Cambridge University Press.

Carmona, C., Buunk, A. P., Peiró, J. M., Rodríguez, I., & Bravo, M. J. (2006). Do social comparison and coping styles play a role in the development of burnout? cross-sectional and longitudinal findings. *Journal of Occupational and Organizational Psychology, 79*(1), 85–99.

Carra, C., Lavelli, M., & Keller, H. (2014). Differences in practices of body stimulation during the first 3 months: Ethnotheories and behaviors of Italian mothers and West African immigrant mothers. *Infant Behavior and Development, 37*(1), 5–15.

Cheah, C. S., & Chirkov, V. (2008). Parents' personal and cultural beliefs regarding young children: A cross-cultural study of aboriginal and Euro-Canadian mothers. *Journal of Cross-Cultural Psychology, 39*(4), 402–423.

Cicchetti, D. (2013). An overview of developmental psychopathology. *The Oxford handbook of developmental psychology, 2*, 455–480.

Craig, T. K., & Boardman, A. P. (1997). ABC of mental health: Common mental health problems in primary care. *British Medical Journal, 314*(7094), 1609–1612.

Crittenden, P. M. (1985). Maltreated infants: Vulnerability and resilience. *Journal of Child Psychology and Psychiatry, 26*(1), 85–96.

Davidov, M., & Khoury-Kassabri, M. (2013). Recollections of harsh discipline in childhood and depressive feelings in adulthood: The roles of culture and gender. *Children and Youth Services Review, 35*(6), 1007–1014.

Dean, L. G., Kendal, R. L., Schapiro, S. J., Thierry, B., & Laland, K. N. (2012). Identification of the social and cognitive processes underlying human cumulative culture. *Science, 335*(6072), 1114–1118.

Dixon, S., Tronick, E., Keefer, C., & Brazelton, T. B. (2014). Mother-infant interaction among the Gusii of Kenya. In T. M. Field, A. M. Sostek, P. Vietze, & P. H. Leiderman (Eds.), *Culture and early interactions (psychology revivals)* (pp. 149–169). New York, NY: Psychology Press.

Duncan, L. G., Coatsworth, J. D., & Greenberg, M. T. (2009). A model of mindful parenting: Implications for parent-child relationships and prevention research. *Clinical Child and Family Psychology Review, 12*(3), 255–270.

Durrett, M. E., Otaki, M., & Richards, P. (1984). Attachment and the mother's perception of support from the father. *International Journal of Behavioral Development, 7*(2), 167–176.

Egeland, B. (1991). A longitudinal study of high-risk families: Issues and findings. In R. Starr & D. A. Wolfe (Eds.), *The effects of child abuse and neglect: Issues and research* (pp. 33–56). New York, NY: Guilford Press.

Elwick, S., Bradley, B., & Sumsion, J. (2014). Infants as others: Uncertainties, difficulties and (im) possibilities in researching infants' lives. *International Journal of Qualitative Studies in Education, 27*(2), 196–213.

Engert, V., Plessow, F., Miller, R., Kirschbaum, C., & Singer, T. (2014). Cortisol increase in empathic stress is modulated by emotional closeness and observation modality. *Psychoneuroendocrinology, 45*, 192–201.

Feldman, R., Eidelman, A. I., & Rotenberg, N. (2004). Parenting stress, infant emotion regulation, maternal sensitivity, and the cognitive development of triplets: A model for parent and child influences in a unique ecology. *Child Development, 75*(6), 1774–1791.

Feldman, R., Gordon, I., Influs, M., Gutbir, T., & Ebstein, R. P. (2013). Parental oxytocin and early caregiving jointly shape children's oxytocin response and social reciprocity. *Neuropsychopharmacology, 38*(7), 1154–1162.

Fonagy, P., Steele, M., & Steele, H. (1991). Intergenerational patterns of attachment: Maternal representations during pregnancy and subsequent infant-mother attachments. *Child Development, 62*, 891–905.

Fonagy, P., Target, M., Steele, H., & Steele, M. (1998). *Reflective-functioning manual, version 5.0, for application to adult attachment interviews*. London, UK: University College London.

Forman, D. R., & Kochanska, G. (2001). Viewing imitation as child responsiveness: A link between teaching and discipline domains of socialization. *Developmental Psychology, 37*(2), 198–206.

Fox, N. A., Henderson, H. A., Marshall, P. J., Nichols, K. E., & Ghera, M. M. (2005). Behavioral inhibition: Linking biology and behavior within a developmental framework. *Annual Reviews of Psychology, 56*, 235–262.

Freel, K. S. (1996). Finding complexities and balancing perspectives: Using an ethnographic viewpoint to understand children and their families. *Zero to Three, 16*, 1–7.

Frick, P. J., & Morris, A. S. (2004). Temperament and developmental pathways to conduct problems. *Journal of Clinical Child and Adolescent Psychology, 33*(1), 54–68.

Goodnow, J. J. (1988). Parents' ideas, actions, and feelings: Models and methods from developmental and social psychology. *Child Development, 59*(2), 286–320.

Greenfield, P. M. (1994). Independence and interdependence as developmental scripts: Implications for theory, research, and practice. In P. M. Greenfield & R. R. Cocking (Eds.),

Crosscultural roots of minority child development (pp. 1–37). Hillsdale, NJ: Lawrence Erlbaum.

Greenfield, P. M., Keller, H., Fuligni, A., & Maynard, A. (2003). Cultural pathways through universal development. *Annual Review of Psychology, 54*(1), 461–490.

Greenfield, P. M., Suzuki, L. K., & Rothstein-Fisch, C. (2006). Cultural pathways through human development. In *Handbook of child psychology*. New York, NY: Wiley.

Greenspan, S. I., & Wieder, S. (2007). *Infant and early childhood mental health: A comprehensive developmental approach to assessment and intervention*. Washington, DC: American Psychiatric Publications.

Grossmann, K. E., & Grossmann, K. (1991). Attachment quality as an organizer of emotional and behavioral responses in a longitudinal perspective. In C. M. Parkes, J. Stevenson-Hinde, & P. Marris, (Eds.). (2006), *Attachment across the life cycle* (pp. 93–114). Oxford, UK: Routledge.

Harkness, S., & Super, C. M. (Eds.). (1996). *Parents' cultural belief systems: Their origins, expressions, and consequences*. New York, NY: Guilford Press.

Harris, P. L., Donnelly, K., Guz, G. R., & Pitt-Watson, R. (1986). Children's understanding of the distinction between real and apparent emotion. *Child Development, 57*, 895–909.

Hay, D. F., & Cook, K. V. (2007). The transformation of prosocial behavior from infancy to childhood. In C. Brownell & C. Kopp (Eds.), *Socioemotional development in the toddler years: Transitions and transformations* (pp. 100–131). New York, NY: Guilford Press.

Hertsgaard, L., Gunnar, M., Erickson, M. F., & Nachmias, M. (1995). Adrenocortical responses to the strange situation in infants with disorganized/disoriented attachment relationships. *Child Development, 66*(4), 1100–1106.

Homer, B. D., & Nelson, K. (2009). Naming facilitates young children's understanding of scale models: Language and the development of symbolic understanding. *Journal of Cognition and Development, 10*(1–2), 115–134.

Johow, J., & Voland, E. (2014). Family relations among cooperative breeders: Challenges and offerings to attachment theory from evolutionary anthropology. In H. Otto & H. Keller (Eds.), *Different faces of attachment: Cultural variations on a universal human need* (pp. 27–49). Cambridge, UK: Cambridge University Press.

Kawakami, K., Takai-Kawakami, K., & Kanaya, Y. (1994). A longitudinal study of Japanese and American mother-infant interactions. *Psychologia: An International Journal of Psychology in the Orient, 37*(1), 18–29.

Kawasaki, C., Nugent, J. K., Miyashita, H., Miyahara, H., & Brazelton, T. B. (1994). The cultural organization of infants' sleep. *Children's Environments, 11*(2), 135–141.

Keller, H. (2013). *Cultures of infancy*. New York, NY: Psychology Press.

Keller, H., Lohaus, A., Kuensemueller, P., Abels, M., Yovsi, R., Voelker, S., … & Mohite, P. (2004). The bio-culture of parenting: Evidence from five cultural communities. *Parenting: Science and Practice, 4*(1), 25–50.

Khoury-Kassabri, M. (2010). Attitudes of Arab and Jewish mothers towards punitive and non-punitive discipline methods. *Child & Family Social Work, 15*(2), 135–144.

Khoury-Kassabri, M., Attar-Schwartz, S., & Zur, H. (2014). Understanding the mediating role of corporal punishment in the association between maternal stress, efficacy, co-parenting and children's adjustment difficulties among Arab mothers. *Child Abuse & Neglect, 38*(6), 1073–1082.

Koren-Karie, N., Oppenheim, D., Dolev, S., Sher, E., & Etzion-Carasso, A. (2002). Mothers' insightfulness regarding their infants' internal experience: Relations with maternal sensitivity and infant attachment. *Developmental Psychology, 38*(4), 534–542.

Lamb, M. E., & Sternberg, K. J. (1990). Do we really know how day care affects children? *Journal of Applied Developmental Psychology, 11*(3), 351–379.

Lancy, D. F. (2014). *The anthropology of childhood: Cherubs, chattel, changelings*. Cambridge, UK: Cambridge University Press.

Lillard, A. S., Lerner, M. D., Hopkins, E. J., Dore, R. A., Smith, E. D., & Palmquist, C. M. (2013). The impact of pretend play on children's development: A review of the evidence. *Psychological Bulletin, 139*(1), 1–34.
Lubiewska, K. (2013). Intergenerational congruence of attachment: Limitations of findings. In I. Albert & D. Ferring (Eds.), *Intergenerational relations* (pp. 85–100). Bristol, UK: Policy Press.
Maccoby, E. E. (1992). The role of parents in the socialization of children: An historical overview. *Developmental Psychology, 28*(6), 1006–1017.
Maccoby, E. E., & Martin, J. A. (1983). Socialization in the context of the family: Parent-child interaction. In P. H. Mussen (Series Ed.) & E. M. Hetherington (Vol. Ed.), *Handbook of child psychology: Vol. 4. Socialization, personality, and social development* (4th ed., pp. 1–101) New York: Wiley.
Meltzoff, A. N., & Moore, M. K. (1998). Infant intersubjectivity: Broadening the dialogue to include imitation, identity and intention. In S. Bråten (Ed.), *Intersubjective communication and emotion in early ontogeny* (pp. 47–62). Cambridge, UK: Cambridge University Press.
Mercer, R. T. (1981). A theoretical framework for studying factors that impact on the maternal role. *Nursing Research, 30*(2), 73–77.
Miller, W. B., Feldman, S. S., & Pasta, D. J. (2002). The effect of the nurturant bonding system on child security of attachment and dependency. *Social Biology, 3–4*, 125–159.
Moore, C. (2007). Understanding self and others in the second year. In C. Brownell & C. Kopp (Eds.), *Socioemotional development in the toddler years: Transitions and transformations* (pp. 43–65). New York, NY: Guilford.
Moore, C., & Dunham, P. (Eds.). (2014). *Joint attention: Its origins and role in development.* New York, NY: Psychology Press.
Mundy, P., Block, J., Delgado, C., Pomares, Y., Van Hecke, A. V., & Parlade, M. V. (2007). Individual differences and the development of joint attention in infancy. *Child Development, 78*(3), 938–954.
Nelson, K. (2009). Wittgenstein and contemporary theories of word learning. *New Ideas in Psychology, 27*(2), 275–287.
Oppenheim, D., & Koren-Karie, N. (2002). Mothers' insightfulness regarding their children's internal worlds: The capacity underlying secure child–mother relationships. *Infant Mental Health Journal, 23*(6), 593–605.
Ordway, M. R., Sadler, L. S., Dixon, J., & Slade, A. (2014). Parental reflective functioning: Analysis and promotion of the concept for paediatric nursing. *Journal of Clinical Nursing, 23* (23–24), 3490–3500.
Otto, H. (2009). *Culture-specific attachment strategies in the Cameroonian Nso: Cultural solutions to a universal developmental task.* Unpublished doctoral dissertation.
Otto, H., & Keller, H. (Eds.). (2014). *Different faces of attachment: Cultural variations on a universal human need.* Cambridge, UK: Cambridge University Press.
Over, H., & Carpenter, M. (2012). Putting the social into social learning: Explaining both selectivity and fidelity in children's copying behavior. *Journal of Comparative Psychology, 126*(2), 182–192.
Owen, D. J., Slep, A. M., & Heyman, R. E. (2012). The effect of praise, positive nonverbal response, reprimand, and negative nonverbal response on child compliance: A systematic review. *Clinical Child and Family Psychology Review, 15*(4), 364–385.
Perez, S. M., & Gauvain, M. (2007). The sociocultural context of transitions in early socioemotional development. In C. Brownell & C. Kopp (Eds.), *Socioemotional development in the toddler years: Transitions and transformations* (pp. 396–421). New York, NY: Guilford.
Phillips, L. (2013). *Human adaptation and its failures*. New York, NY: Academic.
Ruffman, T., & Perner, J. (2005). Do infants really understand false belief? *Trends in Cognitive Sciences, 9*(10), 462–463.
Rutter, M. (2005). Environmentally mediated risks for psychopathology: Research strategies and findings. *Journal of the American Academy of Child & Adolescent Psychiatry, 44*(1), 3–18.

Sameroff, A. J. (2010). A unified theory of development: A dialectic integration of nature and nurture. *Child Development, 81*, 6–22.

Shonkoff, J., & Philips, D. (2000). *From neurons to neighborhoods: The science of early childhood development*. Washington, DC: National Academies Press.

Slade, A. (2005). Parental reflective functioning: An introduction. *Attachment & Human Development, 7*(3), 269–281.

Sroufe, L. A. (2000). Early relationships and the development of children. *Infant Mental Health Journal, 21*(1–2), 67–74.

Super, C. M., & Harkness, S. (1982). The infant's niche in rural Kenya and metropolitan America. In L. L. Adler (Ed.), *Cross-cultural Research at Issue* (pp. 47–55). New York, NY: Academic Press.

Takahashi, K. (2005). Toward a life span theory of close relationships: The affective relationships model. *Human Development, 48*(1–2), 48–66.

Taylor, C. A., Lee, S. J., Guterman, N. B., & Rice, J. C. (2010). Use of spanking for 3-year-old children and associated intimate partner aggression or violence. *Pediatrics, 126*(3), 415–424.

Thompson, R. A., & Goodvin, R. (2007). Taming the tempest in the teapot. In C. Brownell & C. Kopp (Eds.), *Socioemotional development in the toddler years: Transitions and transformations* (p. 320). New York, NY: Guilford Press.

Tomasello, M. (1999). *The cultural origins of human cognition*. Cambridge, MA: Harvard University Press.

Triandis, H. C. (1989). The self and social behavior in differing cultural contexts. *Psychological Review, 96*(3), 506–520.

Tronick, E. Z. (2013). The mutual regulation model: The infant's self and interactive regulation and coping and defensive. In T. M. Field, P. M. McCabe, & N. Schneiderman (Eds.), *Stress and coping across development* (pp. 47–68). New York, NY: Psychology Press.

Van IJzendoorn, M. H., Juffer, F., & Duyvesteyn, M. G. (1995). Breaking the intergenerational cycle of insecure attachment: A review of the effects of attachment-based interventions on maternal sensitivity and infant security. *Journal of Child Psychology and Psychiatry & Allied Disciplines, 36*, 225–248.

Van IJzendoorn, M. H., & Kroonenberg, P. M. (1988). Cross-cultural patterns of attachment: A meta-analysis of the strange situation. *Child Development, 59*, 147–156.

Weisner, T. S. (2002). Ecocultural understanding of children's developmental pathways. *Human Development, 45*(4), 275–281.

Whiten, A. (Ed.). (1991). *Natural theories of mind: Evolution, development and simulation of everyday mindreading*. Oxford, UK: Basil Blackwell.

Woodward, A. L. (2005). The infant origins of intentional understanding. *Advances in Child Development and Behaviour, 33*, 229–262.

Zahn-Waxler, C. (1995). Introduction to special section: Parental depression and distress: Implications for development in infancy, childhood, and adolescence. *Developmental Psychology, 31*(3), 347–348.

Zahn-Waxler, C. (2002). Caregiving, emotion, and concern for others. *Behavioral and Brain Sciences, 25*(1), 48–49.

Chapter 4
The Nature-Versus-Nurture Controversy and Its Implications for Infant and Early Childhood Mental Health

Introduction

Researchers have grappled continuously with the question of how to identify the factors which contribute to child development and infant and early childhood mental health. The models which have been proposed range from simplistic to abstract, narrative to statistical, theoretical to translational, and static to dynamic (Sameroff, 2009). Originally the most simplistic designs were dichotomous and research focused on explanations regarding factors stemming from the biological makeup of the child and those related to the experiences the child is exposed to through the environment in which development occurs. This was referred to as the "nature versus nurture" controversy. The questions which were discussed in this controversy revolved around whether determinants of an individual's behavior could be found in intrinsic characteristics of the child or in extrinsic properties of experience. In most cases questions such as these arise when something goes wrong developmentally and the child or the parents experience difficulties. It is not easy to untangle the possible components contributing to specific problems. Some possible causes originate in the child (constitutional), some in the parents (environment), some in the interaction between them and some in other environmental factors.

This chapter is about the difficulty in investigating the various elements involved in behavioral outcomes for young children. It is an attempt to address whether the interaction between nature and nurture is deterministic and to discuss some of the research methodologies which are trying to cull out the proportionate contributions of nature and nurture in any outcome behavior, as well as to appreciate the nature-nurture controversy in terms of developmental change, environmental context, and the transactional relationship between them in order to enhance our understanding of the complexities of development. These issues are particularly pertinent to the field of infant mental health, as one of its main goals is to understand the components which contribute to the wellbeing of children and optimal behavioral and

C. Shulman, *Research and Practice in Infant and Early Childhood Mental Health*, Children's Well-Being: Indicators and Research 13,
DOI 10.1007/978-3-319-31181-4_4

developmental outcomes, in order to support those young children and their families who are displaying mental health problems and to develop preventative programs for those at risk of developing such problems. Thus, this chapter surveys the models used to understand individual change over time, moving from linear models to interactive multilevel dynamic systems models.

History of the Nature Versus Nurture Controversy

In order to understand change over time, it is necessary to examine general systems models which deal with the principles of organization, through varying levels of abstraction. These can range from mathematical formulations to theories regarding specific behaviors in a given child (Sameroff, 2009). The models which are used to explain the complementary aspects of the biological and environmental components of behavior in young children are all dynamic models (Plomin, 1989, 1995, 2008) wherein the parts cannot be separated from the whole; rather, predictions must be made on the basis of the individual. The applicability of the model in explaining the origins of behavior and development is one prominent way in which its efficacy is evaluated.

In order to understand the nature versus nurture question, Sameroff (2010) reviews its history, beginning with the empirical psychological research of Francis Galton (1876) who first coined the term "nature versus nurture". He strongly supported the notion that inherited characteristics, expressed in inherited differences and traits, were the origins of human nature. Perhaps responding to this biologically determined view of development, John Watson (1914), a leading proponent of the opposite view of the sources of behavior, who founded a new school of psychology called behaviorism, explained individual human differences in terms of learning theory. Like the behaviorists, the psychoanalysts also felt that behavior was determined by experience. Despite their different overall orientations, both behaviorists and psychoanalysts proposed that child development was the result of external factors – very simply put, behaviorists believed that children's behavior was a result of reinforcement and psychoanalysts assumed that the parents and quality of interaction with caregivers determined children's course of development.

As it became clear that many complex behaviors did not need reinforcement, and that some responses seemed impervious to experience (Seligman, 1970), another explanation was needed. The field of behavioral genetics (Plomin, 1994) began looking at individual differences in large samples, which made it possible to use statistical models to find patterns of influence on development. These models seemed to provide evidence that some behavior was influenced by genes and some by experience, and that it might be possible to separate them (DeFries, 1967). Even findings from cognitive psychology lent support to the fact that certain skills could not be learned until biological maturation had transpired (Piaget, 1952), which seemed to support a biological base for development. Experience was necessary but could not fully explain individual differences.

Once again, a shift in orientation transpired, perhaps as a result of advances in the social sciences. With the war on poverty and intervention programs such as Head Start, the concept of social ecology was generated (Bronfenbrenner, 1979). Rather than simply focusing on theorizing about reinforcement and performance, social ecology supplemented learning with environmental conditions, specifically economic circumstances, noting that similar individuals from different social classes would have different outcomes, as the developmental environments of the poor put them at a disadvantage in comparison to those of the affluent. At this point, as the social ecology model became an interactive rather than a linear model, it became possible to differentiate distinct levels of influence on the developing child.

Placing the child in the center of co-centric circles, Bronfenbrenner and Morris (2006) incorporated the child's biological constitutional factors, which are affected by the more distal environmental influences of family, school, community, and culture, providing a more comprehensive empirical model for predicting individual differences in development. As a result of technical advances in the fields of neuroscience and molecular biology, the focus has returned once again to the centrality of the child's biological traits. By imaging the brain and manipulating the genome, it has become possible to map brain functioning onto areas of the brain and to link brain functioning to the individual differences found in young children. These individual differences and the search for understanding their basis is the theoretical foundation for behavioral genetics.

It is quite striking that the theories which address the nature-nurture question have alternated between nature and nurture respectively and may continue to do so, as many unanswered questions remain. The fact that there are still so many unexplained individual differences means that exploration must continue. This repetitive pattern, moving from an emphasis on nature to one on nurture and back again, points to a seemingly unresolvable conundrum, which may continue to characterize the understanding of infant behavior and its outcome. Before addressing the lessons to be learned from the nature-nurture question, however, it is important to understand the centrality of individual differences in the field of infant mental health and the gene-environment interplay in relation to infant mental health and emotional and behavioral disturbance. The chapter will end with an analysis of what can be learned about infant development and its outcomes from the nature-nurture controversy.

Individual Differences in Infancy and Early Childhood and Behavioral Genetics

In order to deal with the challenge of understanding the role of genetics and environmental factors in infant and early childhood development, the field of behavioral genetics formulated an innovative methodology for research. Whereas the traditional study of behavior focused on comparisons of the means of the variables being investigated, the preferred methodology in behavioral genetics is the study of variance which focuses on individual differences. Behavioral genetics theory and methods provide a unique perspective on nature and nurture during infancy and early childhood, combining the search for environmental influences on behavior and the exploration of the role of heredity in explaining behavior. This field uses two statistical models to investigate the interactions between nature and nurture. The first is the components of variance approach and the second is model-fitting analyses, both of which often indicate that both biological and environmental factors are significant in understanding individual differences in children.

The methodology which is used in the data analyses focuses on the analysis of the variation (or standard error) which is conceptualized as a measure of individual differences, defined as continuous variation among individuals within a population. Variance is an index of individual differences because it is the squared deviation from the mean. Therefore the measurement used in behavioral genetics is a measurement of each individual's difference from the expected mean as opposed to the study of differences between groups, in which group membership is considered an independent variable and the measurement is of group means, which do not relate to the individual. It is possible to investigate the range of scores by relating to individual differences in this model, because there is a continuously distributed difference among individuals (Silberg, Rutter, Neale, & Eaves, 2001). This is particularly important when looking into attentional abilities and behavior issues and their relationship to genetic and/or environmental factors, because it is not a diagnostic categorical group issue but a dimensional one. Information can be lost, when measurements are collapsed into an average mean score upon which group comparisons are based.

Research Methods for Studying Behavioral Genetics

Analyzing differences in variance as opposed to differences based on group means allows for investigation of interactions among variables and is therefore most pertinent for infant mental health research regarding high risk families, where there are many possible interactions among different variables at different ages. Furthermore it is possible to study individual differences within groups, such as individual differences among boys or girls, or among children at different ages. In the Colorado Adoption Project (CAP: Plomin & DeFries, 1985, Plomin, 1994; 2013), these differences were studied to investigate associations between gene and environment and parent-offspring resemblance. Behavioral measures were compared in infancy and early childhood in order to detect possible differences in the etiology of individual differences. Thus, the behavioral variance is translated into the genetic and the environmental components of the overall statistical variance. Furthermore, the environmental component is broken down into elements shared by family members (similar home environments) and those not shared.

Research in which unrelated children raised together in the same adoptive home participate is the most powerful tool for understanding the influence of growing up together. Investigating the impact of heredity and environment in adoptive families in which family members share environmental but not genetic influences can shed light on environment-development associations and genotype-phenotype interactions and correlations. This distinction between shared and nonshared environments is important because different profiles of relationships emerge in the two environments. For example, in CAP, it was found that adopted children and biological children were more alike in their cognitive abilities in infancy and that adopted children were more like their own biological parents and other biological siblings in other domains of development, such as personality traits, e.g. shyness.

Findings from Behavioral Genetics Research

The aim of research in the field of behavioral genetics is to understand the role of genetic and environmental factors in creating individual differences in child development. This field of study puts forth a conceptual reorganization of genetic influences on infant behavior, moving away from the notion that genes are static, with a straight, uni-dimensional pathogenesis, toward a hypothesis that there are genetic etiologies to developmental change which can be identified in longitudinal research beginning in infancy. Because the Louisiana Twin Study examined identical twins, fraternal twins and non-twin siblings for over 20 years, researchers were able to investigate various levels of genetic closeness and their influences on development. The longitudinal research model can address developmental change and continuity, and by focusing on specific samples, such as twins and adoptees, it is possible to address the relatedness between genetic and environmental factors in shaping a child's behavior.

Researchers in CAP, mentioned above, were able to address genetic and environmental factors in development and behavior through parent-child comparisons by virtue of having four groups in their sample. They researched biological parents and their own biological children who were living together, biological parents living with their adopted children, and the biological parents of those adopted children who were not living together, along with the non-adopted siblings of the parents who had adopted children.

Extrapolating from CAP, Harold et al. (2013) studied the gene-environment interaction in adoptive samples, focusing on the association between maternal hostility, a specific feature of children's rearing environment, and child attention deficit hyperactivity disorder (ADHD) symptoms, while analyzing genetic and environmental variables in biological and adoptive parents of children with ADHD. The adoptive mothers were genetically unrelated to the children, controlling for possible confounding biological effects across the analyses. Findings revealed significant associations between maternal hostility in biologically unrelated adoptive mothers and children's symptoms of ADHD, and between all mothers' ADHD symptoms and child ADHD symptoms, which highlight the salience of maternal parenting behavior in the course of the children's ADHD symptoms. A second key finding of this study was that the biological mother's ADHD symptoms signaled heightened genetic risk for child ADHD, which had an indirect effect on maternal hostility in adoptive mothers only. Significantly, the path from biological mother ADHD symptoms to child impulsivity/activation suggests that such child behaviors might be among the earliest manifestations of genetic influences on child ADHD, and might provide a clue to the mechanisms underlying biologically-based intergenerational transmission of ADHD within families.

Intervention Strategies Based on Behavioral Genetics

Because behavioral genetics deals with variance within the individual, the findings often provide practical implications for intervention, particularly in the field of infant and early childhood mental health. The association between adoptive mothers' parenting hostility and child ADHD symptoms suggests that early interventions targeting mothers' hostility directed towards children may bolster the effectiveness of intervention programs aimed at reducing child ADHD symptom levels in the general population. Numerous existing evidence-based programs targeting child conduct problems include such a focus (e.g. Dishion et al., 2008; Webster-Stratton, Reid, & Hammond, 2001), and National Institutes for Health and Care Excellence (NICE, UK; Birchwood et al., 2014) and European guidelines recommend such programs for the initial treatment of ADHD, but the findings from such studies suggest that earlier intervention might be even more successful. Concomitantly, it may be possible to help parents understand which child traits trigger their hostility, which as a result may decrease subsequent ADHD symptoms. In summary, genetic and environmental factors contributing to young children's ADHD symptoms were successfully separated and studied. Alongside the association between maternal and child ADHD symptoms, it is evident from these findings that these associations cannot be explained solely by common genetic factors.

Gene-Environment Interplay

The field of infant mental health is rapidly assimilating conclusions from research in the area of gene-environment interactions. Almost all gene-environment interaction research has been guided, implicitly if not explicitly, by the diathesis stress model of environmental action (Ingram & Luxton, 2005; Monroe & Simons, 1991), which stipulates that some individuals are more susceptible to the negative consequences of adverse experiences than others (Burmeister, McInnes, & Zöllner, 2008). The two receptors which have been identified as affecting emotional behavior and activity level are a dopamine receptor and a serotonin transmitter, which have been postulated as being associated with the mechanisms for some key individual differences in behaviors such as approach behavior, inhibition, attention and novelty seeking (Auerbach, Benjamin, Faroy, Geller, & Ebstein, 2001). For example, infants with a short allele of the dopamine receptor gene were rated higher in negative emotionality by their mothers at ages 2 and 12 months, and infants with short alleles of the serotonintransmitter gene were found to display heightened fear and inhibition (Auerbach, Faroy, Ebstein, Kahana, & Levine, 2001).

Research also suggests an additive effect across the dopamine and serotonin genes, with infants showing short alleles in both dopamine and serotonin displaying more negative reactivity then infants who carry only one risk allele (Auerbach et al., 1999). While these genes were identified as playing a role in infant behavioral variation, it is important to consider the critical influence of early social experience on gene functioning. Environmental factors can either improve or intensify genetically based behavior (Caspi et al., 2003; Fox, Henderson, Marshall, Nichols, & Ghera, 2005). The expectation, then, is that individuals who carry 'risk alleles' or 'vulnerability genes' function more poorly than those without the identified vulnerability under conditions of contextual adversity, such as child maltreatment, or other negative life events. Examples of this include children who carried the serotonin allele risk gene and had experienced childhood abuse, who were more likely to develop depression, but only when their caregivers were under heightened stress (Kaufman et al., 2006). Similarly, behaviorally inhibited infants who carried the serotonin risk allele were at higher risk for behavioral inhibition later in life, but only when their caregivers reported low social support systems (Fox et al., 2005). Poulton et al. (2002) investigated a functional X-linked variant of the gene encoding a neurotransmitter metabolizing enzyme which was found to moderate subsequent effects of physical abuse, thereby explaining some variability in outcome. Those with higher levels of this enzyme were less likely to develop violent and other deviant behaviors associated with anti-social behavior.

These findings were replicated and extended in two other studies of neglected and abused white children (Nilsson et al., 2007; Widom & Brzustowicz, 2006), although another study with a more diverse sample failed to replicate this effect (Huizinga et al., 2005). Silberg et al. (2001) found that the presence of a short allele of the serotonin transporter gene, in combination with life stress, was a risk factor for depression. Specific inherited gene variants may thus augment risk for adverse reactions to traumatic life experiences and cause the organism to follow one or another developmental path (Fisher & Gunnar, 2010).

In addition to the diathesis-stress model of environmental action (Ingram & Luxton, 2005), Belsky, Bakermans-Kranenburg and Van IJzendoorn (2007) proposed the differential-susceptibility framework, which posits that some individuals are generally more susceptible and may react more strongly negatively to adverse environmental influences and also react more strongly positively to optimal ones. A corollary of this hypothesis is to broaden the idea of vulnerability to susceptibility and encapsulate this characteristic as plasticity (Belsky & Pluess, 2013). In order to test this plasticity hypothesis, Belsky et al. (2009) suggested alternative statistical criteria for discriminating the gene-environment interactions which reflect differential susceptibility from ones reflecting the diathesis-stress model. Traditional regression analyses were added in order to evaluate regions of significance (Aiken & West, 1991; Preacher, Curran, & Bauer, 2006), and even more rigorous statistical criteria were employed for testing differential susceptibility (Ellis, Boyce, Belsky, Bakermans-Kranenburg, & van Ijzendoorn, 2011).

Belsky, Pluess and Widaman (2013) proposed performing a confirmatory statistical analysis that explicitly evaluates alternative theoretical models. This method systematically varies the number of parameters included in a regression equation in order to contrast alternative conceptual frameworks, most notably parameters specifying where on the continuum of environmental measurement regression lines reflecting the association between environmental predictors and the outcome for different genetic subgroups will cross. This analysis can distinguish between the diathesis-stress theory and the differential susceptibility theory, because according to the diathesis stress theory, an ordinal interaction with regression lines crossing at or above the most positive observed value for the measured environment would be predicted, whereas results revealing a non-ordinal or cross-over interaction with regression lines would provide evidence for the differential susceptibility theory.

The utility of this method of analysis and the differential susceptibility theory was tested using data from the large-scale NICHD Study of Early Child Care (NICHD Early Child Care Research Network, 2005a), because all prior analyses of these data were unable to reveal main effects of childcare quality (Belsky et al., 2007; NICHD Early Child Care Research Network, 2005b). The dopamine allele became the focus, as it was identified in a meta-analysis of ten studies as a main source of variations in genes related to signaling in the brain which influences children's sensitivity to both sensitive/responsive and harsh/unresponsive parenting (Bakermans-Kranenburg & van Ijzendoorn, 2011), and because experimental evidence indicated that children carrying the specific dopamine allele targeted in this study benefited more than others from interventions which emphasized skilled parenting (Bakermans-Kranenburg, van IJzendoorn, Pijlman, Mesman, & Juffer, 2008).

These findings supported the differential susceptibility theory because they revealed that children carrying the dopamine allele were the most socially competent and had the fewest behavior problems when they experienced high-quality child care, and those same children were the least socially competent and exhibited the most behavior problems when they experienced low-quality care. Those without the dopamine allele were not affected by quality of childcare. Thus, it seems possible that by using statistical models it may be possible to decide between alternative models and that all models should be subjected to this vigorous statistical analysis, which implies that genetic expression can moderate environmental influences on child behavior (Belsky et al., 2013).

Studies which focused on very young children have likewise investigated the ways in which individual biology interacts with environmental characteristics in shaping the course of development. For example, parental caregiving can alter the social developmental course of children who have genetic vulnerability for shy and inhibited temperamental traits (Fox et al., 2005), and maternal sensitivity towards a child at 7 months was significantly related to attachment security only for children with a short allele in the serotonin transmitter (Kochanska, Boldt, Kim, Yoon, & Philibert, 2014). Similarly, Burt, Klahr, Neale and Klump (2013) found that maternal warmth and directiveness jointly moderate the etiology of child conduct problems, reflecting the fact that genetic influences may sometimes be positive and support optimal outcomes.

In the new millennium, these alternative theories investigating individual differences in young children's development and behavior attempt to include aspects of both nature and nurture in explaining the origins of individual difference among children. They reveal the interplay between constitutional and environmental factors in childhood outcomes and their goal is to identify which biological factors are associated with one another (gene-environment correlations), and which are interrelated (gene-environment interaction). It is clear that adequate understanding of the processes involved in behavioral problems will require the identification of the many mechanisms involved, and progress will depend on the recognition that susceptibility genes not only affect the individual in an adverse manner but can also augment positive outcomes, thus addressing some of the issues in the study of the nature and nurture interplay in infant mental health (Rutter & Silberg, 2002).

General Models of the Nature-Nurture Controversy

Gene-environment interaction research has grown dramatically over the last decade, as scholars have discussed and debated whether and how the genetic make-up of individuals moderates their susceptibility to environmental influences (Belsky et al., 2013; Risch et al., 2009; Uher & McGuffin, 2010). Sameroff (2010) proposed a unified theory of development based on the dialectical perspective on gene environment interaction as an expression of the debate on nature and nurture. Tracing the history of the question of nature and nurture leads to the recognition that they co-exist in a mutual system of human development. Acknowledging this interrelatedness between them has brought support to more complex interpretations and has highlighted the need for more complex analyses to understand differential influences on behavior. Although they seem to be opposites, in fact development cannot occur without both of them, and nature changes as a result of nurture and nurture is modified as a result of nature, as captured in Sameroff's (2009) transactional model. There is continuous joint regulation between the organism's constitutional character and experiential factors through which development takes place. Neither has priority over the other and the ever-present tension between cultural and constitutional change is the foundation for reciprocal processes affecting behavioral and developmental outcomes (Boyce, Sokolowski, & Robinson, 2012).

It is important to appreciate that there is a recurring and ongoing re-examination of nature and nurture in an attempt to answer the question of what lies at the origins of human behavior. A single answer from the proponents of nurture or those who believe in nature would not suffice. It would be too simplistic, too linear and too causal. No matter what measures of nature have been posited, there will always be individual differences, such that two children with the same biological characteristic can have different outcomes and two children with two different characteristics can have the same outcome. Similarly, two children with the same experiences can have different outcomes and two children with quite different experiences can have the same outcome. Because of the interface, interdependence and unending interactions between nature and nurture, they cannot be understood in isolation.

Current research trends for studying nature and nurture are based on new biological measures of individual differences in a multi-disciplinary model (Bronfenbrenner & Ceci, 1994). Advances in molecular genetics, neurology and behavior genetics are being integrated into infant and early childhood mental health models, which are based on multidirectional models for development with growing emphasis on gene-environment interaction, epigenome-experience transactions and brain plasticity. These advances require increasingly complex systems analyses to understand the complexity and interrelatedness underlying developmental changes. A large amount of unexplained variance remains and so the pendulum swings back from a preoccupation with nature to nurture. There is consensus that successful developmental predictions are highly contingent on the social and biological context.

Infant mental health is an interdisciplinary field, based on the assumption that development is embedded in relationships and in social networks that either constrain or foster different aspects of development. Families and educational frameworks are social institutions in which development occurs and must be taken into consideration in understanding development. Neither nature nor nurture will provide ultimate truths nor be an end unto itself; rather, each can explain the influences of the other and they must be integrated in order to explain the complexities of development.

References

Aiken, L. S., & West, S. G. (1991). *Multiple regression: Testing and interpreting interactions* (pp. 75–87). London, UK: Sage Publications.

Auerbach, J. G., Benjamin, J., Faroy, M., Geller, V., & Ebstein, R. (2001). DRD4 related to infant attention and information processing: A developmental link to ADHD? *Psychiatric Genetics, 11*(1), 31–35.

Auerbach, J. G., Faroy, M., Ebstein, R., Kahana, M., & Levine, J. (2001). The association of the dopamine D4 receptor gene (DRD4) and the serotonin transporter promoter gene (5-HTTLPR) with temperament in 12-month-old infants. *Journal of Child Psychology and Psychiatry, 42* (06), 777–783.

Auerbach, J., Geller, V., Letzer, S., Shinwell, R., Belmaker, R., Levine, J., & Ebstein, R. (1999). Dopamine D4 receptor (D4DR) and serotonin transporter promoter (5-HTTLPR) polymorphisms in the determination of temperament in two month old infants. *Molecular Psychiatry, 4*, 369–373.

Bakermans-Kranenburg, M. J., & Van Ijzendoorn, M. H. (2011). Differential susceptibility to rearing environment depending on dopamine-related genes: New evidence and a meta-analysis. *Development and Psychopathology, 23*(01), 39–52.

Bakermans-Kranenburg, M. J., Van IJzendoorn, M. H., Pijlman, F. T. A., Mesman, J., & Juffer, F. (2008). Differential susceptibility to intervention: Dopamine D4 Receptor Polymorphism (DRD4 VNTR) moderates effects on toddlers' externalizing behavior in a randomized control trial. *Developmental Psychology, 44*, 293–300.

Belsky, J., Bakermans-Kranenburg, M. J., & Van IJzendoorn, M. H. (2007). For better and for worse differential susceptibility to environmental influences. *Current Directions in Psychological Science, 16*(6), 300–304.

Belsky, J., Jonassaint, C., Pluess, M., Stanton, M., Brummett, B., & Williams, R. (2009). Vulnerability genes or plasticity genes & quest. *Molecular Psychiatry, 14*(8), 746–754.

Belsky, J., & Pluess, M. (2013). Beyond risk, resilience, and dysregulation: Phenotypic plasticity and human development. *Development and Psychopathology, 25*(4pt2), 1243–1261.

Belsky, J., Pluess, M., & Widaman, K. F. (2013). Confirmatory and competitive evaluation of alternative gene-environment interaction hypotheses. *Journal of Child Psychology and Psychiatry, 54*(10), 1135–1143.

Birchwood, M., Lester, H., McCarthy, L., Jones, P., Fowler, D., Amos, T., … & Marshall, M. (2014). *The UK National evaluation of the development and impact of early intervention services* (The National Eden Studies): Study rationale, design and baseline characteristics. Early intervention in Psychiatry, *8*(1), 59–67.

Boyce, W. T., Sokolowski, M. B., & Robinson, G. E. (2012). Toward a new biology of social adversity. *Proceedings of the National Academy of Sciences, 109*(Suppl 2), 17143–17148.

Bronfenbrenner, U. (1979). Contexts of child rearing: Problems and prospects. *American Psychologist, 34*(10), 844–850.

Bronfenbrenner, U., & Ceci, S. J. (1994). Nature-nurture reconceptualized in developmental perspective: A bioecological model. *Psychological Review, 101*(4), 568–586.

Bronfenbrenner, U., & Morris, P. A. (2006). The bioecological model of human development. In R. M. Lerner (Ed.), *Handbook of child psychology: Vol. 1. Theoretical models of human development* (6th ed., pp. 793–828). New York, NY: Wiley.

Burmeister, M., McInnes, M., & Zöllner, S. (2008). Psychiatric genetics: Progress amid controversy. *Nature Reviews Genetics, 9*, 527–540.

Burt, A. S., Klahr, A. M., Neale, M. C., & Klump, K. L. (2013). Maternal warmth and directiveness jointly moderate the etiology of childhood conduct problems. *Journal of Child Psychology and Psychiatry, 54*(10), 1030–1037.

Caspi, A., Sugden, K., Moffitt, T. E., Taylor, A., Craig, I. W., Harrington, H., … & Poulton, R. (2003). Influence of life stress on depression: Moderation by a polymorphism in the 5-HTT gene. *Science, 301*(5631), 386–389.

DeFries, J. C. (1967). Quantitative genetics and behavior: Overview and perspective. In J. Hirsch (Ed.), *Behavior-genetic analysis* (pp. 322–339). New York, NY: McGraw-Hill.

Dishion, T. J., Shaw, D., Connell, A., Gardner, F., Weaver, C., & Wilson, M. (2008). The family check-up with high-risk indigent families: Preventing problem behavior by increasing parents' positive behavior support in early childhood. *Child Development, 79*, 1395–1414.

Ellis, B. J., Boyce, W. T., Belsky, J., Bakermans-Kranenburg, M. J., & van Ijzendoorn, M. H. (2011). Differential susceptibility to the environment: An evolutionary–neurodevelopmental theory. *Development and Psychopathology, 23*(01), 7–28.

Fisher, P. A., & Gunnar, M. R. (2010). Early life stress as a risk factor for disease in adulthood. In R. A. Lanius, E. Vermetten, & C. Pain (Eds.), *The impact of early life trauma on health and disease* (pp. 133–141). Cambridge, UK: Cambridge University Press.

Fox, N. A., Henderson, H. A., Marshall, P. J., Nichols, K. E., & Ghera, M. M. (2005). Behavioral inhibition: Linking biology and behavior within a developmental framework. *Annual Reviews of Psychology, 56*, 235–262.

Galton, F. (1876). The history of twins, as a criterion of the relative powers of nature and nurture. *Journal of the Anthropological Institute of Great Britain and Ireland, 5*, 391–406.
Harold, G. T., Leve, L. D., Elam, K. K., Thapar, A., Neiderhiser, J. M., Natsuka, M. N., ... & Reiss, D. (2013). The nature of nurture: Disentangling passive genotype–environment correlation from family relationship influences on children's externalizing problems. *Journal of Family Psychology, 27*(1), 12–21.
Huizinga, D., Haberstick, B. C., Smolen, A., Menard, S., Young, S. E., & Corley, R. P. (2005). Childhood maltreatment, subsequent antisocial behavior, and the role of monoamine oxidase: A genotype. *Biological Psychiatry, 60*, 677–683.
Ingram, R. E., & Luxton, D. D. (2005). Vulnerability-stress models. In B. L. Hankin & J. R. Z. Abela (Eds.), *Development of psychopathology: A vulnerability-stress perspective* (pp. 32–46). Thousand Oaks, CA: Sage Publications.
Kaufman, J., Yang, B. Z., Douglas-Palumberi, H., Grasso, D., Lipschitz, D., Houshyar, S., ... & Gelernter, J. (2006). Brain-derived neurotrophic factor–5-HTTLPR gene interactions and environmental modifiers of depression in children. *Biological Psychiatry, 59*(8), 673–680.
Kochanska, G., Boldt, L. J., Kim, S., Yoon, J. E., & Philibert, R. A. (2014). Developmental interplay between children's biobehavioral risk and the parenting environment from toddler to early school age: prediction of socialization outcomes in preadolescence. *Development and Psychopathology, 27*(3), 1–16.
Monroe, S. M., & Simons, A. D. (1991). Diathesis-stress theories in the context of life stress research: Implications for the depressive disorders. *Psychological Bulletin, 110*(3), 406–425.
NICHD Early Child Care Research Network. (2005a). Early child care and children's development in the primary grades: Follow-up results from the NICHD Study of Early Child Care. *American Educational Research Journal, 42*(3), 537–570.
NICHD Early Child Care Research Network. (2005b). *Child care and child development: Results from the NICHD study of early child care and youth development*. New York, NY: Guilford Press.
Nilsson, K. W., Sjoberg, R. L., Wargelius, H., Leppert, J., Lindstrom, L., & Oreland, L. (2007). The monoamine oxidase A (MAO-A) gene, family function and maltreatment as predictors of destructive behaviour during male adolescent alcohol consumption. *Addiction, 102*, 389–398.
Piaget, J. (1952). *The origins of intelligence in children* (Vol. 8, No. 5, p. 18). New York, NY: International Universities Press.
Plomin, R. (1989). Environment and genes: Determinants of behavior. *American Psychologist, 44* (2), 105–111.
Plomin, R. (1994). *Genetics and experience: The interplay between nature and nurture*. London, UK: Sage Publications, Inc.
Plomin, R. (1995). Genetics and children's experiences in the family. *Journal of Child Psychology and Psychiatry, 36*(1), 33–68.
Plomin, R. (2008). *Behavioral genetics*. New York, NY: Macmillan.
Plomin, R., & DeFries, J. C. (1985). *Origins of individual differences in infancy: The Colorado Adoption Project*. Orlando, FL: Academic.
Plomin, R., DeFries, J. C., Knopik, V. S., & Neiderhiser, J. (2013). *Behavioral genetics* (6th ed.). New York, NY: Worth Publishers.
Poulton, R., Caspi, A., Milne, B. J., Thomson, W. M., Taylor, A., Sears, M. R., & Moffitt, T. E. (2002). Association between children's experience of socioeconomic disadvantage and adult health: A life-course study. *Lancet, 360*, 1640–1645.
Preacher, K. J., Curran, P. J., & Bauer, D. J. (2006). Computational tools for probing interactions in multiple linear regression, multilevel modeling, and latent curve analysis. *Journal of Educational and Behavioral Statistics, 31*(4), 437–448.
Risch, N., Herrell, R., Lehner, T., Liang, K. Y., Eaves, L., Hoh, J., ... & Merikangas, K. R. (2009). Interaction between the serotonin transporter gene (5-HTTLPR), stressful life events, and risk of depression: A meta-analysis. *Journal of the American Medical Association, 301*(23), 2462–2471.

Rutter, M., & Silberg, J. (2002). Gene-environment interplay in relation to emotional and behavioral disturbance. *Annual Review of Psychology, 53*(1), 463–490.

Sameroff, A. (2009). *The transactional model.* Washington, DC: American Psychological Association.

Sameroff, A. (2010). A unified theory of development: A dialectic integration of nature and nurture. *Child Development, 81*(1), 6–22.

Seligman, M. E. (1970). On the generality of the laws of learning. *Psychological Review, 77*(5), 406–418.

Silberg, J., Rutter, M., Neale, M., & Eaves, L. (2001). Genetic moderation of environmental risk for depression and anxiety in adolescent girls. *The British Journal of Psychiatry, 179*(2), 116–121.

Uher, R., & McGuffin, P. (2010). The moderation by the serotonin transporter gene of environmental adversity in the etiology of depression: 2009 update. *Molecular Psychiatry, 15*(1), 18–22.

Watson, J. B. (1914). *Behavior: An introduction to comparative psychology.* New York, NY: H. Holt.

Widom, C. M., & Brzustowicz, L. M. (2006). MAOA and the cycle of violence: Childhood abuse and neglect, MAOA genotype, and risk for violent and antisocial behavior. *Biological Psychiatry, 60*, 684–689.

Chapter 5
Risk Factors in Infant and Early Childhood Mental Health

Introduction

The previous chapter dealt with the interrelatedness of constitutional and environmental variables and the differential susceptibility model (Belsky & Pluess, 2009), which highlighted the fact that individual children respond differently to risk factors, resulting in diverse outcomes. Risk factors are those factors which are associated with a lower likelihood of positive outcomes. The model of human development and mental health, particularly infant mental health, which is presented here, incorporates a multi-factorial way of thinking about developmental outcomes. The assumptions of this approach force the researcher and clinician to move beyond the traditional medical model. For example, traditionally medical models are causal and they are presumed to be linear, moving in a relatively straightforward manner from the cause to the effect, focusing on the search for core causal agents that can account for developmental or behavioral outcomes. By contrast, the models presented here are concerned with the search for dynamic mediating processes that account for growth, adaptation and maturation over time.

The models are transactional, or mediational, with bi-directional, reciprocal patterns of effect among the multiple elements of the model accounting for children's functioning and development over time, similarly to the models presented in the previous chapter. In order to grapple with the complexity of the issues involved in risk in infant and early childhood mental health, it is necessary to emphasize dynamic processes of interaction between multiple biological, internal characteristics of the child and external interactional and environmental factors, thus requiring the study of process and not simply the investigation of the presence or absence of certain features.

The study of infant mental health entails the examination of multiple domains and responses that may mediate relations between variables that have an impact on development and child outcomes. Ultimately the study of process is dependent on the appropriateness and the accuracy of the measurement of the factors which are

C. Shulman, *Research and Practice in Infant and Early Childhood Mental Health*,
Children's Well-Being: Indicators and Research 13,
DOI 10.1007/978-3-319-31181-4_5

assessed empirically to understand the processes through which change occurs in the developing child.

Contextual features associated with person-environment interactions can also be taken into consideration and each element can be analyzed to assess its part in the overall model. For example, marital conflict has been extensively studied and it has been found that children respond differently to their exposure to parents' arguing. Children seem to show few negative effects from frequent marital conflict, even if their parents are quite emotional while arguing, if the children feel that the arguments result in resolution of the disagreements (Cummings, Davies, & Campbell, 2002). However, if children feel that the occurrence of conflict has serious consequences for the future intactness of the family, the outcome is usually negative for the children even if their parents do not fight openly or argue only infrequently (Laumakis, Margolin, & John, 1998). Thus, different child behavioral outcomes may be associated more with patterns of events rather than with the occurrence of a particular event.

Infant mental health includes the study of developmental processes underlying both typical development and the development of maladaptive behavior, as illustrated by the example of children's response to marital conflict. Specific types and intensities of conflict have been shown to elicit different responses from children, and therefore concentrating on just one aspect of the conflict reveals limited information about the effects of a particular phenomenon, such as marital conflict, on children. It is necessary to examine a continuum of effects in order to achieve a more comprehensive understanding of key mediating processes and developmental sequelae, and it is likewise important to remember that processes in the study of risk factors in infant and early childhood mental health are dynamic pathways.

The Conceptualization of Risk

Risk factors are those factors which predispose individuals to negative or non-optimal outcomes. The magnitude of risk is measured as the probability of a specific negative outcome when the risk factor is present, compared to the probability of that same outcome when the factor is not present. Alternatively it can be conceptualized statistically as a correlation between risk and outcomes, as a continuous dimensional variable rather than a categorical one. When risk factors are present in an infant's life they may result in poor socialization, later problems with mental health, and poor academic achievement.

Traditionally risk was seen as a stressor, any factor that increases a person's psychological or physical stress, and efforts were made to define discrete events which predicted adverse outcomes. Today, however, risk is seen as a process which is not defined by the variable itself, but rather by the consequences which result from the variable, because the presence of an identified discrete event does not always result in the predicted outcome. Therefore, risk is currently seen as a set of links or associations between specific risk conditions and specific negative outcomes, and not the result of discrete stressors. Unfortunately, even the broadening of the concept of risk to that of linkage does not always relate to the reality of what is observed in young children's developmental outcomes. Empirical research seems to point to the fact that for very young children, risks and outcomes are not necessarily specifically linked, so one avenue of research strives to investigate the pathways through which factors are associated with particular outcomes, and from what age. In infancy, similar outcomes can be the result of very different risk conditions. In addition, it seems that a number of diverse outcomes can result from a single risk factor, leading to research into the possible pathways from one risk factor to the various associated outcomes.

This observed variability in infant and early childhood developmental outcomes is the rationale for the outpouring of research into identifying risk and protective factors in infant and early childhood mental health. Understanding the developmental processes among children who do not develop problems despite growing up in seemingly high risk environments and among those who do not develop optimally despite their living in apparently low risk environments may shed light on seminal processes so that intervention programs can focus on specific factors to help develop protective factors in young children or, alternatively, prevention programs can be established in order to combat the high risk factors so prevalent in many young children's lives.

The complexity inherent in investigating risk factors in young children and the sometimes contrasting results have led researchers along different paths. Instead of looking for direct relationships between factors and outcomes, two other research methodologies have been adopted when studying risk. The first is that instead of looking for the linear causal effect, an additive model has been implemented. The conclusion from this line of research has demonstrated that often the number of risk factors is more predictive of adverse outcomes than any particular risk factor or even specific combination of risk factors. This seemingly counterintuitive finding has evolved into the cumulative model of risk which is widely accepted today. Given the lack of specificity in risk factors and their correlates, research investigating risk factors and outcomes is typically longitudinal, and assimilates numerous child, parent, interactional and environmental factors into a single research paradigm, bringing us to the second line of research, which studies mediational and moderating variables. The purpose of these types of research designs is to assess which factors influence the main effects (mediating variables) and which group effects have an effect on the interaction between variables (moderating variables).

In any event, risk factors most often occur in combination and possibly interact with one another to lead to negative outcomes even more severe than the outcomes expected from each risk factor individually. This additive quality of risk makes research in the area of risk, particularly in very young children, quite complicated. The risk factors which have been identified through longitudinal research will be presented here, along with the methodological considerations to be taken into account when investigating risk. Understanding individual differences in adaptation within broad categories of risk is the emphasis in current research. Simply conceptualizing links between a particular risk factor, or even a combination of risk factors, and child outcomes is only a first step in formulating transactional risk models. Before presenting the results from some of these complex research designs, singular risk factors will be discussed in order to specify factors which have been identified as risk factors and as such can be considered as contributory factors in the cumulative risk model. Furthermore, many intervention programs target specific risk factors, and populations which share common characteristics may respond to specific treatment programs.

Identifying Risk Factors

Longitudinal Research

Sameroff, Seifer, Zax, and Barocas (1987) were among the first investigators of risk factors in one of the most comprehensive longitudinal studies called the Rochester Longitudinal Study (RLS), which examined the intergenerational transmission of mental health between parents with psychiatric diagnoses and their offspring. Children's cognitive, psychomotor, emotional, and social development and functioning were measured and followed from birth through adulthood. The study continues today and the individuals who participated when they were children are now parents who are raising their own families. The effects of environmental risk scores were examined at different points in time.

The original sample included 337 pregnant women with and without a history of psychiatric disorder. Their offspring were followed at 4, 12, and 30 months, and 4, 13 and 18 years of age, thus encompassing the developmental stages of infancy, early childhood, adolescence, and young adulthood. At each time point, appropriate measures of personality, intelligence, school performance and mental health status were collected regarding the children, while family measures including parental mental illness, parenting values and attitudes, family functioning and the quality of mother-child interaction were also gathered. Peer conflict and characteristics of the neighborhood were included as measures of distal environment. Finally, stressors such as stressful life events and environmental risks such as exposure to violence and poverty, as well as measures of social support, were also included. In general, results revealed that a mother's specific psychiatric diagnosis was not related to early child outcomes but general factors such as severity of symptoms and chronicity were.

This extensive study was among the first to provide empirical support for the concept of a cumulative risk model, in which cumulative environmental risk was related to child outcome at each time period, and it was found that the number of risk factors was a better predictor of child outcomes than any specific single risk factor or characteristic of the child. Summarizing the risk factors identified in the Rochester study, Sameroff and Fiese (2000) identified anxiety, parental perspectives, occupation, education and minority status as possible risk factors ranging from low to high risk. Environmental factors included minority status, family support, stressful life events and family size, whereas variables related to the child included physical health problems, prenatal exposure to drugs, temperament, poor social competence and depression.

Changes in Familiar Situations as a Risk Factor

Some risk factors involve experiences that occur more or less by chance and can appear in the lives of high or low risk infants. These incidental risk factors may affect the infant or both the family and the infant. Incidental risk factors involve stress for the infant, and in many cases the stress is the result of a change from a familiar to an unfamiliar situation which is either too rapid or too frequent. Such events could be as devastating as losing a parent or as mundane as having a new baby sibling. Stressful events also have an additive impact on young children even when none is particularly severe. The passage of time between such events has been found to contribute to improvement after a stressful occurrence.

Significant stress is also the result of separation from attachment figures after attachment has transpired. It is important to remember that very young infants have not yet become attached and so separation from familiar people seems less stressful for them. When separations are gradual and do not last long, attached infants might protest but seem basically unaffected. Risk is present when the separation is abrupt and prolonged. When this happens, infants and toddlers generally respond in three stages, which may take up to a year to complete (Keren, 2015). The initial response to an abrupt separation is protest and the child cries, appears anxious and searches actively for the missing attachment figure. The child becomes vigilant and responds immediately when someone approaches, even if it is not the attachment figure. Play, eating and sleeping patterns may become disrupted. If the separation continues the child enters a stage of despair and appears to be in mourning. Sad affect and passivity towards other people characterize the young child at this phase. It seems hard for the child to accept comfort, and even if the attachment figure returns the child remains anxious. However, if the separation continues, the child moves into a stage of detachment. If reunited with the adult at this point the child is angry and ambivalent and may even ignore the adult. Reestablishing the relationship at this time may be difficult. Continued separation after the detachment phase results in the child's resolution of grief and readiness to form a new attachment relationship with an alternative caregiver. It has been proposed that children who have suffered this type of loss in early childhood are at high risk for developing depression in adolescence.

It is important to note that, similarly to other risk factors, separation does not operate independently. It may combine with other risk factors to increase the stress or it may be buffered by factors which can reduce the negative effects. For example, infants' stress response to separation as measured by andrenocortical responses was reduced when a warm, responsive substitute caregiver interacted with the baby. Surprisingly, this pattern was especially effective with infants with a difficult temperament (Gunnar, Larson, Hertsgaard, Harris, & Brodersen, 1992). The most serious separation may occur as a result of violence or war. If the young child has seen one parent kill the other, nightmares, fears and aggressive behavior may result (Appleyard & Osofsky, 2003; Holt, Buckley, & Whelan, 2008; Lieberman, 2011; Osofsky & Osofsky, 2010).

Parental Characteristics and Risk

In addition to risk factors which come from the child or the external environment, some risks can originate in parental characteristics. These risks can include biological or physiological problems which make it difficult for the parent to respond in a sensitive manner to the infant or toddler. Examples of such parental risk factors include parental schizophrenia, depression or impulsivity which might be a behavioral characteristic of hyperactivity. Concerns regarding substance abuse such as the overuse of use of alcohol or drugs are also considered parental risk factors (Anda et al., 2007). Mothers who use drugs have been described as easily frustrated and emotionally detached, on the one hand, while, on the other hand, other mothers who have substance additions have been described as having a tendency to overstimulate the baby. Because of their need for the substance to which they are addicted, they are not able to protect their children and keep them safe or to be consistent caregivers. Disorganized patterns of attachment are common in children of addicted mothers.

Mental illness and depression may also lead to neglect of the infant or toddler. Goodman et al. (2011) studied infants of clinically depressed mothers and found that the infant's capacity to experience joy and excitement is markedly reduced, especially if the maternal depression lasts beyond the first year. Experience affects the child's emotional activation and it seems that the absence of positive shared emotional states for children with depressed parents is a risk factor which can adversely affect emotional development and expression.

Other risk factors for the infant and young child growing up with a depressed mother have been studied and will be addressed later in this chapter. Other general familial risk factors include characteristics of the household such as marital status. Although single parent families used to be seen as a risk factor in themselves, today it is recognized that single parent families are often associated with other risk factors such as poverty and living in violent neighborhoods. Single parent families are quite diverse, and specifically mother-only families fall into two separate categories. The first group is composed of mothers who had an unplanned child, typically without being married, often early in their life, and the other group includes mothers who planned the pregnancy because they were older and thought they would probably not marry. These two groups of single mothers are different in educational level and income but may be similar in the difficulties they experience in raising an infant alone and coping with the never-ending needs that an infant or toddler has, as well as the feelings of loneliness for other adults and grief for lost dreams. Single parents who are divorced or widowed also experience stress and other deep emotions which may include anger or depression, depending on the circumstances of the divorce. Despite the findings reviewed above which seem to indicate a direct cause and effect relationship between the presence of risk and subsequent adverse outcomes, it is important to remember that exposure to risk does not determine the outcome, as risk will not necessarily translate itself into a specific adverse outcome for a particular child or for children as a group.

Research Methodologies for Studying Risk

Factors such as these as well as others may in turn add to or account for risk that children experience. In order to unravel the multidimensional complexities of risk factors, it is necessary to use complex statistical models, looking for pathways and associations. For example, the manifestations of depression differ and each child's experience with parental depression varies as a function of timing in development, parental behavior, child characteristics, and environmental factors. Trying to understand the variations in the underlying organization of the multidimensional risk model requires complex path analyses which are one of many methods for analyzing different implications for developmental outcome (NICHD Early Child Care Research Network, 2001). In a similar vein, many of the conceptualizations of environmental influences on development simply compare and contrast different features of the environment in which young children are growing, including geographical location, ethnicity, family structure, and social background (Bronfenbrenner, 1986). In summary, a better understanding of the factors and processes that might account for risk requires a broad focus in order to map the multivariate nature of risk contexts while simultaneously focusing on distinguishing between diverse constellations of risk processes.

Moderator models assume that the nature of the relationship between risk and child outcome is not uniform across different conditions or people; they search for statistical analyses which will be able to describe the differences which emerge from using more traditional linear models, such as correlations. Moderators relate to the strength and the direction of relations between the independent variables being investigated (e.g, parental depression) and the salient outcome variables (e.g, child adjustment), and because the results are not identical in each case, they reflect the influences that variables can have on one another. For example, a child's age when first exposed to marital strife may serve as a moderator of relations between family functioning associated with conflict and child adjustment. This may be one reason why siblings who experience the "same" household and are witnesses to the "same" interactions between their parents can interpret them so differently. Similarly, gender may be a moderator in that interaction as well. Thus, moderator models can identify who is at risk and when they are most at risk. So moderator models move beyond documenting the direct relationship between two variables, in that they specify the conditions under which risk factors most powerfully predict children's developmental outcomes (Kraemer, Stice, Kazdin, Offord, & Kupfer, 2014). The two most powerful moderator models are the organism–environment interaction (e.g., Rutter, 1987, 2005; discussed in chapter 4), and the synergistic or additive effects model discussed in this chapter.

In order to work towards identifying under what circumstances risk factors have their most powerful effects, synergistic models specify that the co-occurrence of two or more factors incurs a greater deleterious effect than the sum of the factors considered in isolation (Monk, Georgieff, & Osterholm, 2013; Rutter & Silberg, 2002; Shonkoff et al., 2012). As a result, one or more factors may exponentially increase the risk associated with another factor. Rutter, Tizard, and Whitmore (1970) were among the first to demonstrate this claim when their research findings regarding the relationship between six familial risk factors – severe marital distress, low socioeconomic status (SES), large family size or overcrowding, paternal criminality, maternal psychiatric disorder, and admission of the child to foster care – and child psychopathology revealed that the probability that a child experiencing a solitary risk factor (any of the individual factors investigated) and subsequently developing child psychopathology was comparable to the probability of a child who experienced no risk factors going on to develop psychopathology. However, experiencing two or three of the risk factors together increased the incidence of child psychopathology threefold (2 % versus 6 %), with an even larger increase in children's psychiatric disturbance with exposure to four factors (20 %). These findings have been replicated and found to be robust (e.g., Evans, Li, & Whipple, 2013; Myers, 2009; Rutter, 2009).

Although the synergistic aspect of risk models has been reinforced by empirical evidence supporting the additive effect of risk factors on child psychiatric problems, it does not specify the exact nature of the synergism (Rutter, Thapar, & Pickles, 2009). While the Rutter et al. (1970) study showed that none of the six family risk factors could be considered a risk factor in and of itself, it is clear that interaction effects occur and must be examined. It has been proposed that perhaps there is a hierarchical effect of the risk factors, with one specific risk factor being necessary for the others to adversely affect the others. Alternatively, it is possible that some factors "provoke" others by having a direct, precipitating impact on the development of psychopathology in children, while another proposal posits that there are vulnerability factors which have no direct effect on their own but when combined with others have a negative effect on other risk factors. For example, it has been found that lack of a confiding relationship is a vulnerability factor in the development of depression in women (but not in men), which poses no risk in isolation but seems to catalyze the potent impact of stressful life events which can result in depression (Goodyer, 1990).

The diathesis-stress framework discussed in chapter 4 is the basis from which the organism-environment interaction model grew. This model also attempts to address questions regarding who is at risk and from what factors, and they can be investigated using mediational statistical models. The organism component consists of vulnerable personal characteristics, such as temperament and coping patterns (Windle & Tubman, 1999), but these are not genetic defects; rather, they are seen as individual differences (Sameroff, 2010; Sroufe, Egeland, Carlson, & Collins, 2005). In contrast, the stress or environment component reflects exposure to stressful life experiences.

When the stress from the environment and the constitutional makeup of the individual are integrated, this model posits that individuals with certain intrapersonal attributes respond differently or more specifically with greater difficulty to similar environmental contexts. For example, research which focused on the link between parental depression and child outcomes proposed that children with difficult temperamental styles (i.e., diathesis – a constitutional tendency towards a specific problem) may exhibit greater vulnerability in depressive family contexts (i.e., stress situations) than children with easy temperamental styles, simply because one element of difficult temperament is greater reactivity to environmental conditions, in this case the negative family characteristic of parental depression (Cummings & Davies, 1999). Complementing the organism-environment model is the "goodness of fit" model, which suggests that certain personal characteristics become particularly potent risk factors when they are inconsistent with the expectations, demands or pressures of the context (Windle & Lerner, 1986). For example, greater discrepancies between the child's behavior and the parents' expectations for behavior are linked to lower social competence and academic achievement (Lerner, 1991).

In an attempt to understand why some people are vulnerable only in certain circumstances, it is necessary to integrate the moderator model, which addresses the question who is at risk, with the mediation model, which addresses when the risk is most potent. The moderator model can serve as a foundation for answering such questions as "who is more at risk?" while the mediator model can address why people possessing certain characteristics are more vulnerable to adverse outcomes. Thus, statistical analysis of moderation in risk research can determine whether certain groups are more or less affected by a particular environmental event or other influences in the prediction of adjustment. In other words, by grouping people together (e.g., children who have experienced trauma versus children who have not experienced trauma) such analyses can help establish differential risk in the context of a process oriented model.

Employing Statistical Models to Explain Risk

There are two models of statistical analysis which can help coordinate the mediation and moderation effects in process models. In order to accomplish the conceptual goals which involve analyzing multi-layered variables affecting various outcome measures which are the basis for models of risk and vulnerability, the challenge is to go beyond examining simple relationships between variables towards understanding the complex processes underlying these relationships. Structural equation modeling (SEM) is a model which shows the proportional effects of different variables on different outcomes (Bullock, Harlow, & Mulaik, 1994). This methodology uses the correlations among all the measures being investigated in a study to estimate the specific pathways predicted by the hypotheses of the study. A good fit between a model and the theory means that the pathways predicted by the theory correspond to the pathways resulting from the observed correlations. Using this method it is also possible to compare the proposed model with alternative models that add or remove relationships among the constructs. When used appropriately this statistical approach can determine how well purported measures of a psychological variable relate to an underlying construct, thus addressing issues raised by mediation models, longitudinal models and group differences inherent in moderation models.

The second statistical model which can address the complexity of research into risk factors is growth curve modeling or hierarchical linear modeling, which can address issues in longitudinal research concerning change over time that cannot be readily tackled by other statistical methods (Raudenbush & Bryk, 2002). This procedure merits special consideration because of the importance of pathways of development in infant mental health research. Specifically, this method can be used to examine inter-individual differences in intra-individual change, which is different from multivariate repeated measures approaches which are limited to examining average intra-individual change across participants in a study (Maxwell & Delaney, 1990).

Clearly the issues which can be addressed by these statistical methodologies are pertinent to the field of infant and early childhood mental health. Returning to the example of child outcomes from marital conflict, if measures of child behavioral and developmental status were assessed yearly over a 5 year period and if marital conflict was measured at the same time periods over the same 5 year period, it would be possible to investigate inter-individual differences in the developmental trajectories of children exposed to marital conflict over a 5 year period. Using the hierarchal linear modeling technique, it would also be possible to investigate the effects of changes in marital conflict on changes in the child's behavior. The encounter of the researcher with the clinical complexity of risk factors and child adverse and optimal outcomes is challenging. Advanced statistical and theoretical models require precise measurement of multilayered variables in order to deal with the understanding of developmental trajectories and pathways which lead to different outcomes for the young child. Examining specific research in the area of risk factors may be helpful in understanding the complexity and the challenge of infant and early childhood mental health.

Environmental Risk Factors in Infancy: Poverty

Despite the fact that it is nowclear that risk factors most often occur in combination and that the cumulative effect is much more deleterious than any one isolated factor, it is important both clinically and for research purposes to discuss what is known about individual risk factors leading to adverse outcomes and the necessity for infant mental health services. Perhaps the most commonly identified and researched risk factor in infant mental health is poverty, which rarely occurs in isolation. Poverty involves multiple risk factors and processes, including limited family resources and parental stress which contributes to the parents' less than optimal emotional wellbeing. Instead of presenting individual risk factors, research in risk factors and possible outcomes will be reviewed in a multi-layered fashion, surveying the processes through which these risks develop as well as the clusters of risk conditions. In clinical settings, it is less important to understand the risk factors, as the fact that the family, child or parents have already arrived for services means that they are no longer merely at risk for problems; hence, the focus changes to identifying the factors which are contributing to the disturbed behavior and moves to identifying those which can be treated.

Environment plays an important role in shaping development from the newborn period throughout life. Many individual environmental risk factors may impinge on development, including poverty, which can come along with mental illness, minority status, and other identified risk factors, therefore resulting in a situation in which multiple risk factors act on a single developing infant. This is of particular interest because early mental health can be predictive of later mental health. If behavior at a later stage is dependent on earlier mental health, then attention must be paid to the multiple contexts that support development of infant and early childhood mental health in the family, the school, and the community from infancy through childhood. Few studies have directly tested the premise that it is continuing environmental adversity that undermines development. Duncan, Brooks-Gunn and Aber (1997) found the best predictor of competence during early childhood to be not the current economic circumstance of the family but rather the number of years that the family had previously spent in poverty. Sameroff (1998) also reported that the longer the continuities in poverty, which is just one example of environmental risks, the more adverse the outcome on children.

In order to focus on environments it is important to assess the variables to be investigated. To examine the effects of the environment on early emotional behavior and on later mental health, it is necessary to identify the child factors to be used subsequently as outcome factors, as well as other environmental characteristics such as poverty. A robust finding from the Rochester Longitudinal Study was that family socioeconomic status (SES) was associated with the most deleterious child outcomes. Children from the poorest families exhibited the poorest development, with poorer obstetric status, more difficult temperaments, and lower developmental test scores at 4 months, less responsivity during the home and laboratory observations at 12 months, and less adaptive behavior in the home and laboratory at 30 and 48 months of age. At the end of 4 years of development, the multi-layered, cumulative model of risk explained different outcomes. For example, when the developmental risk for a child was a mother with an emotional problem *or* one who lacked social support *or* had a low educational level, the child was usually doing fine; but when, on the other hand, the child had a mother who was mentally ill *and* poor *and* uneducated *and* without social supports, that child was doing poorly, supporting the importance of attending to the combination of environmental adversity factors in the social context of children. In order to better understand the role of contextual factors, researchers have taken a more differentiated approach to environmental influences in order to discover what was different about the experiences of children raised in different socioeconomic environments.

Although SES may be the best single variable for predicting children's cognitive competence and a predictor of the child's social–emotional functioning, researchers have begun to realize that SES is not just level of income but also includes psychological, interactional and social variables (Bornstein & Bradley, 2014; Brooks-Gunn, Duncan, & Aber, 1997). Poverty affects many levels of the ecology in which children are living and growing, including parenting, parental attitudes and beliefs, family interactions, and institutions in the community. Yeung, Linver and Brooks-Gunn (2002) presented a conceptual model based on 30 years of research. Their work is an attempt to clarify poverty's effect on young children's social-emotional and behavioral health. The model describes the pathways through which poverty has an impact on the parenting process in which the child is developing and the structure of the environment in which the child is being raised, and the manner in which both the process and the structure influence the young child's mental health.

Their model integrated findings from two theories, one from research in economics and the other from the family process model. Adler et al. (1994) postulated that the main pathways through which poverty affects children's future outcomes are time and money. With more money parents can buy more stimulating toys, can access higher quality child care and can live in a safer neighborhood and have more time to spend with their children. The family process model claims that the main mediators of poverty on children's outcome are the emotional well being of the parents and the quality of family interactions, particularly the manner in which stress is handled. The integration of the economics and family perspectives contributes significantly to the understanding of how poverty affects young children. Similarly to the resolution of the nature-nurture debate discussed in chapter 4, it is clear that both the economics of time and money and the quality of the family environment affect the mental health of the developing child. It appears that the interaction between these two perspectives provides evidence that both the structural characteristics, such as having accessibility to high quality child care and stimulating toys, and experiencing the affective quality of the child's environment, are critical. In order to distinguish among these variables and trace pathways, research has begun to focus on defining different aspects of poverty, such as how to rank poverty and how to incorporate the length of time – including how many generations – a family has experienced poverty.

Researchers, using some the methodological strategies described above, are looking into different ways in which the child can be affected, including direct and indirect effects – moderational and mediational effects. Research looking into the direct effects of poverty shows relatively small effects (Dearing, McCartney, & Taylor, 2006), which first emerge in toddlerhood (Ryan, Fauth, & Brooks-Gunn, 2006), but research into the indirect effects of poverty on children's mental health has identified parenting as the most significant mediator of poverty. In addition, the quality of early child care and broader neighborhood characteristics mediate poverty's deleterious effects on young children. There is evidence that children growing up in poverty are exposed to more risk factors and that the effects of these risk factors are more negative than for children who are not growing up in poverty.

In order to investigate the moderating effects on poverty, Dearing et al. (2006) calculated a new proportional variable measuring the ratio of income to needs which addresses what they called relative poverty. For example, income is divided by the number of members in a particular household. In addition this research project focused on very young children, examining the effects of poverty in the first 5 months of life. The infants were divided into three categories: (1) chronically poor; (2) transiently poor; and (3) never poor. The association between family income and externalizing behaviors was considerably larger for children living in chronic poverty. In other words, the chronicity of poverty during infancy moderated the direct effect of family income on externalizing behavior. Similarly, Sameroff (1998) created a multiple risk score that was the total number of risks for each individual family. As the number of risk factors increased, performance decreased for children at 4 years of age. The combination of risk factors resulted in a nearly threefold increase in the magnitude of differences found in groups of children relative to the effect of single variables. Researchers also identified a set of risk factors, including the family's resources for coping with stress, the number of children that share resources and the parents' flexibility in understanding and dealing with their children, as the variables which moderated poverty's effect on young children.

Research addressing the gene-environment nexus also lends support to the moderating effects of poverty in the study of risk. For example, Gunnar and Donzella (2002) investigated the physiological underpinnings of poverty and found that exposure to excessive amounts of stress during the first years of life can actually change the architecture of the developing brain and result in permanent changes in the infant's stress response (National Scientific Council on the Developing Child, 2005; Rifkin-Graboi, Borelli, & Bosquet, 2009; Siegel, 2012).

Parental Risk Factors: Depression

In addition to poverty, which is a complex, multi-faceted environmental variable, risk factors associated with the parents can affect the developing child adversely and must be examined. Depression in mothers of infants has consistently raised concern, as it is not clear that a mother with depression can care for an infant's physical and emotional needs. Research has focused on the issues involved in depression in mothers while pregnant, at birth, and after giving birth. In addition, the investigation of the infant's developmental trajectories has elucidated some of the risks involved developmental pathways toward psychopathology. The prevalence of depression in pregnant women ranges from 8 to 51 % (Bennett, Einarson, Taddio, Koren, & Einarson, 2004), which reflects the problems with specificity in the definition of the condition and differences in sampling.

Estimating the prevalence of depression in mothers of infants is similarly plagued with definitional and sampling inconsistencies. Gavin et al. (2005) performed a meta-analysis and found that as many as 19 % of women reported major or minor depressive symptoms during the first 3 months after giving birth. When only including major depressive episodes the prevalence decreases to 7 %, revealing that not an insignificant number of woman experience depression which might have adverse effects on their infant.

Depression in mothers puts the infant at risk for mental health in early childhood and later. Many studies have found that maternal depression was significantly related to lower rates of secure attachment styles (Lyons-Ruth, Zoll, Connell, & Grunebaum, 1986). Looking for moderators and mediators of this association, McMahon, Barnett, Kowalenko and Tennant (2006) found that insecure states of mind in mothers strengthened the association between maternal depression and infant insecure attachment. Infant physical status is also a moderating factor in the association between maternal depression and insecure attachment. This is particularly salient in the case of premature births (Poehlmann & Fiese, 2001). In addition to insecure attachment, children of depressed mothers display less positive affect and more negative affect than other children and have more difficulty regulating their emotions and behaviors (Huot, Brennan, Stowe, Plotsky, & Walker, 2004). The mechanisms for these associations are not clear but they include the possibility of heritability, perhaps linked with other environmental risk factors, which merits further study.

There are several possible pathway models which address the risk mechanisms related to maternal depression and negative child outcomes in infancy and early childhood. If the mother is depressed during pregnancy, it is possible that the fetus has absorbed high levels of the stress enzyme cortisol from the depressed mother, and research findings suggest that fetal exposure to cortisol produces lasting damage to the hippocampal area of the brain, increasing the risk of infants being born with dysfunctional neuroregulatory systems (Goodman, 2007). In Goodman's work, maternal anxiety and stress in the third trimester were significantly related to higher fetal heart rate, which is associated with lower neonatal arousal (Field, Diego, & Hernandez-Reif, 2006). Parenting qualities that are associated with infant mental health are warmth and sensitivity, and it is possible that maternal depression affects the mother's ability to respond with positive affect to the infant. Depressed mothers have been characterized as neglectful (Bifulco, & Moran, 2002), unresponsive, (Murray, Fiori-Cowley, Hooper, & Cooper, 1996), intrusive and hostile (Cohn, Matias, Tronick, Connell, & Lyons-Ruth, 1986) or unpredictable (Field, Diego, & Hernandez-Reif, 2006), all of which have been identified as risk factors for the developing infant. Research regarding maternal depression as a risk factor for adverse outcomes in infant mental health is still focused on establishing links and has not yet fully investigated moderating and mediating models.

Child Risk Factors: Prematurity

Finally, prematurity, a child factor which has already been mentioned as a risk factor for depressed mothers, will be covered more comprehensively. Giving birth prematurely is a complex condition which has received attention because of the physical risk to the child's survival. With technological advances, babies are surviving after shorter and shorter gestation periods. This state of affairs leads to intense emotions in the parents which can have an effect on the parent-infant relationship. Thus, physiological, developmental, social and emotional factors are involved in prematurity and need to be addressed in order to understand the risk mechanism.

Outcomes of prematurity have been investigated in correlational research designs, but it is difficult to compare results from different studies as they sometimes report contradictory results, perhaps as a result of different methodologies or more likely as a result of different sampling definitions. Some define prematurity by gestation date and others by weight. Children born prematurely often display subtle neurodevelopmental disabilities, such as developmental language disorders, learning disabilities, attention deficit disorder with or without hyperactivity, sensorimotor problems and emotional difficulties, which have all been associated with later cognitive impairment and social-emotional problems (Bayer, Hiscock, Ukoumunne, Price, & Wake, 2008). Behavioral problems at home have also been reported (Salt & Redshaw, 2006). Focusing on the emotional and behavioral outcomes of preterm delivery, premature babies have been described at age 6 months as more stressed, having less social approach behavior and more problems with self–regulation (Wolf et al., 2002), and in early childhood as more difficult, with less adaptive behavior, than full term infants (Tu et al., 2007). Research has focused on the parents' traumatic response to the premature birth as a mediating factor in understanding the risk pathways of infant and child mental health outcomes. Becoming a parent is a challenging and emotional experience, which can be positive, difficult or overwhelming even for those parents whose children are born full term and in good health.

It is important to understand the impact of a premature birth as a risk factor, with particular attention paid to the parental traumatic response to the birth. Premature birth is recognized as a stressful event, and parents' experience can be filled with anxiety regarding the baby and the difficulties the family faces (Miles, Holditch-Davis, Schwartz, & Scher, 2007). Mothers report more stress and poorer adjustment than fathers do (Jackson, Ternestedt, & Schollin, 2003). Stressors influence parents' abilities to cope with the challenges. Miles et al. (2007) have reported that mothers can suffer from anxiety and depression for months after coming home from the hospital with the baby. As the traumatic aspect of this experience is recognized and examined, it has become clear that some parents continue to have symptoms of trauma reactions up to a year after the premature birth (De Mier et al., 2000).

Qualitative research methods have analyzed the parental narrative, helping to define the factors which might warrant more quantitative research, while empirical data collected through standardized questionnaire and open-ended interviews have supplied researchers with an understanding of parents' subjective experience (Udry-Jørgensen et al., 2011). These narratives provide researchers with a view of themes and variables which merit additional investigation. Parents' experiences and behavior and infant characteristics must be analyzed in order to understand the mediating or moderating factors. Maternal distress has been associated with less positive mother infant interactions and has been conceptualized as a moderating factor in infant mental health outcomes for premature infants (Singer et al., 2003). Another moderating factor investigated by Muller-Nix et al. (2004) was the quality of interaction between mothers of high risk premature babies and it was found mothers of full-term babies tended to be less controlling and more sensitive in dyadic play with their children than mothers of pre-term babies. Interestingly, maternal trauma was found to mediate maternal and infant interactional quality in that association. Pursuing research on prematurity is of critical importance, as more prematurely born infants are surviving and it appears that this creates a different parenting experience, with different outcomes for the parents and the child, than full term birth.

Risk Factors for Early Infant and Child Mental Health in Developing Countries

The study of risk factors has particular salience for mental health in developing countries, as developmental neuroscience shows how early biological and psychosocial experiences affectbrain development. Walker et al. (2011) identified inadequate cognitive stimulation, stunting, iodine deficiency, and iron deficiency as key risks for children growing up in developing countries. Risk factors can account for some of the discrepancies between child outcomes in developing and developed countries which prevent millions of young children from attaining their developmental potential. Recent research (e.g., Grantham-McGregor et al., 2007; Walker et al., 2007) emphasizes the importance of these risks and strengthens the evidence for other risk factors, including intrauterine growth restriction, malaria, lead exposure, HIV infection, maternal depression, institutionalization, and exposure to societal violence, particularly wars. Evidence on risks resulting from prenatal maternal nutrition, maternal stress, and families affected with HIV is emerging (Dunkel Schetter, 2011). Biological and psychosocial risk factors associated with poverty will lead to inequalities in early child development, not just among children in the same country but also among more developed and less developed countries around the world.

In middle and low income countries children are exposed to many risk factors, making it difficult for them to attain optimal developmental outcomes. Because exposure to biological and psychosocial risks affectsthe developing brain, it compromises the development of children, the next generation of these countries, thus perpetuating inequality between and within populations. At least one cause of the disparity among children has its origins in adverse early experiences. These inequalities in child development begin prenatally and continue during the first years of life, and with cumulative exposure to developmental risks, disparities widen and trajectories become more firmly established. Poverty and associated health, nutritional, and social factors prevent millions of children in developing countries from attaining optimal outcomes. Since risks occur together or cumulatively, with concomitant increased adverse effects, the development of the world's poorest children is severely compromised.

References

Adler, N. E., Boyce, T., Chesney, M. A., Cohen, S., Folkman, S., Kahn, R. L., et al. (1994). Socioeconomic status and health: The challenge of the gradient. *American Psychologist, 49*(1), 15–24.

Anda, R. F., Brown, D. W., Felitti, V. J., Bremner, J. D., Dube, S. R., & Giles, W. H. (2007). Adverse childhood experiences and prescribed psychotropic medications in adults. *American Journal of Preventive Medicine, 32*(5), 389–394.

Appleyard, K., & Osofsky, J. D. (2003). Parenting after trauma: Supporting parents and caregivers in the treatment of children impacted by violence. *Infant Mental Health Journal, 24*(2), 111–125.

Bayer, J. K., Hiscock, H., Ukoumunne, O. C., Price, A., & Wake, M. (2008). Early childhood aetiology of mental health problems: A longitudinal population-based study. *Journal of Child Psychology and Psychiatry, 49*(11), 1166–1174.

Belsky, J., & Pluess, M. (2009). Beyond diathesis stress: Differential susceptibility to environmental influences. *Psychological Bulletin, 135*(6), 885–908.

Bennett, H. A., Einarson, A., Taddio, A., Koren, G., & Einarson, T. R. (2004). Prevalence of depression during pregnancy: Systematic review. *Obstetrics & Gynecology, 103*(4), 698–709.

Bifulco, A., & Moran, P. (2002). *Wednesday's child: Research into women's experience of neglect and abuse in childhood and adult depression.* London: Routledge.

Bornstein, M. H., & Bradley, R. H. (Eds.). (2014). *Socioeconomic status, parenting, and child development.* London: Routledge.

Bronfenbrenner, U. (1986). Ecology of the family as a context for human development: Research perspectives. *Developmental Psychology, 22*(6), 723–742.

Brooks-Gunn, J., Duncan, G., & Aber, J. L. (Eds.). (1997). *Neighborhood poverty, Volume 2: Policy implications in studying neighborhoods.* New York: Russell Sage Foundation.

Bullock, H. E., Harlow, L. L., & Mulaik, S. A. (1994). Causation issues in structural equation modeling research. *Structural Equation Modeling, 1*(3), 253–267.

Cohn, J. F., Matias, R., Tronick, E. Z., Connell, D., & Lyons-Ruth, K. (1986). Face-to-face interactions of depressed mothers and their infants. *New Directions for Child and Adolescent Development, 1986*(34), 31–45.

Cummings, E. M., & Davies, P. T. (1999). Depressed parents and family functioning: Interpersonal effects and children's functioning and development. In T. Joiner & J. Coyne (Eds.), *The interactional nature of depression: Advances in interpersonal approaches* (pp. 299–327). Washington, DC: American Psychological Association.

Cummings, E. M., Davies, P. T., & Campbell, S. B. (2002). *Developmental psychopathology and family process: Theory, research, and clinical implications.* New York: Guilford Press.

Dearing, E., McCartney, K., & Taylor, B. A. (2006). Within-child associations between family income and externalizing and internalizing problems. *Developmental Psychology, 42*(2), 237–252.

DeMier, R. L., Hynan, M. T., Hatfield, R. F., Varner, M. W., Harris, H. B., & Manniello, R. L. (2000). A measurement model of perinatal stressors: Identifying risk for postnatal emotional distress in mothers of high-risk infants. *Journal of Clinical Psychology, 56*(1), 89–100.

Duncan, G., Brooks-Gunn, J., & Aber, J. L. (1997). *Neighborhood poverty: Context and consequences for children* (Vol. I and II). New York: Russell Sage.

Dunkel Schetter, C. (2011). Psychological science on pregnancy: Stress processes, biopsychosocial models, and emerging research issues. *Annual Review of Psychology, 62*, 531–558.

Evans, G. W., Li, D., & Whipple, S. S. (2013). Cumulative risk and child development. *Psychological Bulletin, 139*(6), 1342–1396.

Field, T., Diego, M., & Hernandez-Reif, M. (2006). Prenatal depression effects on the fetus and newborn: A review. *Infant Behavior and Development, 29*(3), 445–455.

Gavin, N. I., Gaynes, B. N., Lohr, K. N., Meltzer-Brody, S., Gartlehner, G., & Swinson, T. (2005). Perinatal depression: A systematic review of prevalence and incidence. *Obstetrics & Gynecology, 106*(5, Part 1), 1071–1083.

Goodman, S. H. (2007). Depression in mothers. *Annals Reviews of Clinical Psychology, 3*, 107–135.

Goodman, S. H., Rouse, M. H., Connell, A. M., Broth, M. R., Hall, C. M., & Heyward, D. (2011). Maternal depression and child psychopathology: A meta-analytic review. *Clinical Child and Family Psychology Review, 14*(1), 1–27.

Goodyer, I. M. (1990). *Life experiences, development, and childhood psychopathology*. New York: Wiley.

Grantham-McGregor, S., Cheung, Y. B., Cueto, S., Glewwe, P., Richter, L., Strupp, B., et al. (2007). Developmental potential in the first 5 years for children in developing countries. *The Lancet, 369*(9555), 60–70.

Gunnar, M. R., & Donzella, B. (2002). Social regulation of the cortisol levels in early human development. *Psychoneuroendocrinology, 27*, 199–220.

Gunnar, M. R., Larson, M. C., Hertsgaard, L., Harris, M. L., & Brodersen, L. (1992). The stressfulness of separation among nine-month-old infants: Effects of social context variables and infant temperament. *Child Development, 63*, 290–303.

Holt, S., Buckley, H., & Whelan, S. (2008). The impact of exposure to domestic violence on children and young people: A review of the literature. *Child Abuse and Neglect, 32*(8), 797–810.

Huot, R. L., Brennan, P. A., Stowe, Z. N., Plotsky, P. M., & Walker, E. F. (2004). Negative affect in offspring of depressed mothers is predicted by infant cortisol levels at 6 months and maternal depression during pregnancy, but not postpartum. *Annals of the New York Academy of Sciences, 1032*(1), 234–236.

Jackson, K., Ternestedt, B. M., & Schollin, J. (2003). From alienation to familiarity: Experiences of mothers and fathers of preterm infants. *Journal of Advanced Nursing, 43*(2), 120–129.

Keren, M. (2015). Perspectives in infant mental health. *Infant Mental Health Journal, 36*(1), 78–87.

Kraemer, H. C., Stice, E., Kazdin, A., Offord, D., & Kupfer, D. (2014). How do risk factors work together? Mediators, moderators, and independent, overlapping, and proxy risk factors. *The American Journal of Psychiatry, 158*, 848–856.

Laumakis, M. A., Margolin, G., & John, R. S. (1998). The emotional, cognitive and coping responses of preadolescent children to different dimensions of marital conflict. In G. W. Holden, R. Geffner, & E. Jouriles (Eds.), *Children exposed to marital violence: Theory, research, and applied issues* (pp. 257–288). Washington, DC: American Psychological Association.

Lerner, R. M. (1991). Changing organism-context relations as the basic process of development: A developmental contextual perspective. *Developmental Psychology, 27*(1), 27–32.

Lieberman, A. F. (2011). Infants remember: War exposure, trauma, and attachment in young children and their mothers. *Journal of the American Academy of Child & Adolescent Psychiatry, 50*(7), 640–641.

Lyons-Ruth, K., Zoll, D., Connell, D., & Grunebaum, H. U. (1986). The depressed mother and her one-year-old infant: Environment, interaction, attachment, and infant development. *New Directions for Child and Adolescent Development, 1986*(34), 61–82.

Maxwell, S. E., & Delaney, H. D. (1990). *Designing experiments and analyzing data: A model comparison approach*. Belmont, CA: Wadsworth.

McMahon, C. A., Barnett, B., Kowalenko, N. M., & Tennant, C. C. (2006). Maternal attachment state of mind moderates the impact of postnatal depression on infant attachment. *Journal of Child Psychology and Psychiatry, 47*(7), 660–669.

Miles, M. S., Holditch-Davis, D., Schwartz, T. A., & Scher, M. (2007). Depressive symptoms in mothers of prematurely born infants. *Journal of Developmental & Behavioral Pediatrics, 28* (1), 36–44.

Monk, C., Georgieff, M. K., & Osterholm, E. A. (2013). Research review: Maternal prenatal distress and poor nutrition—mutually influencing risk factors affecting infant neurocognitive development. *Journal of Child Psychology and Psychiatry, 54*, 115–130.

Muller-Nix, C., Forcada-Guex, M., Pierrehumbert, B., Jaunin, L., Borghini, A., & Ansermet, F. (2004). Prematurity, maternal stress and mother–child interactions. *Early Human Development, 79*(2), 145–158.

Murray, L., Fiori-Cowley, A., Hooper, R., & Cooper, P. (1996). The impact of postnatal depression and associated adversity on early mother-infant interactions and later infant outcome. *Child Development, 67*(5), 2512–2526.

Myers, H. F. (2009). Ethnicity-and socio-economic status-related stresses in context: An integrative review and conceptual model. *Journal of Behavioral Medicine, 32*(1), 9–19.

National Scientific Council on the Developing Child. (2005). *Maternal depression can undermine the development of young children* (Working paper 8). Harvard University, Center for the Developing Child: Harvard University http://developingchild.harvard.edu/wp-content/uploads/2009/05/Maternal-Depression-Can-Undermine-Development.pdf

NICHD Early Child Care Research Network. (2001). Child care and children's peer interaction at 24 and 36 months: The NICHD study of early child care. *Child Development, 72*, 1478–1500.

Osofsky, J. D., & Osofsky, H. J. (2010). Understanding and helping traumatized infants and families. In B. M. Lester & J. D. Sparrow (Eds.), *Nurturing children and families: Building on the legacy of T. Berry Brazelton* (pp. 254–263). New York: Blackwell Scientific.

Poehlmann, J., & Fiese, B. H. (2001). Parent-infant interaction as a mediator of the relation between neonatal risk status and 12-month cognitive development. *Infant Behavior and Development, 24*(2), 171–188.

Raudenbush, S. W., & Bryk, A. S. (2002). *Hierarchical linear models: Applications and data analysis methods* (Vol. 1). London: Sage.

Rifkin-Graboi, A., Borelli, J. L., & Bosquet, M. (2009). Neurobiology of stress in infancy. In C. R. Zeanah (Ed.), *Handbook of infant mental health* (3rd ed., pp. 59–79). New York: Guilford Press.

Rutter, M. (1987). Psychosocial resilience and protective mechanisms. *American Journal of Orthopsychiatry, 57*(3), 316–331.

Rutter, M. (2005). Environmentally mediated risks for psychopathology: Research strategies and findings. *Journal of the American Academy of Child & Adolescent Psychiatry, 44*(1), 3–18.

Rutter, M. (2009). Understanding and testing risk mechanisms for mental disorders. *Journal of Child Psychology and Psychiatry, 50*(1–2), 44–52.

Rutter, M., & Silberg, J. (2002). Gene-environment interplay in relation to emotional and behavioral disturbance. *Annual Review of Psychology, 53*(1), 463–490.

Rutter, M., Thapar, A., & Pickles, A. (2009). Gene-environment interactions: Biologically valid pathway or artifact? *Archives of General Psychiatry, 66*(12), 1287–1289.

Rutter, M., Tizard, J., & Whitmore, K. (1970). *Education, health, and behaviour*. London: Longman.

Ryan, R. M., Fauth, R. C., & Brooks-Gunn, J. (2006). Childhood poverty: Implications for school readiness and early childhood education. In B. Spodek & O. N. Saracho (Eds.), *Handbook of research on the education of young children* (2nd ed., pp. 323–346). Mahwah, NJ: Lawrence Erlbaum Associates Publishers.

Salt, A., & Redshaw, M. (2006). Neurodevelopmental follow-up after preterm birth: Follow up after two years. *Early Human Development, 82*, 185–197.

Sameroff, A. J. (1998). Environmental risk factors in infancy. *Pediatrics, 102*(Suppl E1), 1287–1292.

Sameroff, A. (2010). A unified theory of development: A dialectic integration of nature and nurture. *Child Development, 81*(1), 6–22.

Sameroff, A. J., & Fiese, B. H. (2000). Transactional regulation: The developmental ecology of early intervention. In J. P. Shonkoff & S. J. Meisels (Eds.), *Handbook of early childhood intervention* (pp. 135–159). New York: Cambridge University Press.

Sameroff, A., Seifer, R., Zax, M., & Barocas, R. (1987). Early indicators of developmental risk: Rochester longitudinal study. *Schizophrenia Bulletin, 13*(3), 383–394.

Shonkoff, J. P., Garner, A. S., Siegel, B. S., Dobbins, M. I., Earls, M. F., McGuinn, L., … & Wood, D. L. (2012). The lifelong effects of early childhood adversity and toxic stress. *Pediatrics, 129*(1), e232–e246.

Siegel, D. J. (2012). *The developing mind: How relationships and the brain interact to shape who we are*. New York: Guilford Press.

Singer, L. T., Fulton, S., Davillier, M., Koshy, D., Salvator, A., & Baley, J. E. (2003). Effects of infant risk status and maternal psychological distress on maternal-infant interactions during the first year of life. *Journal of Developmental & Behavioral Pediatrics, 24*(4), 233–241.

Sroufe, L. A., Egeland, B., Carlson, E., & Collins, W. A. (2005). *The development of the person: The Minnesota study of risk and adaptation from birth to adulthood*. New York: Guilford Press.

Tu, M. T., Grunau, R. E., Petrie-Thomas, J., Haley, D. W., Weinberg, J., & Whitfield, M. F. (2007). Maternal stress and behavior modulate relationships between neonatal stress, attention, and basal cortisol at 8 months in preterm infants. *Developmental Psychobiology, 49*(2), 150–164.

Udry-Jørgensen, L., Pierrehumbert, B., Borghini, A., Habersaat, S., Forcada-Guex, M., Ansermet, F., et al. (2011). Quality of attachment, perinatal risk, and mother–infant interaction in a high-risk premature sample. *Infant Mental Health Journal, 32*(3), 305–318.

Walker, S. P., Wachs, T. D., Gardner, J. M., Lozoff, B., Wasserman, G. A., Pollitt, E., … & International Child Development Steering Group. (2007). Child development: risk factors for adverse outcomes in developing countries. *The Lancet, 369*(9556), 145–157.

Walker, S. P., Wachs, T. D., Grantham-McGregor, S., Black, M. M., Nelson, C. A., Huffman, S. L., … & Richter, L. (2011). Inequality in early childhood: risk and protective factors for early child development. *The Lancet, 378*(9799), 1325–1338.

Windle, M., & Lerner, R. M. (1986). Reassessing the dimensions of temperamental individuality across the life span: The Revised Dimensions of Temperament Survey (DOTS-R). *Journal of Adolescent Research, 1*(2), 213–229.

Windle, M., & Tubman, J. G. (1999). Children of alcoholics. In W. K. Silverman & T. H. Ollendick (Eds.), *Developmental issues in the clinical treatment of children* (pp. 393–414). Needham Heights, MA: Allyn & Bacon.

Wolf, M. J., Koldewijn, K., Beelen, A., Smit, B., Hedlund, R., & Groot, I. D. (2002). Neurobehavioral and developmental profile of very low birthweight preterm infants in early infancy. *Acta Paediatrica, 91*(8), 930–938.

Yeung, W. J., Linver, M. R., & Brooks-Gunn, J. (2002). How money matters for young children's development: Parental investment and family processes. *Child Development, 73*, 1861–1879.

Chapter 6
The Relational Context of Infant and Early Childhood Mental Health

Relationships as a Bridge Between Theory and Intervention

This is the pivotal chapter in this book on the topic of infant and early childhood mental health, not merely because it is the middle chapter dividing the book between its first and second halves, but more significantly because this is the chapter which transitions between theory and practice, between what is known and what can be done with that knowledge, between scientific knowledge and its translation into applied settings and real life. The bulk of what was covered in the initial chapters related to social and emotional development and the centrality of the quality of the relationship between young developing children and their caregivers was consistently highlighted, as was the case in the chapter regarding the larger social cultural context in which development occurs. The interaction between the characteristics which the child brings to development, the relationship with primary caregivers and the parent characteristics was expounded upon in the chapter regarding the larger contextual framework of acceptable and appropriate social behavior, of beliefs and expectations from the child and his or her surroundings including the neighborhood, the available services, and cultural mores.

The Committee on Integrating the Science of Early Childhood Development (Shonkoff & Phillips, 2000) conceptualized this idea as "from neurons to neighborhoods", reflecting the importance of understanding that children are influenced by contextual variables such as socioeconomic status, exposure to violence, and cultural norms, as well as by constitutional variables such as temperament. This multi-level model of the ecology of social development (Bronfenbrenner, 1979, 1986) emphasizes that development cannot be understood without taking into account the multiple levels of context in which it occurs. Finally, grasping the interactions between child and environmental variables, which has been conceptualized in terms of the nature-nurture controversy, gene-environment interaction, or the study of biogenetics, has led to the understanding that some children have

C. Shulman, *Research and Practice in Infant and Early Childhood Mental Health*,
Children's Well-Being: Indicators and Research 13,
DOI 10.1007/978-3-319-31181-4_6

vulnerabilities which put them at higher risk for having mental health issues in infancy or early childhood (Rutter, 2009). This chapter stresses the centrality of the relationship with significant caregivers in the early life of the developing child which was emphasized throughout the topics discussed previously in this book.

Brain development is responsive to environmental influences which shape the emerging structure and functioning of the brain, particularly in the early years of development. Siegel (2012) posits that although there is broad consensus regarding the premise that experience shapes the neural pathways within the brain, it is also important to recognize that experience early in life may be especially crucial in organizing the basic regulatory structures of the brain. This chapter organizes scientific findings regarding the premise that the mind develops as relationships and the brain change over time, supporting Sameroff's (2009) transactional theory of development, and that the mind progresses within the context of neurophysiological processes and interpersonal relationships. The manner in which infants experience relationships has a dominant influence on the mind because the pathways in the brain which are involved in social cognition are also those involved in the creation of meaning, the modulation of emotions and the capacity for interpersonal communication.

The role of interpersonal experience in development seems to be multifaceted, especially in the early years. The findings from studies investigating attachment cross-culturally (Otto & Keller, 2014) reveal the crucial nature of this relational context. After presenting results which support this imperative, this chapter will provide the basis for the second half of the book, which deals with interventions in the field of infant and early childhood mental health from a relational perspective. The topics covered in this chapter include defining the special role that interpersonal relationships play for the young child, while emphasizing parents, parenting, and assessment of the quality of the dyadic interaction (e.g., the dyad consisting of the mother and the infant). In addition, an introduction to the principles which will be at the base of the infant and early childhood mental health relational interventions which constitute the second half of this book will be presented.

The Relational Imperative in Infant Mental Health

The environment provided by the developing child's first caregivers has a profound effect on every facet of the child's development. For example, the health and physical state of the newborn are dependent on the state of the mother during pregnancy, which will have implications for the infant's continued development (Shonkoff & Phillips, 2000). The first years of life are remarkable for the rapid transformations which take place in both the social and emotional developmental domains, and the field of infant mental health has long since realized that social and emotional competencies emerge from the dynamic interplay which comprises the relationship between the infant and his or her primary caregivers, who regulate, support and facilitate development. Early development is intricately related to the most proximal, interpersonal relationship which occurs with primary caregivers.

The child is profoundly affected by the relationship with parents and the behavior of the parents or any other adult figure in the life of the young child who gives consistent care, attention and affection, the three variables constantly posited as the foundation of the relational context (Gerhardt, 2006; Hartup & Rubin, 2013; Stern, 2009).

Zero-to-Three Diagnostic System

This relational context has been operationalized as the dyadic interaction between parent and infant, and is so central in the field of infant mental health that it has been incorporated in the Diagnostic Classification of Mental Health and Developmental Disorders of Infancy and Early Childhood – Revised (DC: 0-3R) by Zero to Three (2005), which is used to understand the developmental and transactional aspects of the relational context. The seminal purpose of the DC: 0-3R was to help recognize mental health and developmental challenges in young children and to understand how relationships and environmental factors contribute to mental health and developmental disorders, in order to work more effectively with parents and other professionals to develop effective treatment plans when necessary. The DC: 0-3 was the first developmentally based system for diagnosing mental health and developmental disorders in infants and toddlers and supplemented other diagnostic systems (e.g., DSM-IV-TR: APA, 2000; DSM 5: APA, 2013) which were seen as inappropriate for use with very young children. In addition, it has been used to specify behavioral and developmental profiles without establishing a diagnosis. The expanded and revised DC: 0-3 (2005) is an extension of the original DC: 0-3 reflecting empirical research and clinical practice that have taken place worldwide since 1994.

DC: 0-3 is a multi-axial, categorical diagnostic system. Its first axis deals with diagnosis and is not pertinent for discussion in this chapter; rather, the focus will be on Axis II and Axis V, both of which deal with the evaluation of relationships. Axis II reflects a basic premise in the field of infant mental health: infants and young children develop in the context of their primary emotional relationships and the quality of these relationships has a profound influence in shaping the child's developmental course towards mental health or disorder. Understanding the quality of the infant parent relationship, therefore, is an important part of developing a behavioral profile for infants and young children, which may or may not lead to a diagnosis. Clinicians can be assisted in understanding the meaning of behaviors systematically within the young child's primary relationship(s), and interventions can then be formulated and focused on both individual and relationship levels. Axis II can also lead to the establishment of a primary diagnosis, as it assesses the possible presence of a clinical problem in the child's relationship with the primary caregiver, usually the parent. In order to meet diagnostic criteria for a diagnosis of relationship disorder, the problem must be specific to a relationship, meaning that the child's behavioral disturbances while interacting with a particular caregiver are not observed in the child's relationships with other caregivers. If the relationship disorder does not affect the child's functioning in other domains, then the child would be characterized only on Axis II and not on Axis I.

Functional and emotional developmental level is scored on the Axis V of the DC: 0-3 system, which deals with the child's ability to function socially and emotionally, and is an indication of how much support the child and/or the family may need. This system is based on Greenspan and Weider's (1993, 2007) social emotional interactional development model and organizes information which is garnered from observation of the child–parent relationship when they play together in natural situations with familiar toys and objects. Interactions with the clinician, with whom the child becomes increasingly comfortable through the course of the evaluation, are also noted. The domains of functioning which are assessed include mutuality as expressed in shared attention, which is noted at all ages. The milestones are developmental and as such each is an elaboration of the previous ones.

From birth to 3 months one is expected to observe attention and regulation; then mutual engagement and purposeful two-way communication, which should be readily observable by 3–10 months; subsequently, interactive intentionality and growing reciprocity in interactions, expressed in complex gestures and beginning problem-solving abilities, should be observable. These are extensions of mutual engagement and appear around 10–18 months. Representational and affective communication, which appears around 18 months of age, follows, and is a meshing of cognitive abilities with the play interaction between the infant and caregiver. It is followed by representational elaboration (around 30 months) and by representational differentiation (around 36 months – 48 months), which includes symbolic and emotional themes and continues to develop.

Since Axis V is a functional score it is coded on a 5-point scale that results in a summary of the child's overall functional emotional developmental level (http://www.zerotothree.org/child-development/early-childhood-mental-health/dc-0-3r-multi-axial-system). Counterintuitively, the lower the score the less help needed: a score of "1" means that the child has reached expected levels; "2" signifies abilities at expected levels but with some constraints; "3" reflects developmental maturity, measured by the fact that the child has achieved all prerequisite skills but not yet achieved expected levels; "4" indicates that the child has not achieved current expected level but has achieved some prior levels; while a code of "5" means that the child has not mastered expected levels nor prerequisite skills. This summary is based primarily on direct observation of and interaction with the child, but it is also important to ask about the child's functioning at home, in other salient settings, and at other times. The summary level is based on the child's best functioning, even if the child does not reach this optimal level of functioning with this level consistently or with all caregivers.

These developmental milestones are assessed in a relational context, comprising unstructured interactions between the parent and the child. Depending on the age and preferences of the child, different toys are offered. This developmentally appropriate framework allows observations of the parent's ability to catch and maintain the child's interest in addition to observations of interactions with objects and to observe interactions with the caregiver. Some examples of possible toys for different uses, preferences and ages include sensory toys, such as textured balls, puppets and musical toys; symbolic toys such as toy telephones, dolls, toy cars, and a dollhouse with furniture; and movement toys, such as a rotating spinning board or a jump rope. The quality of interaction is noted in the different play settings, which provide a variety of contexts for interactions. It is pertinent to observe when the child is best able to achieve self-modulation, and to note over- or under-responsiveness from child or parent, as well as the emotional valence of the interaction. Likewise it is essential to remember that the rating is not categorical; rather, it ranges from "not present" to "age appropriate functioning, even when under stress and presents an appropriate range of affective states" (Zero to Three, 2005, page 5).

Emotional Availability

The quality of the relationship between the primary caregiver and the infant affects developing children in a myriad of ways. What they learn, how they behave, what they expect from others around them, what they believe in and how they approach others are only a few examples of the ways in which the relationship between a sensitive adult and a young child can affect which developmental pathway any given child will follow. Longitudinal research designs which track salient developmental variables of young children over time can inform us about trajectories, pathways and outcome variables. By following the unfolding of behavior for a specific child over time, it is possible to find associations between relational variables and child outcomes. This research is multi-disciplinary and is based on an attempt to understand whether it would be possible to change the course of development by focusing on specific variables which have been identified as supporting infant mental health or as having deleterious effects.

One of the relational variables which has been studied longitudinally is emotional availability (EA), which is not a general reference to good parental qualities but a well-defined multifaceted perspective and a scientifically rigorous assessment of dyadic or relational capacity for mutual emotional awareness, perception, experience, and expression (Biringen, 2000). It stresses the importance of emotional communication and of maternal sensitivity for successful adaptation (Sorce & Emde, 1981). Maternal sensitivity refers to a mother's ability to understand her young child's behaviors and to infer meaning from them. After perceiving her infant's signals, the sensitive mother will then respond promptly and appropriately (Feldman, Eidelman, & Rotenberg, 2004). This framework provides an integration of attachment (Ainsworth, Blehar, Waters, & Wall, 1978) and affective availability (Emde & Sameroff, 1989) perspectives. Bowlby (1969, 1988) and Ainsworth et al. (1978) utilized the concept of sensitivity to describe the clarity with which the mother perceives her child's signals and the way in which she responds to them. Sensitivity as a concept has become the centerpiece of attachment research (van IJzendoorn & Tavecchio, 1987). In addition to attachment theory, the emotional availability theoretical framework is based on the family systems approach, which underscores the importance of all family members as parts of an interwoven whole that cannot be explained simply by looking at the individuals.

This view integrates the transactional perspective (Sameroff & Fiese, 2000), which emphasizes both the child's contribution to the interaction and the dynamic change in the system over time. But EA moves beyond these theories and modifies both attachment and family systems perspective, with somewhat different emphases. Firstly, the EA system focuses more on positive emotions than the attachment framework. Secondly, there are differences in the contexts in which attachment and EA are observed. Attachment behavior is elicited and coded in the context of stress and fear (e.g., the strange situation paradigm), whereas EA can be coded across a broader range of contexts. Thirdly, the measurement of attachment takes into account primarily the behavior of one individual (the child) in inferring the relationship with the attachment figure. Similarly, traditional measurement of maternal sensitivity considers individual characteristics of the adult in the relationship, so that an individual caregiver might appear to be sensitive with no consideration for the child's interaction. In contrast, the conceptualization and operationalization of EA via the EA Scales (EAS: Biringen, 2004; Biringen, Robinson, & Emde, 1998; Biringen et al., 2012) incorporate a dyadic or relational perspective on interactions and recognize the mutual effect that partners in an interaction have on one another. In the EA scales (Biringen, Robinson, & Emde, 2000; Pipp-Siegel & Biringen, 1998), interpretation of the adult's behavior is dependent upon the behavior of the child. In addition, each interaction is seen as unique and specific, with each partner dynamically influencing the other. Although the EA scales distinguish the adult dimensions from the child dimensions, the EA of both adult and child are assessed relationally.

These concepts are evaluated through the assessment of a dyad's capacity for emotional connection and the extent to which the connection is genuine, affectively positive, and healthy. The result of such an interaction is that the dyadic participants accommodate and regulate negative affect successfully in order to continue to interact (Barone & Biringen, 2007; Biringen, 2000, 2004; Biringen & Easterbrooks, 2008, 2012; Biringen et al., 1998; Easterbrooks & Biringen, 2000, 2005, 2009; Emde & Easterbrooks, 1985). The coding of EA on the emotional availability scales is based on the facial, vocal, and physical signals of both partners, emphasizing the displays of positive and negative emotion which are the components by which the quality of a relationship is measured. EA is operationalized as comprising four adult components (sensitivity, structuring, nonintrusiveness, and nonhostility) and two child components (responsiveness and involvement) that describe global relational quality. Each of the six dimensions is scored on Likert-type scales (e.g., 1–7, with 7 reflecting optimal availability).

The EA scales have been employed cross-culturally and have demonstrated both reliability and validity across contexts (Easterbrooks & Biringen, 2009). The ability to use this measurement across contexts that can be selected according to cultural applicability is a strength (e.g., Aviezer, Sagi, Joels, & Ziv, 1999, in Israel; Ziv, Aviezer, Gini, Sagi, & Koren-Karie, 2000, in Israel; Oyen, Landy, & Hilburn-Cobb, 2000, in Canada; Salo et al., 2009, in Finland). Because the EA scales assess the "emotional connection" between partners in a relationship, they have been shown to be predictive of child and parent outcomes in almost all the cultures in which they have been utilized (Easterbrooks & Biringen, 2009). The six dimensions assessed by the EA Scales (sensitivity, structuring, nonintrusiveness, nonhostility, child responsiveness, and child involvement) capture the affective tone of a dyadic relationship under any set of contexts and in everyday life interactions.

In addition to cross cultural research, the EA scales have been applied in research into the quality of interactions with children at risk and children with disabilities, such as mental retardation syndromes, autism, and hearing impairments (for a review see Biringen, Fidler, Barrett, & Kubicek, 2005). The risk factors studied using the EA scales include dyads from high-risk, low-income backgrounds and the effects of international adoption. In longitudinal research, Stack et al. (2012) evaluated EA in two independent, at-risk, low-income Canadian samples of mothers and children. In their first study, Stack et al. evaluated dyads when children were preschool aged and again during middle childhood. In the second study, they evaluated dyads when children were 6 months, 12 months, and 18 months of age, and again when the children were in preschool and in elementary school.

Results from both studies showed that mothers with a personal history of aggression and social withdrawal during their own childhoods exhibited higher levels of maternal hostility with their children at preschool age, but surprisingly not at other ages. Findings revealed that mothers with a history of social withdrawal during childhood had preschoolers who were less responsive to and involving of them during social interaction, and more significantly, that a higher level of appropriate maternal structuring was associated with greater child responsiveness, and more maternal sensitivity and structuring were linked to more child involvement of the mother. Moreover, when age was controlled, better maternal psychosocial functioning (i.e., more maternal support and less maternal stress) and a higher quality home environment were related to more optimal patterns of EA. These results highlight that a maternal history of psychopathological symptoms can affect patterns of dyadic EA in high-risk dyads of preschoolers, and they contribute to our understanding of the intergenerational transmission affecting EA.

Likewise, Killeen and Teti (2012) examined whether measures of maternal responsiveness to changing infant emotions were associated with behavioral measures of maternal EA during mother–infant play at 6 months. They collected self-report measures from the mothers about their subjective interpretations of the interactions they had with their infant. Specifically, the focus was on maternal reports of anxiety and depressive symptoms and on maternal reports of their own emotional experience in response to their infant's communicative cues. The findings seem to suggest that measures of mothers' capacity for flexibility in emotional contexts may provide the strongest assessment of maternal empathetic response to infant distress, a particularly difficult challenge to grapple with when there is depression or severe anxiety on the part of the mother.

The EA of mothers and their young children who had experienced maternal abuse and those who had been subject to abuse by their mothers and had been exposed to marital conflict (cumulative risk factors) was assessed using the EA Scales (Timmer, Thompson, Culver, Urquiza, & Altenhofen, 2012); significant interactions between physical abuse and exposure to parental violence were observed but, surprisingly, only in the child-directed context. Mothers in the abuse-only group exhibited the least sensitivity and the most hostility, compared to mothers in the other groups, and their children exhibited the least responsiveness and involvement. The dyads in the abuse group who had also been exposed to marital violence demonstrated signs of over-responsiveness in the face of mothers' low EA, a pattern which is characteristic of relating to children with a disorganized attachment style. The authors suggested that measures of participants' mental representations of their relationships should be included in future studies with maltreated children, along with additional behavioral measures.

Easterbrooks, Bureau, and Lyons-Ruth (2012) investigated EA and its correlates in a small longitudinal sample of high risk, low-income mother–child dyads followed from infancy to middle childhood (7 years of age) and results revealed that mothers' behavior with their infants during infancy (e.g., maternal hostility and disrupted communication) predicted EA during middle childhood (e.g., maternal sensitivity and nonhostility). This was particularly important as maternal EA indices were found to be correlated with children's adaptive functioning (e.g., externalizing and total behavior problems in school; depressive symptoms). These results provide preliminary support for the relative coherence of different measures of the mother–child relationship from infancy to middle childhood, despite small sample sizes. Such studies should be replicated in order to provide validity for the longitudinal use of EA scales measuring adult–child interactions from infancy to middle childhood.

Parenting Across Cultures

Emotional availability is only one aspect of the relationship which develops between children and the significant adults with whom they interact. In addition to being affectively attentive to the child, another role that the parent fulfills for infants, toddlers and preschoolers is raising them to be productive, successful and happy adults. Parenting is a focused and differential relationship that adults have with young children. The adults are emotionally invested in the child and consistently available. Adults fulfilling this role for young children become significant attachment figures for them. One demonstration of the importance of the relationship which develops between the adult and child is that the adult is not readily exchangeable with others. The child looks specifically for this adult when distressed and in need of comfort or soothing. The field of inquiry which investigates various multi-layered dimensions of parenting reflects the belief that raising a child shapes the child's developmental trajectory.

The study of infant mental health revolves around the premise that parents and the quality of the relationship which develops between parents and their child are central to the child's subsequent social and emotional development. At first research focused on styles of parenting, until it became clear that although various associations emerged, parenting styles are more complex and conditional that what was once thought (Shonkoff & Phillips, 2000). Parenting style could be redefined as the ability of parents to adjust to their child's needs and characteristics and the conditions and circumstances of their lives (Cowan, Cohn, Cowan, & Pearson, 1996; Holden & O'Dell, 1995). Whereas parenting was once studied in isolation, today's research paradigms investigate parenting in relational context, recognizing the fact that, for example, authoritarian parents may be less authoritarian while on vacation or when with extended family members. Thus research which investigates parenting often assesses parenting styles across contexts and gathers data about parenting at home, around issues in childcare, with peers and with neighbors. It has become clear that children contribute to their childrearing environment, influencing the parenting that they receive, just as they influence emotional availability in the relational, dyadic context.

Creating research designs which address the complexity of the ways in which parenting intersects with the child's inherited strengths and vulnerabilities is quite challenging (Rutter & Silberg, 2002). In addition to cross-cultural research into emotional availability, other aspects of parenting and the establishment of a meaningful relationship have been studied in various cultures. The specific, differentiated relationship between children and their parents has been well documented, and is conceptualized as a universal feature of child development and of parent-infant relationships across ethnic and cultural groups. Nugent (1995) stresses the importance of understanding not just the similarities in this collective phenomenon but also the areas of variability, so research now goes beyond descriptions of similarities and differences in child development in different cultural settings to topics that are central to infant mental health practitioners. For example, in addition to emotional availability, there have been many studies focusing on parameters such as maternal sensitivity and maternal responsivity in differing cultures. In addition there is an increasing number of studies conducted by scholars indigenous to the cultural group under consideration (Grossmann, Grossmann, Spangler, Suess, & Unzner, 1985; Miyake, Chen, & Campos, 1985; Nakagawa, Lamb, & Miyake, 1989), and as presented in previous chapters there are now theoretical models which strive to understand the influence of culture and the broader ecological context on infant development and caregiver behavior (Carlson & Harwood, 2014; Keller & Otto, 2009).

The psychology of different cultures affects the role of parenting in each culture in ways that depend on the values and belief systems of that culture. Each culture has its own view of the adult into which the child should grow (Rosenthal & Roer-Strier, 2006), with gender differences and differences as a result of locality (rural versus urban) only two of the variables which influence parents in their parenting.

The physical environment and the historical circumstances are also determinants of a societal maintenance system, delineating the social structure, economy and household type of a particular culture. Group differences in child-rearing techniques are predicated on the cognitive, linguistic, motivational, and social competencies desired by the cultural group. There is a hierarchy of goals that begins with basic physical survival and proceeds to the inculcation in the child of the cultural group's social behavioral and moral standards. Cultural and transcultural theoretical frameworks highlight the complex contributions made by the culture at multiple levels of the child and caregiving environment, and focus on identifying the levels and the specific characteristics of different cultures.

Improved conceptualization of maternal sensitivity, taking into account and being sensitive to cultural diversity, would help to give a better understanding of the role of maternal behavior as an antecedent to attachment quality (Otto & Keller, 2014). Maternal sensitivity can be defined by three different aspects of behavior: promptness, consistency and appropriateness, all of which are subjectively defined. Additional aspects of maternal sensitivity include the global qualities of warmth and acceptance. Stams, Juffer, and van IJzendoorn (2002) suggest that these may not be the core elements for maternal sensitivity cross-culturally and posit that it is necessary to reconceptualize maternal sensitivity in order to discriminate among the disparate elements, especially because sensitivity can change according to the context in which the interaction occurs (Keller et al., 2004). Results from the few empirical studies that have examined the role of parental beliefs in parental sensitivity and responsive behaviors suggest significant variability in maternal sensitivity and contingent responsiveness to infants' cues based on the parents' beliefs with regard to children (Harwood, Handwerker, Schoelmerich, & Leyendecker, 2001).

The results from cross cultural studies of maternal sensitivity are mixed. Nakagawa et al. (1989) investigated maternal behavior in terms of the accessibility, acceptance, cooperation and sensitivity of the mother, and found no significant correlations between maternal behavior and attachment classifications in Japanese mother-infant interactions, while Miyake et al. (1985), who also investigated attachment styles and maternal sensitivity in Japanese mothers and their infants, reported that maternal sensitivity was a significant factor in establishing secure attachment. Grossmann et al. (1985) reported that North German mothers' maternal sensitivity was shaped by the cultural goals of the importance of independence and preference for a non-clingy child.

van IJzendoorn and Tavecchio (1987) cite evidence for two independent dimensions of maternal sensitivity – one for affective behaviors and one for instructional behaviors. In their study both the mother's affective (smiling, distance from the child and encouragement) and cognitive (hints, feeding and instruction) behaviors during joint problem solving tasks were rated, and their findings indicated that affective and cognitive maternal behaviors varied independently and formed two orthogonal (i.e., statistically independent) factors in a factor analysis, suggesting that some mothers provide adequate instruction and some supply affective interaction, while some do both. Thus, despite structural similarities between the two concepts which suggest a global construct of sensitivity, in actuality sensitive caregiving behavior may be specific to various maternal parenting styles and cultural mores. The finding that individuals varied orthogonally along two dimensions of maternal sensitivity lent support to Schaffer and Collins's position that the construct of sensitivity must not be approached as a unitary entity.

These findings suggest that the conceptualization of the behaviors which constitute sensitivity in a mother may vary cross-culturally and even intra-culturally, which highlights the need for a reconceptualization of the construct of maternal sensitivity from an ecological and cultural perspective (Belsky & Isabella, 1988; Nicholls & Kirkland, 1996). It appears that addressing parental beliefs as a mediating factor would add to our understanding of maternal sensitivity. Korbin (1994) was among the few researchers who explored the range of child-rearing attitudes in diverse cultures. In order to study child maltreatment across cultures, she included an assessment of parental beliefs about children, childhood and their parental role, and feels that such a variable is necessary in cross-cultural research of parenting. Parental beliefs are a more fundamental construct than simple observations of parental style and may serve as a more robust mediator between parents' inner states and their behaviors.

Attachment

The special relationship which develops between very young children and their parents has been conceptualized as resulting, among other things, from the attachment style which develops between parent and child from a very young age. Attachment figures provide the confidence, security, and trust that other adults cannot, although children can benefit from close relationships with different caregivers (Shonkoff & Phillips, 2000). Unfortunately, attachment researchers have neglected the identification of sociocultural antecedents to caregiver-child attachment relationships within minority and immigrant populations in the US and other countries. It is important to examine sociological factors, such as racial group membership, socioeconomic status, parental beliefs, socialization goals, emotion display rules, linguistic socialization, and the structure of the caregiving environment in order to understand the expression of the quality of the attachment relationship (Goh, 2013). Ethnicity may serve as the foundation for the parents' culturally driven belief system. The ethnicity of the caregiver is a new area of exploration to better understand the role of culture and psychology of the caregiver and its part in the relational context in which the young child develops.

Interrelational Context

Child Characteristics in the Relational Context

The investigation of infant core abilities as revealed during dyadic and triadic interactions and their relationship to later social cognitive abilities, as well as of the role environment plays in this relationship, has until recently relied on behavioral data (Legerstee, 2005); but as a result of technological and methodological advances merging with developmental, social, and cognitive neuroscience, new light has been shed on important aspects of the developing infant brain which influence the interactional relationship which develops between the infant and the caregiver. Feldman (2007) reviewed the factors that promote the perception and conception of social stimuli and studied temporally matched interactions, called synchrony, between mothers and infants, suggesting that they are underpinned by biological rhythms and are one of the first expressions of the infant-parent relationship.

Although there is increasing biological evidence for infants' sensitivity to social stimuli which reinforces the developing interactions and relationships with adults, questions remain about the domain specificity of emotions and the role that environment plays in the establishment of the relationships which are the foundation of infant and early childhood mental health. de Haan and Gunnar (2009) investigated the progressive emergence of relationships and the social abilities of the maturing infant, with the goal of specifying developmental pathways. They proposed that in order to understand the child's contribution to the relational context of early interactions between mothers and their infants it is necessary to focus on the subcomponents of and precursors to adult behavior.

Jealousy

An example of this type of research design, of extrapolating downward and studying in infants and young children abilities which have been specified in adults, was the study of jealousy in children in the first year of their life (Legerstee, Ellenbogen, Nienhuis, & Marsh, 2010). Jealousy is defined as an aversive reaction that results from fear of losing a loved one to a third party, who is perceived as a rival. In adults, jealousy is a complex emotion with complicated accompanying feelings, including sadness from a sense of loss; anger as a result of a feeling of betrayal; and fear/anxiety as a consequence of feeling marginalized and alone. In adults, the degree of intensity which the feeling of jealousy incurs is linked to the subcortical emotional networks, and, as a result, variations in human jealousy may be a function of different cognitive capabilities and environmental circumstances (Markova, Stieben, & Legerstee, 2010).

Although most investigators denied the possibility that infants have the prerequisite abilities to feel jealousy, Legerstee et al. (2010) began their investigation of jealousy in infants by focusing on a specific subcomponent of jealousy that adults and infants have in common. Legerstee proposed that the attachment bond could be conceptualized as the existence of a differentiating social bond and that infants responded in a fearful manner when faced with the possibility or reality of losing that bond, from which she insinuated that the infant felt social exclusion. Because of the existence of the attachment bond, according to Legerstee and others, it might be possible that infants are born with an innate desire for a social bond, and jealousy could be viewed as a response to someone who threatens that bond (Fivaz-Depeursinge, Favez, Scaiola, & Lopes, 2010; Hart & Legerstee, 2010; Panksepp, 2010). Thus, the ability to experience jealousy in infants probably develops during early infancy, and might even vary as a function of the quality of the social bond infants have with their caregivers.

Working with this premise, Legerstee systematically specified the skills that an infant or young child would need in order to apprehend jealousy, and set out to investigate when these abilities develop. First, infants would have to recognize social stimuli and differentiate them from nonsocial stimuli. In addition, because jealousy- evoking situations rely on the perceived separation from a loved one, infants would need to have established a social bond. The social bond is the primary relationship within the interpersonal system of jealousy. Furthermore, in order to experience jealousy infants would have to be aware of another, secondary relationship, the one between the caregiver and the rival. Thus infants would need to have developed an understanding of triadic relationships revolving about the self, the caregiver and the rival. Finally, infants would need to have some understanding of why they are being excluded, or, more clearly, that there are goals and intentions which provide the motivation for people's actions. Through examining these intersubjective transactions, it should be possible to establish whether infants have the capabilities necessary to experience jealousy within the first months of life.

Panksepp (2010) concludes that the brain is evolutionarily prepared for jealousy (and other similar emotions) to emerge in early brain development; and if we accept the definition of jealousy as "a fearful emotion that is felt when one loses a loved one to a rival" (Legerstee & Haley, 2013, p. 237), it has been demonstrated that infants as young as 5 months get upset when their mothers ignore them and play with another child (Draghi-Lorenz, 2010) or even play with a doll (Hart, Carrington, Tronick, & Carroll, 2004). However, although this may seem like jealousy, the infants' distress responses may simply be the result of not getting the attention that they want from their mothers.

In order to investigate whether the infants in fact responded out of jealousy and not from lack of stimulation, an experimental paradigm was used in which the infant had to behave in a manner which provided evidence of understanding that there was a rival who was getting the mother's attention. Four experimental conditions were used to distinguish between distress resulting from insufficient maternal attention and from jealousy. The first interaction was natural and the second was the traditional still face paradigm (Tronick, Als, Adamson, Wise, &

Brazelton, 1979), where the child reacts with sadness and gaze aversion as the mother maintains eye gaze but stops talking and interacting with the infant. The two remaining conditions employed modified still face paradigms, in which the experimenter had a lively conversation with the mother after disrupting the interaction with the baby. During one condition the experimenter spoke to the mother about the experiment, and during the other condition the mother and the experimenter spoke in an animated fashion about the baby, although excluding the baby. The results confirmed that infants between 3 and 6 months perceived an animated conversation between their mother and another person which excluded them as a threat to the social bonds that they have with their mothers. Their approach and protest responses in this condition were different than their emotional responses during all other conditions, supporting the claim that there is a behaviorally distinct response which could be understood as jealousy by age 6 months.

Social Cognition in Infants

This attachment bond between mothers and their children is seen by Dunbar (2013) as the biological basis of social relationships, and is a result of the evolution of the bondedness which can be seen in primates, who all form close emotional ties. It has been posited that parental care and bonding can shape the brain structure (Siegel, 2012), and therefore, establishing and maintaining social relationships may be hardwired into the infant's brain. In order to maintain social relationships, which are often complex, it is necessary to have flexible social cognitive abilities, because in order to be successful in the complex social world, people need to adjust and conform to others. To do this they need to read others' minds (i.e., mentalizing), which has been postulated as developing by the age of 4, not in the first year of life. On the other hand, newborn babies can imitate tongue protrusions and mouth opening, which requires some cognitive ability (Meltzoff & Moore, 1998).

One hypothesis is that the mirror neuron system is the foundation for intersubjectivity and social cognition. These neurons have been investigated in primates and they fire when a specific action is executed or perceived. Similar processes are hypothesized to take place when human infants reproduce facial expressions. Gallese (2011) suggests that this early imitation, accompanied by the firing of mirror neurons, mediates the infant's capacity to share the meaning of actions, intentions, feelings and emotions with others, and serves as the basis for the connectedness among people from a very early age. Mirror neurons also seem to play an important part in intersubjectivity in infancy (Gallagher & Meltzoff, 1996). For example, when someone is crying, the areas in the brain associated with those feelings become activated. Such empathic sharing, referred to as emotional contagion, can be elicited in very young infants (Hoffman, 1975). Mirror neurons do more than automatically reproduce actions; when there are two social agents interacting, the activation of the mirror neurons creates a shared representation (Gallese, Rochat, & Berchio, 2013). These shared representations allow people to understand not simply what others are doing but also why they are doing it, thereby producing an awareness of their intentional state.

Additional empirical research supports this very basic, early onset social cognition. Research findings show that newborns discriminate between faces of their mothers and strangers, even when potential olfactory cues are masked (Bushnell, Sai, & Mullin, 1989). Infants also begin to recognize their own faces and others' voices as familiar social stimuli, discriminate them from inanimate objects and sounds, and become better at it between 5 and 8 months (Legerstee, 1998). In general, infants smile and vocalize more towards social (e.g., faces and sounds) stimuli than towards nonsocial stimuli. By 6 months infant brains react differently to upright and inverted faces in a way that is similar to the way adults process the difference, using event-related potential methods (de Haan & Carver, 2013).

Recognizing faces and voices indicates that infants are familiar with these stimuli, and this familiarity provides the opportunity for establishing social bonds with the mother. Not only does the ability to recall information improve rapidly during infancy, but emotionally salient events are better remembered than others. Bornstein, Arteberry and Mash (2004) investigated long term memory in 20 month old infants who had participated in a social interaction in which an adult looked at them but refrained from communicating, a distressing experience, at 5 months. The infants who had experienced the still face paradigm with a novel person at 5 months fixated on the face of that person significantly less than on the faces of two other novel persons at 20 months. The infants who were in the comparison group and were matched for age fixated longer overall or equally on the face which infants in the experimental group avoided. Thus, toddlers almost 2 years old were able to remember something that had happened to them when they were 5 months old. Overall, these findings suggest that infants recognize social cues and signals from a very young age. This sensitivity so early in life may be the mechanism which promotes bonding and through which infants become familiar with their caregivers, thus preparing infants to engage in communication with other people and to learn from them.

So infants have a proclivity for social stimuli and a mirror neuron system which is activated by social signals. This tendency to prefer social stimuli should result in them having different responses to people than they do to nonsocial objects. From birth, infants smile, vocalize, and alternate their gaze more when facing people than when facing objects (Gelman & Spelke, 1981; Legerstee, 1992). By 5 weeks infants make communicative noises and movements with people and not with objects (Legerstee, Pomerleau, Malcuit, & Feider, 1987). Between 2 and 3 months, infants imitate movements of opening the mouth and protrusion of the tongue when people are the models, but not when inanimate objects that simulate these movements are the models. Imitative responsiveness in infancy to people and not to physical objects supports the contention that there is a differentiation between people and objects from a very young age. In addition, infants seem to expect that adults will share their affective states with them, and seemingly have no such expectation from objects.

Affect is relational by nature and it is the earliest emotional information that is shared between the infant and other people (Stern, 1995). This animate / inanimate distinction is also apparent in early categorization skills of infants, because by 7–8 months of age infants respond differently to animate and inanimate stimuli (Jeschonek, Marinovic, Hoehl, Elsner, & Pauen, 2010). Thus the social brain has systems for recognizing and understanding people and for discriminating people from inanimate objects.

Differentiating between animate and inanimate stimuli does not mean that infants are aware of people's thoughts, feelings and intentions. Mentalizing refers to the ability to read the mental states of others and has been conceptualized as the ability to represent mental states of self and other, and evidence for this ability exists from age 5 months, when infants recognize other's eye gaze as intentional. At this same age infants begin to use social signals, such as their own gaze patterns, to share attention about interesting toys with people and not with inanimate objects. Grossman and Johnson (2010), using near infra-red spectroscopy, examined 5 month old infants' ability to follow gazes of adults, and found that the prefrontal cortex was activated during dyadic and, most interestingly, during triadic interactions. Infants seem to be aware of the difference between people and objects from a very young age and to distinguish between social and non-social worlds.

Thus far evidence suggests that newborns have the predispositions that allow them to recognize other human beings at birth. There are two positions as to the manner in which this recognition leads the infant to establish meaningful relationships with other people. The first hypothesis is that infants are born with reflexes that react to incoming social stimulation, which becomes the basis for connectedness (Gergely & Watson, 1999; Meltzoff, 2007; Piaget, 1952). According to this theory, infants connect with the social world because they are sensitive to social contingencies. Around age 3 months, infants begin to be sensitive to the type of contingent interactions provided by people. It is suggested that infants establish intersubjective connections with people by detecting similarities between their own and others' actions through imitation games. Imitation is an attention getter and through it infants begin to perceive others as like themselves. Thus, according to these authors, infants are not capable of connecting with their caregivers in a meaningful way in the first few months of their lives.

Alternatively, according to Legerstee (2005, 2009), infants perceive others to be like them because they are born with an affect sharing device that is made up of three components that act together: (1) the ability to recognize people as similar to themselves; (2) the ability to be sensitive to their own and others' emotions and (3) the ability to perceive whether adults are attuned to their needs and emotions. The interplay among these three predispositions results in affectively attuned relationships that are important mechanisms for infants' social cognitive development. Infants seem to have an innate sense of people which is activated through sympathetic emotions, through which they learn about themselves and others and establish ongoing relationships, during which infants progress toward an increased knowledge about shared meaning which is formed not through social contingencies (nurture), but rather through other beings with whom they can share experiences and establish social attunement (nature).

Contingencies and imitation seem to draw infant attention to others, while affective communication appears to lay the foundation for infants' social awareness and subsequent social relationships. The premise is that infants are innately prepared to connect to their caregivers not only through imitation but also through affective attunement (Gallese, Rochat, & Berchio, 2013; Legerstee, 2005; Markova & Legerstee, 2006). Social bonds are fundamental for human beings because social connections with others ensure the satisfaction of physiological needs (food and shelter) but also of social needs. Swain, Lorberbaum, Kose, and Strathearn (2007) studied the effects of environmental adversity on the emotional wellbeing of parents and how this affected subsequent behavior in their infants. They found that in mother-infant dyads, the infants' behavior activated particular interacting transmitters such as oxytocin, prolactin, vasopressin and dopamine in the mother. For example, oxytocin released during breast feeding was associated with lower levels of anxiety and stress in infants, which elicited more attuned behaviors of the mothers. However, when mothers became less attentive to infant signals because of substance abuse or depression, identified risk factors for problems in infant mental health, this affected social bonding.

Attunement

Attunement can be conceptualized as the dynamic adaptation of two partners, who after sensing one another's affective state adjust their own behavior accordingly (Bornstein, 2013). Mothers bond with their infants and infants bond with their caregivers, and the quality of that relationship is at the base of infant and early childhood mental health. The quality of the infant-caregiver relationship has been characterized by terms such as mutuality, reciprocity, responsiveness, intersubjectivity, coherence, contingency, co-regulation, matching, mirroring, synchrony, and many other words, all of which reflect the special character of well-functioning mother infant relationships. Parent and child interactions are often described as intricate patterns of sensitive mutual understanding and the unfolding of synchronous transactions (Bornstein, 2006, 2012, 2013; Feldman, 2007; Kochanska, Murray, & Coy, 1997; Maccoby, 1992). Achieving harmonious dyadic interaction is considered one of the most significant developmental issues of infancy (Sroufe, 2000) and is the cornerstone of infant mental health. The construct attunement has been used to refer to the ability one person has to respond to another's emotional needs and moods. Well attuned parents are able to sense what their infants are feeling and respond appropriately. Attuned parents adapt their language and behaviors in responding to their infants' mental states.

Parenting in an attuned fashion is a job whose primary object of attention and action is the child. Maccoby (1992) observed that in the bi-directionality of parent–child interactions, there will always be asymmetry in the relationship, with caregivers having more interactive skills and adapting themselves to the child's capacities and current status. Thus, even when the participation in interactions is balanced, caregivers are still more responsible for facilitating attunement (Kochanska & Aksan, 2004). Mothers are generally emotionally prepared and positively motivated to engage and care for their children. Parents must be sensitive to their infants' cues and respond appropriately, which means harnessing their sensory, perceptual and affective systems and coordinating them to respond to the infant's needs and desires. Adults' intuitive communicative and empathic behaviors allow for sharing affect and interests (Trevarthen & Aitken, 2001).

Human children cannot grow up as solitary individuals and, as their primary caregivers, parents are their first socializing agents. The more attuned a parent is the more the baby will respond socially. There are a variety of different mechanisms which facilitate attunement to the infant. For example, newborns prefer their mothers' voices (DeCasper & Fifer, 1980); breast fed infants learn their mother's characteristic smells quickly (Porter & Porter, 2004); and infants actively signal and elicit effective parental care by following, clinging, calling and crying (Messer & Vietze, 1984). Mothers experience elevated levels of sympathy and alertness in response to the cries of babies, which is necessary for mother-infant emotional bonding (Feldman, 2012). In attuned interactions infants and mothers experience mutually positive affective exchanges and transition smoothly between activities (Stern, 1995; Tronick & Cohn, 1989). This mutual attention has been demonstrated as early as at birth (Brazelton, Koslowski, & Main, 1974; Greenspan & Wieder, 1993).

Research methodologies for studying attunement include designs that use the same stimuli or tasks with the parent and child, or that compare own-parent versus other-parent stimuli for the child and own-child versus other-child stimuli for the parent, and they apply concordance and sometimes sequential analyses. Concordance describes co-variance in the rank order status of specific mother and infant constructs, structures, functions or processes. In achieving behavioral concordance, for example, mothers who perform one kind of activity relatively more often for longer times, or who manifest a characteristic to a relatively high degree, have infants who perform a specific corresponding characteristic to a relatively high degree. Bornstein (2013) conceptualized attunement as the correlation between mother and infant communicative behaviors. Although correlation approaches are usually employed, related regression approaches are useful and common as well (DeFries, 1967).

References

Ainsworth, M. D., Blehar, M. C., Waters, E., & Wall, S. (1978). *Patterns of attachment: Assessed in the strange situation and at home*. Hillsdale, NJ: Erlbaum.

American Psychiatric Association. (2000). *Diagnostic criteria from DSM-IV-TR*. Washington, DC: American Psychiatric Publications.

American Psychiatric Association. (2013). *Diagnostic and statistical manual of mental disorders: DSM-5*. Washington, DC: American Psychiatric Publications.

Aviezer, O., Sagi, A., Joels, T., & Ziv, Y. (1999). Emotional availability and attachment representations in Kibbutz infants and their mothers. *Development Psychology, 35*, 811–821.

Barone, L., & Biringen, Z. (2007). Le scale per la valutazione della disponibilita' emozionale (Emotional availability scales—EAS). In L. Barone (Ed.), *Emozioni e sviluppo. Percorsi tipici e atipici* (pp. 404–405). Rome: Carocci.

Belsky, J., & Isabella, R. (1988). Maternal, infant, and social-contextual determinants of attachment security. In J. Belsky & T. Nezworski (Eds.), *Clinical implications of attachment* (pp. 41–94). New York: Psychology Press.

Biringen, Z. (2000). Emotional availability: Conceptualization and research findings. *American Journal of Orthopsychiatry, 70*(1), 104–114.

Biringen, Z. (2004). *Raising a secure child: Creating emotional availability between you and your child.* New York: Perigee/Putnam Press.

Biringen, Z., & Easterbrooks, M. A. (2008). Understanding relationships and relationship interventions. *Journal of Early Childhood and Infant Psychology, 4*, 1–3.

Biringen, Z., & Easterbrooks, M. (2012). Emotional availability: Concept, research, and window on developmental psychopathology. *Development and Psychopathology, 24*(01), 1–8.

Biringen, Z., Altenhofen, S., Aberle, J., Baker, M., Brosal, A., Bennett, S., . . . & Swaim, R. (2012). Emotional availability, attachment, and intervention in center-based child care for infants and toddlers. *Development and Psychopathology, 24*(01), 23–34.

Biringen, Z., Fidler, D. J., Barrett, K. C., & Kubicek, L. (2005). Applying the emotional availability scales to children with disabilities. *Infant Mental Health Journal, 26*(4), 369–391.

Biringen, Z., Robinson, J., & Emde, R. (1998). Emotional availability scales (3rd ed.). Unpublished manuscript. Retrieved from http://www.emotionalavailability.com

Biringen, Z., Robinson, J. L., & Emde, R. N. (2000). Appendix B: The emotional availability scales (an abridged infancy/early childhood version). *Attachment & Human Development, 2* (2), 256–270.

Bornstein, M. H. (2006). Parenting science and practice. In A. Renninger & I. E. Sigel (Eds.), *Handbook of child psychology: Vol. 4. Child psychology in practice* (6th ed., pp. 893–949). Hoboken, NJ: Wiley.

Bornstein, M. H. (2012). Cultural approaches to parenting. *Parenting, 12*(2–3), 212–221.

Bornstein, M. (2013). Mother–infant attunement. In M. Legerstee (Ed.), *The infant mind: Origins of the social brain* (p. 266). New York: Guilford Press.

Bornstein, M. H., Arterberry, M. E., & Mash, C. (2004). Long-term memory for an emotional interpersonal interaction occurring at 5 months of age. *Infancy, 6*(3), 407–416.

Bowlby, J. (1969). *Attachment and loss: Vol. 1. Attachment.* New York: Basic Books.

Bowlby, J. (1988). *A secure base: Clinical application of attachment theory.* London, UK: Routledge.

Brazelton, T. B., Koslowski, B., & Main, M. (1974). The origins of reciprocity: The early mother-infant interaction. In M. Lewis & L. A. Rosenblum (Eds.), *The effect of the infant on its caregiver*. Oxford, UK: Wiley-Interscience.

Bronfenbrenner, U. (1979). Contexts of child rearing: Problems and prospects. *American Psychologist, 34*(10), 844–850.

Bronfenbrenner, U. (1986). Ecology of the family as a context for human development: Research perspectives. *Developmental Psychology, 22*(6), 723–742.

Bushnell, I. W. R., Sai, F., & Mullin, J. T. (1989). Neonatal recognition of the mother's face. *British Journal of Developmental Psychology, 7*, 3–15.

Carlson, V. J., & Harwood, R. L. (2014). The precursors of attachment security: Behavioral systems and culture. In H. Otto & H. Keller (Eds.), *Different faces of attachment: Cultural variations on a universal human need* (pp. 278–303). Cambridge, UK: Cambridge University Press.

Cowan, P. A., Cohn, D. A., Cowan, C. P., & Pearson, J. L. (1996). Parents' attachment histories and children's externalizing and internalizing behaviors: Exploring family systems models of linkage. *Journal of Consulting and Clinical Psychology, 64*(1), 53–63.

De Haan, M., & Carver, L. J. (2013). Development of brain networks for visual social-emotional information processing in infancy. In M. Legerstee, D. W. Haley, & M. H. Bornstein (Eds.), *The infant mind: Origins of the social brain* (pp. 123–145). London: Guilford Press.

De Haan, M. & Gunnar, M. R. (2009). The brain in a social environment. Why study development. In *Handbook of developmental social neuroscience* (pp. 3–10). New York: Guilford.

DeCasper, A. J., & Fifer, W. P. (1980). Of human bonding: Newborns prefer their mothers' voices. *Science, 208*(4448), 1174–1176.

DeFries, J. C. (1967). Quantitative genetics and behavior: Overview and perspective. In J. Hirsch (Ed.), *Behavior-genetic analysis* (pp. 322–339). New York: McGraw-Hill.

Draghi-Lorenz, R. (2010). Parental reports of jealousy in early infancy. In S. L. Hart & M. Legerstee (Eds.), *Handbook of jealousy: Theory, research, and multidisciplinary approaches* (pp. 235–266). Chichester, UK: Wiley-Blackwell.

Dunbar, R. I. M. (2013). *Primate social systems*. Bristol, UK: Springer Science & Business Media.

Easterbrooks, M. A., & Biringen, Z. (2000). Mapping the terrain of emotional availability and attachment. *Attachment and Human Development, 2*, 129–135.

Easterbrooks, M. A., & Biringen, Z. (2005). The emotional availability scales: Methodological refinements of the construct and clinical implications related to gender and at-risk interactions. *Infant Mental Health Journal, 26*, 291–294.

Easterbrooks, M. A., & Biringen, Z. (2009). Introduction to the special issue: Emotional availability across contexts. *Parenting: Science and Practice, 9*(3–4), 179–182.

Easterbrooks, M. A., Bureau, J.-F., & Lyons-Ruth, K. (2012). Developmental correlates and predictors of emotional availability in mother-child interaction: A longitudinal study from infancy to middle childhood. *Development and Psychopathology, 24*, 65–78.

Emde, R. N., & Easterbrooks, M. A. (1985). Assessing emotional availability in early development. In W. K. Frankenburg, R. N. Emde, & J. W. Sulivan (Eds.), *Early identification of children at risk* (pp. 79–101). New York: Plenum Press.

Emde, R. N., & Sameroff, A. J. (1989). Understanding early relationship disturbances. In A. J. Sameroff, & R. N. Sameroff (Eds.), *Relationship disturbances in early childhood* (pp. 3–14). New York, NY: Basic Books.

Feldman, R. (2007). Parent–infant synchrony biological foundations and developmental outcomes. *Current Directions in Psychological Science, 16*(6), 340–345.

Feldman, R. (2012). Oxytocin and social affiliation in humans. *Hormones and Behavior, 61*(3), 380–391.

Feldman, R., Eidelman, A. I., & Rotenberg, N. (2004). Parenting stress, infant emotion regulation, maternal sensitivity, and the cognitive development of triplets: A model for parent and child influences in a unique ecology. *Child Development, 75*(6), 1774–1791.

Fivaz-Depeursinge, E., Favez, N., Scaiola, C. L., & Lopes, F. (2010). Family triangular interactions in infancy: A context for the development of jealousy? In S. L. Hart & M. Legerstee (Eds.), *Handbook of jealousy: Theories, research, and multidisciplinary approaches* (pp. 445–476). New York: Wiley-Blackwell.

Gallagher, S., & Meltzoff, A. N. (1996). The earliest sense of self and others: Merleau-Ponty and recent developmental studies. *Philosophical Psychology, 9*(2), 211–233.

Gallese, V. (2011). Embodied simulation theory: Imagination and narrative. *Neuropsychoanalysis, 13*(2), 196–200.

Gallese, V., Rochat, M. J., & Berchio, C. (2013). The mirror mechanism and its potential role in autism spectrum disorder. *Developmental Medicine & Child Neurology, 55*(1), 15–22.

Gelman, R., & Spelke, E. S. (1981). The development of thoughts about animate and inanimate objects: Implications for research on social cognition. In J. H. Flavell & L. Ross (Eds.), *Social cognitive development: Frontiers and possible futures* (pp. 43–66). Cambridge, UK: Cambridge University Press Archives.

Gergely, G., & Watson, J. S. (1999). Early socio-emotional development: Contingency perception and the social-biofeedback model. In P. Rochat (Ed.), *Early social cognition: Understanding others in the first months of life* (pp. 101–136). New York: Psychology Press.
Gerhardt, S. (2006). Why love matters: How affection shapes a baby's brain. *Infant Observation, 9* (3), 305–309.
Goh, E. C. (2013). "You must finish your dinner": Mealtime dynamics between grandparents, parents and grandchildren in urban China. *British Food Journal, 115*(3), 365–376.
Greenspan, S. I., & Wieder, S. (1993). Regulatory disorders. In C. R. Zeanah (Ed.), *Handbook of infant mental health* (pp. 280–290). New York: Guilford Press.
Greenspan, S. I., & Wieder, S. (2007). *Infant and early childhood mental health: A comprehensive developmental approach to assessment and intervention.* Washington, DC: American Psychiatric Publications.
Grossman, T., & Johnson, M. H. (2010). Selective prefrontal cortex responses to joint attention in early infancy. *Biology Letters, 6*, 540–543.
Grossmann, K., Grossmann, K. E., Spangler, G., Suess, G., & Unzner, L. (1985). Maternal sensitivity and newborns' orientation responses as related to quality of attachment in northern Germany. *Monographs of the Society for Research in Child Development, 50*(1-2), 233–256.
Hart, S. L., Carrington, H. A., Tronick, E. Z., & Carroll, S. R. (2004). When infants lose exclusive maternal attention: Is it jealousy? *Infancy, 6*(1), 57–78.
Hart, S. L., & Legerstee, M. (2010). *Handbook of jealousy. Theory, research, and multidisciplinary approaches*. Chichester, UK: Wiley-Blackwell.
Hartup, W. W., & Rubin, Z. (Eds.). (2013). *Relationships and development*. New York: Psychology Press.
Harwood, R. L., Handwerker, W. P., Schoelmerich, A., & Leyendecker, B. (2001). Ethnic category labels, parental beliefs, and the contextualized individual: An exploration of the individualism-sociocentrism debate. *Parenting: Science and Practice, 1*(3), 217–236.
Hoffman, M. L. (1975). Developmental synthesis of affect and cognition and its interplay for altruistic motivation. *Developmental Psychology, 11*, 607–622.
Holden, G. W., & O'Dell, P. C. (1995). *Just how stable is parental behavior? Meta-analysis and reformulation*. Unpublished manuscript, University of Texas at Austin.
Jeschonek, S., Marinovic, V., Hoehl, S., Elsner, B., & Pauen, S. (2010). Do animals and furniture items elicit different brain responses in human infants? *Brain and Development, 32*(10), 863–871.
Keller, H., & Otto, H. (2009). The cultural socialization of emotion regulation during infancy. *Journal of Cross-Cultural Psychology, 40*(6), 996–1011.
Keller, H., Lohaus, A., Kuensemueller, P., Abels, M., Yovsi, R., Voelker, S., … & Mohite, P. (2004). The bio-culture of parenting: evidence from five cultural communities. *Parenting: Science and Practice*, *4*(1), 25–50.
Killeen, L. A., & Teti, D. M. (2012). Mothers' frontal EEG asymmetry in response to infant emotion states and mother–infant emotional availability, emotional experience, and internalizing symptoms. *Development and Psychopathology, 24*(01), 9–21.
Kochanska, G., & Aksan, N. (2004). Development of mutual responsiveness between parents and their young children. *Child Development, 75*, 1657–1676.
Kochanska, G., Murray, K., & Coy, K. C. (1997). Inhibitory control as a contributor to conscience in childhood: From toddler to early school age. *Child Development, 68*(2), 263–277.
Korbin, J. (1994). Sociocultural factors in child maltreatment. In G. B. Melton & F. D. Barry (Eds.), *Protecting children from abuse and neglect: Foundations for a new national strategy* (pp. 182–223). New York: Guilford Press.
Legerstee, M. (1992). A review of the animate-inanimate distinction in infancy: Implications for models of social and cognitive knowing. *Early Development and Parenting, 1*(2), 59–67.
Legerstee, M. (1998). Mental and bodily awareness in infancy: Consciousness of self-existence. *Journal of Consciousness Studies, 5*(5–6), 672–672.

Legerstee, M. (2005). *Infants' sense of people: Precursors to a theory of mind*. Cambridge, UK: Cambridge University Press.

Legerstee, M. (2009). The role of dyadic communication in social cognitive development. *Advances in Child Development and Behavior, 37*, 1–53.

Legerstee, M., Ellenbogen, B., Nienhuis, T., & Marsh, H. (2010). Social bonds, triadic relationships, and goals. In S. L. Hart & M. Legerstee (Eds.), *Handbook of jealousy: Theory, research, and multidisciplinary approaches* (pp. 161–191). Chichester, UK: Wiley-Blackwell.

Legerstee, M., & Haley, D. W. (Eds.). (2013). *Infant mind: Origins of the social brain*. New York, NY: Guilford Press.

Legerstee, M., Pomerleau, A., Malcuit, G., & Feider, H. (1987). The development of infants' responses to people and a doll: Implications for research in communication. *Infant Behavior and Development, 10*(1), 81–95.

Maccoby, E. E. (1992). The role of parents in the socialization of children: An historical overview. *Developmental Psychology, 28*(6), 1006–1017.

Markova, G., & Legerstee, M. (2006). Contingency, imitation, and affect sharing: Foundations of infants' social awareness. *Developmental Psychology, 42*(1), 132.

Markova, G., Stieben, J., & Legerstee, M. (2010). Neural structures of jealousy. In S. L. Hart & M. Legerstee (Eds.), *Handbook of jealousy: Theory, research, and multidisciplinary approaches* (pp. 83–100). Chichester, UK: Wiley-Blackwell.

Meltzoff, A. N. (2007). 'Like me': A foundation for social cognition. *Developmental Science, 10* (1), 126–134.

Meltzoff, A. N., & Moore, M. K. (1998). Infant intersubjectivity: Broadening the dialogue to include imitation, identity and intention. In S. Bråten (Ed.), *Intersubjective communication and emotion in early ontogeny* (pp. 47–62). Cambridge, UK: Cambridge University Press.

Messer, D. J., & Vietze, P. M. (1984). Timing and transitions in mother-infant gaze. *Infant Behavior and Development, 7*, 167–181.

Miyake, K., Chen, S. J., & Campos, J. J. (1985). Infant temperament, mother's mode of interaction, and attachment in Japan: An interim report. *Monographs of the Society for Research in Child Development, 50*(1-2), 276–297.

Nakagawa, M., Lamb, M. E., & Miyake, K. (1989). Psychological experiences of Japanese. *Psychiatry, 32*(12), 13–24.

Nicholls, A., & Kirkland, J. (1996). Maternal sensitivity: A review of attachment literature and definitions. *Early Child Development and Care, 20*, 55–65.

Nugent, P. (1995). *Big men, small boys and politics in Ghana: Power, ideology and the burden of history, 1982–1994*. London: Pinter Publications Ltd.

Otto, H., & Keller, H. (Eds.). (2014). *Different faces of attachment: Cultural variations on a universal human need*. Cambridge, UK: Cambridge University Press.

Oyen, A., Landy, S., & Hilburn-Cobb, C. (2000). Maternal attachment and sensitivity in an at-risk sample. *Attachment and Human Development, 2*, 203–217.

Panksepp, J. (2010). The evolutionary sources of jealousy. In S. L. Hart & M. Legerstee (Eds.), *Handbook of jealousy: Theory, research, and multidisciplinary approaches* (pp. 101–120). Chichester, UK: Wiley-Blackwell.

Piaget, J. (1952). *The origins of intelligence in children* (Vol. 8, No. 5, p. 18). New York: International Universities Press.

Pipp-Siegel, S., & Biringen, Z. (1998). Assessing the quality of relationships between parents and children: The emotional availability scales. *The Volta Review, 100*(5), 237–349.

Porter, L. S., & Porter, B. O. (2004). A blended infant massage-parenting enhancement program for recovering substance-abusing mothers. *Pediatric Nursing, 30*(5), 363–372.

Rosenthal, M. K., & Roer-Strier, D. (2006). "What sort of an adult would you like your child to be?": Mothers' developmental goals in different cultural communities in Israel. *International Journal of Behavioral Development, 30*(6), 517–528.

Rutter, M. (2009). Understanding and testing risk mechanisms for mental disorders. *Journal of Child Psychology and Psychiatry, 50*(1–2), 44–52.

Rutter, M., & Silberg, J. (2002). Gene-environment interplay in relation to emotional and behavioral disturbance. *Annual Review of Psychology, 53*(1), 463–490.

Salo, S., Kivistö, K., Korja, R., Biringen, Z., Tupola, S., Kahila, H., et al. (2009). Emotional availability, parental self-efficacy beliefs, and child development in caregiver-child relationships with buprenorphine-exposed 3-year-olds. *Parenting: Science and Practice, 9*(3–4), 244–259.

Sameroff, A. (2009). *The transactional model.* Washington, DC: American Psychological Association.

Sameroff, A. J., & Fiese, B. H. (2000). Transactional regulation: The developmental ecology of early intervention. In J. P. Shonkoff & S. J. Meisels (Eds.), *Handbook of early childhood intervention* (pp. 135–159). New York, NY: Cambridge University Press.

Shonkoff, J., & Philips, D. (2000). *From neurons to neighborhoods: The science of early childhood development.* Washington, DC: National Academies Press.

Siegel, D. J. (2012). *The developing mind: How relationships and the brain interact to shape who we are.* New York: Guilford Press.

Sorce, J. F., & Emde, R. N. (1981). Mother's presence is not enough: Effect of emotional availability on infant exploration. *Developmental Psychology, 17*(6), 737–745.

Sroufe, L. A. (2000). Early relationships and the development of children. *Infant Mental Health Journal, 21*(1–2), 67–74.

Stack, D. M., Serbin, L. A., Girouard, N., Enns, L. N., Bentley, V., Ledingham, J. E., et al. (2012). The quality of the mother–child relationship in high-risk dyads: Application of the emotional availability scales in an intergenerational, longitudinal study. *Development and Psychopathology, 24*, 93–105.

Stams, G. J. J., Juffer, F., & van IJzendoorn, M. H. (2002). Maternal sensitivity, infant attachment, and temperament in early childhood predict adjustment in middle childhood: The case of adopted children and their biologically unrelated parents. *Developmental Psychology, 38*(5), 806–821.

Stern, D. N. (1995). *Motherhood constellation.* London, UK: Karnac Books.

Stern, D. N. (2009). *The first relationship: Infant and mother.* Cambridge, MA: Harvard University Press.

Swain, J. E., Lorberbaum, J. P., Kose, S., & Strathearn, L. (2007). Brain basis of early parent–infant interactions: Psychology, physiology, and in vivo functional neuroimaging studies. *Journal of Child Psychology and Psychiatry, 48*(3–4), 262–287.

Timmer, S. G., Thompson, D., Culver, M. A., Urquiza, A. J., & Altenhofen, S. (2012). Mothers' physical abusiveness in a context of violence: Effects on the mother–child relationship. *Development and Psychopathology, 24*(01), 79–92.

Trevarthen, C., & Aitken, K. J. (2001). Infant intersubjectivity: Research, theory, and clinical applications. *Journal of Child Psychology and Psychiatry, 42*(1), 3–48.

Tronick, E., Als, H., Adamson, L., Wise, S., & Brazelton, T. B. (1979). The infant's response to entrapment between contradictory messages in face-to-face interaction. *Journal of the American Academy of Child Psychiatry, 17*(1), 1–13.

Tronick, E. Z., & Cohn, J. F. (1989). Infant-mother face-to-face interaction: Age and gender differences in coordination and the occurrence of miscoordination. *Child Development, 60*(1), 85–92.

van Ijzendoorn, M. H., & Tavecchio, L. W. (1987). The development of attachment theory as a Lakatosian research program: Philosophical and methodological aspects. *Advances in Psychology, 44*, 3–31.

Zero to Three (Organization). DC, & 0-3R Revision Task Force. (2005). *DC: 0-3R: Diagnostic classification of mental health and developmental disorders of infancy and early childhood.* Zero to Three.

Ziv, Y., Aviezer, O., Gini, M., Sagi, A., & Koren-Karie, N. (2000). Emotional availability in the mother–infant dyad as related to the quality of infant–mother attachment relationship. *Attachment and Human Development, 2*, 149–169.

Chapter 7
Resilience in Children and Families

Introduction

Risk factors do not fully determine child outcomes, even when there are many risk factors and they appear early in the developing child's life, because in every risk group there will be some children who develop the anticipated negative outcome and others who do not (Kumpfer, 2002; Masten, Best, & Garmezy, 1990). It appears that the balance between risk and protective factors is more salient in determining child outcome than the presence of the risk factor alone (Lester et al., 2002). Protective factors are those conditions that promote resilience (i.e., positive adaptation despite previous exposure to adversity) and increase resistance to later disturbances (Masten & Coatsworth, 1998).

Protective factors, like the risk factors which were discussed in Chap. 5, exist in multiple domains. They may exist within the child, the parent, the child–parent relationship, and/or the environment. Examples of protective factors which are part of the child and come into play when it is necessary for that child to cope with adversity include intelligence, self-regulatory skills, and a calm temperament (Alvord & Grados, 2005), and these factors and others help the child cope positively and function well despite challenging or threatening circumstances (Masten et al., 1999). Protective factors which are located in the parent consist of a strong and clear commitment to the child's needs, sensitive responding to the child, appropriate discipline, consistent monitoring, and relevant supervision (Legge, 2013). In addition to the characteristics inherent in the child and in the parent, a close attachment figure has been identified as a protective factor for children growing up under adversity which gives the child a secure base from which to cope with challenges (Walsh, 2012, 2013; Werner & Smith, 1992).

These factors and relationships also occur within a family system, and a new area of research called family resilience has evolved. Studies in family resilience have identified additional protective factors which are associated with family

C. Shulman, *Research and Practice in Infant and Early Childhood Mental Health*,
Children's Well-Being: Indicators and Research 13,
DOI 10.1007/978-3-319-31181-4_7

functioning, belief system and meaning making (Walsh, 2002, 2006). Research into family resilience has added to our knowledge base of resilience and infant mental health. Environmental factors which support adaptive functioning in the face of adversity in the family system include social support systems, which can be manifested in close relationships that the parents have with other adults, through which they receive needed emotional, informational and concrete resources. Mothers who have more satisfactory social relationships with other adults, particularly stable and supportive marital relationships, manifest better parent–child interactions (Crockenberg, 1981) and feel more competent as parents and less stressed by their parenting responsibilities (Crnic, Greenberg, Robinson, & Ragozin, 1984).

Protective communities have been identified as those which support their weaker members or care for their members when adverse circumstances befall them, and yet some members of such communities are still less resilient than others. Understandably, researching these factors and their interrelatedness is complex, and results are sometimes ambiguous and not always conclusive. This chapter will present definitions of resilience and describe the research being performed today in the field of infant mental health and resilience, including a section on family resilience models.

Resilience Models

Resilience involves the intersection between exposure to a known risk factor and the positive adaptation manifested by individuals in the face of adversity (Luthar, 2006). Inherent in this perspective is a theoretical question: Is risk a prerequisite of resilience? In order to be resilient, must some appreciable risk be present? In order to address this question, professionals have differentiated between two groups of adaptive and competent children. The first is a group of children who cope relatively well with the daily and exceptional challenges which they face, but who after careful evaluation have experienced minimal or no real adversity, whereas the second group of children are also functioning adaptively despite the fact that they have experienced significant risk (Garmezy, 1995; Masten, 2011, 2013). These children are considered resilient as they have come face to face with adverse conditions and still function competently.

It must be made clear that it is not easy to establish which category a child belongs to, as not all children who have a depressive parent, for example, will develop in a maladaptive fashion. This is the reason that adversity has been conceptualized as a risk factor – there is an elevated risk for poorer outcomes but not a one-to-one correspondence between risk factors and negative outcomes for children. It cannot be assumed that children of depressed parents who develop adaptively are resilient (Cicchetti & Garmezy, 1993), as they may in fact not have developed in an adverse environment. It is possible that some of these competent children of a depressed parent who developed along positive adaptive trajectories experienced benign or healthy contexts of development with parental warmth, effective child management strategies, and safe and supportive neighborhoods. In addition, perhaps the extended family was present and supportive, along with high quality educational frameworks. It is not clear whether these factors are protective or whether the child did not experience adversity.

This difficulty is also pertinent for determining the extent of risk in genetic and constitutional factors. Rende and Plomin (1993) discuss the genetic predisposition of children of parents with mental illness to disorders, but the absence of disorder does not necessarily indicate resilience; it is possible that that particular child was not at risk. Similarly, not all children with developmental disorders are at risk, and those who develop adaptively are not necessarily resilient. The severity of the risk factor is determined, among other things, by the values of the family in which the child is being raised and the meaning which the family assigns to the child's disability, a topic which will be elaborated on in the section on family resilience in this chapter. Thus, resilience is not merely competent functioning but rather competent functioning when faced with challenge or stress (Cowan, Cowan, & Schulz, 1996).

The role of relationships in the study of risks and resources in early childhood adaptive functioning is crucial. Whether in the context of adversity or security, early relationships form the foundation for cognitive, affective and neurobiological adaptation. Resilience can be described as a relational process that reflects the establishment of coping strategies among systems and among people. It is not a personality or genetic trait, but rather reflects dynamic processes of adaptation that can be engendered or compromised to a significant degree by the quality of relational processes. Since relationships can support the positive development of young children, and sensitive and supportive relationships are important for optimal developmental and behavioral outcomes, it is important when investigating resilience to assess the relational context in which the child is growing (Peterson & Yates, 2013).

The current focus of many resilience researchers is on identifying both risk and, particularly, protective factors that might modify the negative effects of adverse life circumstances, as well as identifying underlying mechanisms or processes (Luthar, 2006). This type of information allows for the design and testing of intervention programs, the goals of which include strengthening protective factors. Such programs will be discussed in the following chapters, and include components such as promoting the presence of a strong positive relationship with at least one parent or other caring adult, and teaching effective parenting skills that predict positive, resilient trajectories. Similarly, high quality responsive caregiving in childcare can buffer the effects of adversity, such as poverty, on young infants and toddlers (Ghosh-Ippen, Harris, Van Horn, & Lieberman, 2011; Shonkoff et al., 2012).

Research has identified some protective factors, which include maternal sensitivity and the child's security of attachment, which help the child develop optimally despite adversity and stress. Risk factors, such as coercive discipline strategies, child prematurity, family marital discord/divorce and poverty were discussed in Chap. 5, where the additive quality of risk factors was highlighted. The cumulative nature of risk factors guides programming directions in intervention programs, which may target the child directly, or focus on parenting and the parent–child relationship, or support the parent's individual strengths and/or the family ecology and functions. Finally, when researching resilience, it is essential to remember that it is an inferential construct (Luthar & Zelazo, 2003), which is never actually directly measured. It is inferred based on the measurement of the presence of risk and positive adaptations despite those risks, and as such prevention and intervention efforts strive to protect, restore or provide positive relationships in contexts of risk.

Risk and Resilience in a Relational Context

It hasbeen demonstrated that relational vulnerabilities engender distress and maladaptation and, conversely, relational resources have been shown to foster emotional health and competence (Peterson & Yates, 2013). In the context of safe and responsive relationships with caregivers and others, young children can develop regulatory capacities which enable them to develop optimally despite adversity and to effectively negotiate the challenges they encounter. Efforts to identify the relational roots of resilience have revealed that meaningful, quality relationships are positive protective resources which can foster children's capacity to reach age appropriate skills and culturally significant behaviors. Thus relationships are a key focus in resilience research, as they are associated with both positive and non-optimal adjustment patterns.

Research in the field of infant mental health is trying to discover which relationships are important for understanding resilience, which aspects of the relationship are important for resilience, and in what ways they are influential. The roots of relationships and, to a significant degree, of resilience are grounded in the foundational experiences of early childhood. In the context of the early caregiving relationship, children develop regulatory and relational capacities which help them cope with stress if and when they experience stressful and/or adverse circumstances. In addition, the early caregiving relationship is at the base of the child's emerging expectations of the self and others (Stern, 2009). Thus, children's successful adaptation in contexts of adversity (i.e., resilience) reflects the combined influence of multiple relationships, with a unique role accorded to early caregiving experiences.

Resilience research has identified several relational mechanisms by which protective factors operate to increase competence in contexts of adversity. These mechanisms are based on the following four premises: (1) positive relationships contribute to resilient adaptation by promoting resources in the child including higher self-esteem, confidence and coping skills; (2) risk impact is reduced when the child is more protected because of the support and security garnered through positive relationships, such as having alternative caregivers available when the parent is unable to be available; (3) the presence of relational processes may confound the negativity which otherwise would produce chain reactions, such as when the presence of an alternate caregiver may quell the series of negative consequences that might befall a child in the wake of losing a parent; and finally (4) relationships may provide new opportunities for positive adaptation, such as when a friend exposes a young child to positive outlets for expression and connection through new interests (Rajendran, 2008). Developmentally, relationships change as the child grows and is involved with different relational partners (e.g., parents versus peers) and contextually, the content and meaning of relational qualities are influenced by contextual and cultural expectations.

Resilience research highlights the need for a contextually- and culturally-sensitive view of development. Sensitive and responsive caregiving engenders positive development, but there is a need to be aware of the relativity of risk factors. It is clear that factors which are identified with high-quality care in one culture, society or even circumstance may look different in other cultures, in different societies and even under different conditions. In a high risk context, relational factors that would be associated with poor outcomes in low risk contexts may actually engender positive development. For example, studies have shown that authoritarian parenting (i.e., high parental control, low warmth), which may be detrimental in typically developing children, may be associated with better outcomes for children who are at risk due to their environment and/or behavioral profiles. Similarly, although children taking on parental roles at a young age (i.e., parentification) was once considered inherently detrimental, it may be that children's caring for parents and other relatives may be associated with heightened self-esteem and achievement among some cultural and societal groups, depending on the culture and value judgments of family members (Cheah & Chirkov, 2008). Thus, relational processes vary in their importance across different contexts and among individuals, and relational processes associated with competence (i.e., positive adaptation in conditions of normative risk) may be distinct from those associated with resilience (i.e., positive adaptation in conditions of adversity).

Family and Community Resilience

Conceptualizing resilience as an important variable not just for children, or even as a relational construct, but also as a systems value, makes it clear that resilience is a salient construct for families, considered as a unit or system (Walsh, 2006). The evolution of family resilience includes multiple research and clinical interpretations of individual resilience and how they are applied in family settings. Originally the notion of resilience arose from a focus on children and how they functioned in relation to their early life experiences (Masten, 1994, 2001). Over time there was a shift from viewing families as the context for the individual's resilience to regarding the family as a unit of resilience in and of itself, and then to broadening that view and considering resilience at the community level. Historically, Kaplan (2002) based his view that the family was the support system for each individual family member on the individual resilience model, whereas Hawley and de Haan (1996) conceptualized the family as a dynamic system which could be regarded in both positive and negative terms. For example, the family was there to be protective of and support its members, encouraging resilience among family members, while concomitantly, various family components were viewed as risks, including the possibility of abuse and exposure to conflict and violence.

Similarly to research in individual resilience, family resilience research is based on studying the areas of crises and stress, but this research uses family models, such as Hill's (1949, 1971) ABCX model of family strengths research, McCubbin's (1983) double ABCX model and Patterson's (1988) family adjustment and adaption response (FAAR) model. Researchers began only in the 1970s to look at how family members interacted with one another and how they supported one another, what abilities the families called upon in order to adjust and adapt and the role that the community plays in family coping and adaption (McCubbin, McCubbin, Thompson, Sae-Young, & Allen, 1997). The family resilience model is ecologically-based (Bronfenbrenner, 1979) and deals with a range of contexts and influences, including family, extra-family groups, and other affiliate associations such as work or school and larger social systems, and takes into account coping mechanisms across the life span (Bronfenbrenner, 1986).

Community resilience models developed as a result of building on family resilience models and adding social support systems, which had first been seen as a protective factor for individuals. Landau and Saul (2004) integrated four themes into community resilience: (1) building communities and enhancing social connectedness as a basis for resilient growth; (2) employing collective storytelling and validation of crisis experience and response; (3) reestablishing the rhythms and routines of daily life, including engaging in collective healing rituals; and (4) coming up with a collective vision of the future involving renewed hope. This model was used after Hurricane Katrina in New Orleans with families who decided to stay in their community (Rodriguez, Trainor, & Quarantelli, 2006).

Family resilience (Walsh, 2006) refers to coping in an adaptive and functional manner in the family, which is considered a functional unit. The capacity to rebound from adversity is strengthened and resourcefulness is increased when they occur in the family unit. Hawley and de Haan (1996) state that family resilience is "the path a family follows as it adapts and prospers in the face of stress both in the present and over time. Resilient families respond positively to adverse conditions in unique ways, depending on the context, the developmental level, the interactive combination of risks and protective factors and the family's shared outlook" (p. 293). Drawing from research findings in the area of family strengths (Hawley & de Haan, 1996) and family stress (McCubbin & McCubbin, 1993), as well as research focused on children within the framework of developmental psychopathology, Masten (2013) and Rutter (2012) each proposed a definition of family resilience which posited that family resilience describes the path a family follows as it adapts and prospers in the face of stress both in the present and over time. Resilient families respond positively to adverse conditions in unique ways depending on the context, the developmental level, the interactive combination of risk and protective factors and the family's shared outlook.

This definition conceptualizes resilience as the unique paths that families may follow in response to specific stressors, and therefore it is important to consider resilience both in the present and in the long term, as many factors that are initially protective or helpful to families may place these families at risk at a later time. This definition implies that what resilience will actually look like and how it will be assessed will differ according to the particular stressor and the particular family history. For example, positive adaptation to loss of income and job related stress during a farming crisis might include maintaining supportive parenting skills with children (Wu & Thomson, 2001), while parental functioning was found to be less important than a high level of differentiation of self by the mother among children in low income urban environments (Benzies & Mychasiuk, 2009). This definition acknowledges the importance of both the risk and the protective factors that are unique to each family.

Research in Resilience

Individual and contextual factors play a major role in how stressors are responded to and how pathways are developed. Only a few studies have attempted to examine the process-oriented function of family resilience, with one study of family resilience investigating familial responses to child separation and reunification due to maltreatment (Lietz & Strength, 2011). This study used a narrative and qualitative approach to uncover processes of resilience over time in a family experiencing multiple risk conditions. Other examples include short term longitudinal studies examining factors leading to couple resilience in the face of economic pressure (Conger, Rueter, & Elder, 1999) and the effect of various protective factors as predictors of paternal engagement over time (Fagan, Palkovitz, Roy, & Farrie, 2009).

Much of the existing family resilience research has focused on identifying a set of risk or protective factors related to family resilience. This process has its foundation in research on individual childhood responses to stress. Wyman et al. (1992) categorized children as resilient if they were reported to have stable family environments with nurturing relationships with their parents, accompanied by age appropriate and consistent family discipline. More effective family problem-solving and higher levels of communication were found in Hawaiian families of preschoolers categorized as resilient than in the families of those seen as non-resilient (Thompson, McCubbin, Thompson, & Elver, 1995). McCubbin also studied African American military personnel and their spouses to determine factors which affected adjustment to overseas assignments, and the spouse's employment and assessment of family time together emerged as important factors associated with adaptation. Another study investigated resilience in families with internationally adopted children, and it was found that those families identified as more resilient exhibited higher levels of communication and problem solving, maintained a positive outlook, and used spirituality as part of their coping mechanism (Chapin, 2011).

Similar components (positive world view, mobilizing resources and family cohesion) were associated with higher levels of family resilience in families of children with autism (Bayat, 2007). Among single parent families, Greeff and Ritman (2005) identified factors such as perseverance, emotional expression, and self-confidence as individual characteristics of resilience. These studies yield important practical and theoretical results. Although they are cross-sectional in nature, they add an important facet to resilience research, when resilience is defined as a dynamic outcome whose presence or absence characterizes family functioning. These studies attempted to measure family resilience at a given point in time, using standardized instruments that assess characteristics associated with resilience. However, this approach does not regard resilience as a process that changes over time and therefore multiple pathways cannot be researched in this model.

Longitudinal Resilience Research Designs

Researchers, motivated by a desire to examine resilience as a process, began to develop a method of examining family responses to a variety of stressors and situations, with the operationalization of resilience depending on the context and the stressor being investigated. This focus on long-term adaptation called for a longitudinal design which assessed families before, during and after the occurrence of a particular stressor. The goal was to identify common trajectories exhibited by families facing stressful situations, as well as to uncover paths that were associated with adaptive outcomes in the long term. Families which were able to regain or surpass pre-crisis levels of functioning at some point after the stressor were considered resilient.

There are many methodological challenges in the longitudinal study of resilience in families, such as a continuing concern in family research with choosing the proper unit of analysis. One can choose to assess families as units, as opposed to collections of perceptions from individual family members. There are several ways to gather data from more than one family member and transform individual reports into a construct serving as a proxy for family functioning. These range from fairly straightforward difference scores, additive scores, and ratios to slightly more complicated dispersion-based scores and dyadic-level correlations to the social relations model and other covariance-based techniques requiring knowledge of structural equations modeling techniques (for review see Ludbrook, 2002).

Perhaps the biggest problem with these strategies is that they assess perceptions of individual family members rather than assessing the family itself. We can ask families, for example, to report on their perceptions of others or their perceptions of dyadic relationships or their perceptions of triadic relationships or on their perceptions of the family as a whole. Similarly we can ask them to report on their perceptions of other family members' perceptions of the same things. However, we are still obtaining the reports of individuals; we are still gathering data at the individual level and extrapolating to the family level. While such data can be helpful, useful and appropriate for a number of research questions, they are limited in their usefulness for the operationalization of family resilience. As Simon, Murphy, and Smith (2005) argue, not only individual contributions of family members play a role but also "qualities or characteristics of the family unit as a whole can influence resilience" (p. 429). This suggests that the family must be considered as a unit of analysis, for if family resilience is conceptualized as a family level variable, its operationalization must match this theoretical definition.

Longitudinal Resilience Research Statistics

Sothe first change to take place in research methodology, following changes which occurred in research in individual resilience, was the use of the longitudinal research design. In a review of research from developmental psychopathology, Cowan et al. (1996) stated that a "central ingredient of contemporary risk research is its emphasis on moving pictures rather than static snapshots" (p. 7). They went on to suggest that the study of resilience needs to focus on the pathways that individuals follow in response to stressors, which are best captured in longitudinal designs. Patterson (2002) also maintained that longitudinal research designs are needed in order to understand how unique family factors interact over time. The model employed in much current research is one in which resilience is viewed as a process that is visible only over time, which allows us to categorize families according to how they function on the target variable/s. For example, a pattern of high adaptive functioning before crisis, low at crisis and high after crisis is the sign of a resilient family, while a pattern of high before, low during and low after describes a non-resilient family. With this as a goal, statistical methods typically used to assess change over time are problematic. For example, traditional multiple regression designs and path or structural models utilizing autoregressive cross-lag designs (Bollen & Curran, 2006; Falk & Miller, 1991), which are used to analyze data collected more than once on the same individuals over time, in order to provide evidence regarding the direction of causality between variables, allow for the removal of earlier time points from later measures of the same variables but do not allow for the examination of individual family trajectories. Instead these models investigate change between individuals and families, not change within specific individuals and families.

Path or structural models, which are used to describe directed dependencies among a set of variables within developmental designs, are an improvement in some respects (van Montfort, Oud, Satorra, 2010). These designs are not concerned with stability of rank order between families or individuals and do not function under the assumption that the variable of interest will remain stable. While linkages between predictor and outcome variables at a variety of time points emerge, these techniques are applied at a group level and do not allow for the identification of the individual family trajectory that is essential for this perspective.

Repeated measures ANOVA and MANOVA designs allow for the examination of changes in mean levels of variables over time. In addition, the relation of such change to one or more predictor variables also can be examined, but this too can only be done at the aggregate level, making the examination of trajectory on a family-by-family basis impossible. A recently emerging technique is a response to these statistical flaws.

The use of latent growth curves allows for the creation of a latent or measured variable – much like a factor – that represents the average amount of change or growth from one point to another within the data set. Formulas are available that allow for the computation of scores for individual respondents or families that represent the degree of deviation from the group as a whole (see, McArdle & Epstein, 1987, for a more detailed presentation; and see de Haan, Hawley, & Deal, 2002, for an example in family resilience research).

A variation of this technique, the construction of manifest individual growth curves, allows for more direct evaluation of individual level change. As noted by Karney and Bradbury (1995), this technique involves fitting a regression line to the available data points for each individual or family. The slope of this line then represents the best indicator of change for that individual or family over time, and can be reentered into a data set. The predictors of outcome of change become a new variable and their relationship with other variables can be examined. Growth curve models represent a potential improvement in that they allow for the examination of change at the individual or family level. They are limited, however, in that they represent this change with a single variable that is measured by the slope of the particular line fit to the data in use. For example, the slope identifies those families whose trend over time is upward as opposed to those whose trend over time is downwards, but this is not a fine enough differentiation to be useful.

One possible solution to the dilemmas presented by these methods is the use of configural frequency analysis (CFA; von Eye, 1990). Configural frequency analysis is a statistical procedure that analyzes subject data according to their configurations among a group of variables (e.g., high on the first, low on the second, midrange on third versus a different profile for a different person). The variables used can be distinct although conceptually related or they may be the same variable measured at different time points.

To use the procedure the researcher begins by dividing each variable into discrete categories. Each family or individual is then identified by its categorical position on that variable. An observational assessment for family adaptability may be taken at two time points. Using the CFA program, the number of families representing a number of possible configurations would be studied. Statistically, configurations that occur more often than would be expected by chance are identified and termed "types", as are configurations which occur less frequently than would be expected by chance which are termed "antitypes".

Identifying these groups is important for two reasons. Firstly, their identification allows for the detection of categories representing trajectories or relationships that are statistically significant. Secondly, after these configurations are identified they can be used as typological variables for future analyses. Certainly there are limits to CFA, including the need to categorize data before analyzing it. In addition, it may be difficult to determine when to collect the last wave of data, in order to ensure that most families have adequate time to recover from the stressor. It is also important not to err by collecting data at too many points, which would result in the creation of too many identifiable configurations. Finally and most importantly, the use of CFA requires large samples. Without a large enough sample, different types of statistical errors would result, and it is possible that the statistically significant types would account for only a small portion of the total number of subjects and that the majority of the sample would be distributed among statistically insignificant configurations. In Halverson's (2005) study of temperament, he analyzed configurations of four variables in a sample of over 3000 children. The findings yielded only four significant types and one significant antitype, into which only 40 % of the sample fit.

Werner (2013) surveyed the findings from large-scale longitudinal research studies in order to see what can be learned from them about resilience. These longitudinal studies were included in her survey because they all had a core group of at least 100 participants who continued to return at each of the designated time periods for measurement. Some studies maintained over 1000 participants over time. The children were assessed at each time period with multiple and age-appropriate measures and included low-risk comparison groups. The attrition rate was low and several critical time periods were chosen for investigation.

The results were analyzed using several different methods. Since resilience is not an all-or-nothing phenomenon, nor is it a trait like "invulnerability" but rather an abstraction which needs to be operationalized in order to be evaluated empirically, process models can provide an effective method of analysis.

Longitudinal Resilience Research Models

Process models underscore the view that a specified set of factors leads to a particular developmental course and outcome. The goal of these models is to help guide the study of development pathways which lead to more and less adaptive outcomes. In these statistical analyses, protective factors are defined as those variables which reduced the deleterious impact of a stressor while having a negligible association with adaptive behavior in children who were experiencing low risk, whereas compensatory factors are those factors which were identified as having a "main effect", with the factor being investigated predicting greater psychological adjustment regardless of whether the individuals experienced risk (Downey & Walker, 1992).

Mediational models address questions of how and why certain risk conditions lead to maladaptive outcomes. Mediators are the variables that affect the main independent variables and the predicted outcome variables. For example, in an empirical study investigating the relationship between maternal depression (independent variable) and child functioning at age 4 (outcome variable), mediators are those additional variables which partially explain how and why the risk factor leads to maladaptive outcomes. In other words, the basic purpose of mediational research is to delineate the processes which account for the associations between a particular risk factor, or set of risk factors, and behavioral outcomes.

Rather than searching for a single causal mechanism that explains the impact of a single risk factor, the assumption is that there are multiple causal mechanisms which may be operating in tandem. So in the example of maternaldepression, the goal would be to describe the mechanisms by which the depression leads to child behavior problems. It is important in these models to specify what is being studied; otherwise the research can become too broad and uninformative. For example, Cummings and Davies (1994, 1999) studied the effects of maternal depression on child behavior, but instead of investigating biological, genetic, and behavior variables, they narrowed the scope of their model to address interpersonal mechanisms that mediate associations between parental depression and children's adaptive functioning. Field and colleagues (1994, 2006) and Cohn and Tronick (1989) also looked at mediational processes involved in the pathway from parental depression to child maladaptive behavior and developed a multi-level model which addresses sequelae to parental depression including symptomotology, parenting practices, attachment quality, and marital conflict, which all feed into the child's own biological and temperamental characteristics. These relationships also develop and change dynamically over time, culminating in the child's adjustment. Thus, parental depression is perceived as being associated with family characteristics in complex and reciprocal ways.

Multiple mediators are incorporated into these theoretical models, reflecting the array of the pathways of influence on child behavior. Thus, although single mediator models may be useful as exploratory tools in identifying which variables can be of potential significance in complex family processes, it is important to embed these variables in a more comprehensive ecological context of development. For example, single mediator studies of depression discovered that marital discord was a mediator of parental depression, but did not explain the fact that marital discord in a family with depressive symptomotogy affects other aspects of the depression in the household system, and therefore the unitary variable was of limited value in understanding the interrelatedness of various factors in models of depression (Downey & Coyne, 1990).

In order to understand the more complex chain of influence within the family system, mediational models which integrate direct and indirect pathways (Davies & Windle, 1997) are being employed more frequently to investigate the complex relationship between parental depression and marital discord and the manner in which these pathways lead to adaptation and maladaptation in the child. Even within a single conceptual model, key mediating constructs may not be independent and may be multi-determined. Thus, different familial processes may each affect children's specific processes of adaptation to family events. For example, children's attributions of responsibility for parental functioning may be the reason for adjustment problems, rather than parental discord. It may be that children's over-responsibility for others' distress mediates the effects of family discord on their adjustment, even without considering reactions to parental depression. On the other hand, parental depression may also influence children's perceptions of personal responsibility for their parents' functioning. As a result of uncertainty about the pathway of influence, it is necessary to recognize the complex and transactional nature of causality which changes over time, pointing to the need to study children's adaptive behavior over time. The testing of process models of differential risk for different groups is a necessarily complex procedure in the case of an inferential concept such as resilience.

Applications of Resilience Research

Although improvements in statistical methodology are still needed, investigating the factors which contribute to resilience in families has important ramifications for clinical work. The movement towards strengths-based approaches in family therapy recognizes resilience as a key factor in family functioning over time (Walsh, 2011). Moreover, resilient families may not always exhibit characteristics associated with strong families. By definition resilient families have faced potentially overwhelming stressors and have managed to survive and sometimes to thrive. A one-time assessment made in a clinical context may make it appear that such a family is troubled (as in fact it may be), but this does not take into account the progress the family has made over time, nor does it factor in the possibility that the moment at which the family was assessed may have been a low point in their journey toward healthier functioning. Whether a family is overcoming difficult odds in progressing towards a better level of functioning can only be seen through multiple assessments occurring over time.

Clinical research that helps to ascertain factors associated with families who show resilient trends can aid therapists in knowing how best to intervene with families they see in therapy. The research model may provide a useful way to identify the most resilient families and can shed light on what contributes to their ability to be resilient. Walsh has identified a framework for understanding the constructs in family wellbeing. She suggested three broad categories to be studied in order to assess a family's resilience: belief system (what sense the family makes of adversity), organizational patterns (connectedness, flexibility and resources) and communication processes (clarity, emotional expressiveness and problem solving). Researchers employing the model presented here may find these qualities a good starting place to begin their investigations. As process research is less concerned with the final outcomes of therapy and more with the factors that contribute to change, this approach has added benefits, in that it can look at different pathways within the same proposed model, thus examining various associations among experimental variables.

Although understanding the nature of family resilience remains a challenging prospect, its potential payoff is considerable. Learning more about the process by which families in unique environments cope and thrive in the face of stress will help in designing interventions that can be truly effective, particularly for families with young children. In order to uncover process, it is necessary to conduct longitudinal research sensitive to both the context of the family and the unique stressor/s under consideration. The focus should be on identifying differing trajectories commonly traversed by families in the face of crisis and thus identifying the factors which shape those trajectories.

Implications for Intervention

Resilience focuses on strengths rather than on deficits, and assumes that families have the ability not only to survive difficult times, but perhaps even to thrive as they emerge from those experiences. It is an innately appealing concept full of hope and optimism. Resilience tells the story of families who have overcome challenging circumstances to emerge as survivors. It dovetails with approaches to therapy focused on helping families identify strengths as a means of accessing more satisfying ways of functioning. The other side of resilience is about struggles, challenges and risks. It can be conceptualized as a process families engage in when beset by adversity. From this perspective, families do not emerge from their difficulties unscathed. Resilient families are not necessarily those who emerge from crises as bright and shining stars – they are those who struggle well (Walsh, 2010). Theirs is a story of survival in the face of overwhelming odds. Therapy may be less concerned with helping them discover hidden strengths and more with allowing them to process and find meaning in their experiences. An understanding of resilience encompasses both these perspectives. Therapists who adopt a resilience-minded approach need to recognize both the inherent strengths and the challenging struggles of their clients.

Among the strengths identified in the study of family resilience are (1) open communication, (2) good conflict resolution skills, (3) shared time together and (4) a balance between closeness and togetherness (Hampson & Beavers, 1996), all of which can be highlighted in therapy, by searching for ways in which families operated well instead of discovering why they were dysfunctional. Research in resilience reveals strengths, rather than pathology, and has become an important movement in family therapy over the past several decades. Strengths-oriented approaches have become dominant models, and family strengths are frequently equated with resilience (see Hawley, 2013).

Research has stressed the balance of risk and protective mechanisms experienced by individual children and more recently in families as well. Researchers generally agree that there is an interactive effect among risk mechanisms and that exposure to multiple risk factors exponentially increases the probability of maladaptive outcomes. For example, a child with a physical disability who lives in poverty and whose family environment is marked by conflict and instability will be at greater risk that a child with the same disability living in a stable family and economic environment. The effects of risk mechanisms are mediated by protective mechanisms. The basic thesis of this approach suggests that children with strong protective mechanisms are more likely to access them in order to buffer the effects of risk mechanisms and thus more likely to be resilient. Resilience in a family can be conceptualized as a function of how the family members interact and collectively apply their capabilities and definitions of the situation to a given set of stressors. Thus, resilience is conceptualized as an outcome of family functioning. Walsh (2010) adds that resilience is "adaptational pathways over time" (p. 155), spanning events leading up to the crisis event through eventual family reorganization. These paths are influenced by normative events that occur in the course of the family's development but also by individual, familial, social and cultural environmental responses to the stressor (Walsh, 2003). The interplay of all these contexts results in a unique path of resilience for each family.

Translational research, which aims to apply findings generated in the laboratory setting to human behavior in naturalistic settings, or to help adopt best practices into community and clinical settings, by promoting an exchange between basic, preclinical, clinical, epidemiologic, and outcomes research, can lead to guidelines for interventions. For example, after significant associations among variables have been identified in pathways analyses, it is possible to target certain variables for intervention. Since the family of infants and young children experiencing adversity is the context in which they will be treated, it is particularly important to pay special attention to those family processes associated with better outcomes. Firstly, a shared belief system allows the family as a unit to make sense of what is happening to them and lends a sense of coherence (Antonovsky, 1987). Secondly, flexible family organization coupled with leadership can maintain a feeling of stability in the midst of disruption, resulting in connectedness, mutual support, commitment and collaboration among family members. A third process (Walsh, 2006) is family communication. Higher resilience in families is associated with clear communication, including the ability to process and discuss difficult topics. Open expression of emotion is encouraged in the context of discussions during which family members problem solve, make decisions and are able to resolve conflicts and learn from previous decisions that did not work as expected.

Walsh's model provides a useful framework for observing how families deal with challenges over time, before, during and after crises. Because of the complex interaction of risk and protective mechanisms and developmental, social and cultural contexts, there is no formula that concisely measures resilience in families. However, by observing the family belief system, flexibility, connectedness, mobilization of resources and communication patterns as they are manifest over time, a picture emerges of how resilient a given family is when faced with adversity. Family resilience is an emerging concept upon which interventions in infant and early childhood mental health can be predicated. Its hopeful approach and positive orientation are valuable for therapists seeking to help families and their members who are mired in difficulties. Yet there is a complexity to resilience that goes beyond a search for strengths.

Family resilience involves a multifaceted web of risk and protective mechanisms; social, cultural and developmental contexts; and perceptions of adversity. The most resilient families often may not appear to be resilient at all. In some cases they are families who in spite of incredible odds have managed to stay intact. They may be limping along and their strengths may not be readily apparent. This underscores one of the challenges professionals face in applying resilience to families. The variety of ways in which the term is used complicates meaningful discussions which attempt to refine family resilience as a concept. Some perceive resilience as the strengths possessed by all families to various degrees. For others, resilience in families is the exception instead of the rule. Some conceptualize resilience as a quality possessed by families, while others see it as a developmental pathway that can only be observed over time. Continued dialogue aimed at achieving greater definitional clarity would benefit all those who utilize resilience as a concept in their work with families.

In spite of these differing perceptions of resilience, it is a vital lens through which all therapists can view families, and was included in this book on infant mental health for precisely that reason. Before deciding on a particular intervention strategy, a therapist working with a family overwhelmed by adversity should bear in mind that, from a resilience-based perspective, we are searching for strengths which may not be immediately apparent. Helping families balance risk and protective mechanisms and become adaptive, stay connected, utilize their resources, maintain routines and develop shared positive perspectives in the midst of troubles is consistent with almost all therapeutic approaches. Therapists can serve as conduits that allow families in adversity to move forward to new and more satisfying ways of functioning.

References

Alvord, M. K., & Grados, J. J. (2005). Enhancing resilience in children: A proactive approach. *Professional Psychology: Research and Practice, 36*(3), 238–245.

Antonovsky, A. (1987). *Unraveling the mystery of health: How people manage stress and stay well.* New York: Jossey-Bass.

Bayat, M. (2007). Evidence of resilience in families of children with autism. *Journal of Intellectual Disability Research, 51*(9), 702–714.

Benzies, K., & Mychasiuk, R. (2009). Fostering family resiliency: A review of the key protective factors. *Child & Family Social Work, 14*(1), 103–114.

Bollen, K. A., & Curran, P. J. (2006). *Latent curve models: A structural equation perspective* (Vol. 467). New York: Wiley.

Bronfenbrenner, U. (1979). Contexts of child rearing: Problems and prospects. *American Psychologist, 34*(10), 844–850.

Bronfenbrenner, U. (1986). Ecology of the family as a context for human development: Research perspectives. *Developmental Psychology, 22*(6), 723–742.

Chapin, M. (2011). Family resilience and the fortunes of war. *Social Work in Health Care, 50*(7), 527–542.

Cheah, C. S., & Chirkov, V. (2008). Parents' personal and cultural beliefs regarding young children: A cross-cultural study of Aboriginal and Euro-Canadian mothers. *Journal of Cross-Cultural Psychology, 39*(4), 402–423.

Cicchetti, D., & Garmezy, N. (1993). Prospects and promises in the study of resilience. *Development and Psychopathology, 5*(04), 497–502.

Cohn, J. F., & Tronick, E. Z. (1989). Specificity of infants' response to mothers' affective behavior. *Journal of the American Academy of Child and Adolescent Psychiatry, 28*, 242–248.

Conger, R. D., Rueter, M. A., & Elder, G. H., Jr. (1999). Couple resilience to economic pressure. *Journal of Personality and Social Psychology, 76*(1), 54–71.

Cowan, P. A., Cowan, C. P., & Schulz, M. S. (1996). Thinking about risk and resilience in families. In T. A. Wills, E. A. Blechman, G. McNamara, M. Hetherington, & E. A. Blechman (Eds.), *Stress, coping, and resiliency in children and families* (pp. 1–38). New York: Psychology Press.

Crnic, K. A., Greenberg, M. T., Robinson, N. M., & Ragozin, A. S. (1984). Maternal stress and social support: Effects on the mother–infant relationship from birth to eighteen months. *American Journal of Orthopsychiatry, 54*, 224–235.

Crockenberg, S. B. (1981). Infant irritability, mother responsiveness, and social support influences on the security of infant-mother attachment. *Child Development, 52*(3), 857–865.

Cummings, E. M., & Davies, P. T. (1994). Maternal depression and child development. *Journal of Child Psychology and Psychiatry, 35*(1), 73–122.

Cummings, E. M., & Davies, P. T. (1999). Depressed parents and family functioning: Interpersonal effects and children's functioning and development. In T. Joiner & J. Coyne (Eds.), *The interactional nature of depression: Advances in interpersonal approaches* (pp. 299–327). Washington, DC: American Psychological Association.

Davies, P. T., & Windle, M. (1997). Gender-specific pathways between maternal depressive symptoms, family discord, and adolescent adjustment. *Developmental Psychology, 33*(4), 657–668.

De Haan, L., Hawley, D. R., & Deal, J. E. (2002). Operationalizing family resilience: A methodological strategy. *American Journal of Family Therapy, 30*(4), 275–291.

Downey, G., & Coyne, J. C. (1990). Children of depressed parents: An integrative review. *Psychological Bulletin, 108*(1), 50–76.

Downey, G., & Walker, E. (1992). Distinguishing family-level and child-level influences on the development of depression and aggression in children at risk. *Development and Psychopathology, 4*(1), 81–95.

Fagan, J., Palkovitz, R., Roy, K., & Farrie, D. (2009). Pathways to paternal engagement: Longitudinal effects of risk and resilience on nonresident fathers. *Developmental Psychology, 45*(5), 1389–1405.

Falk, R. F., & Miller, N. (1991). A soft models approach to family transitions. In P. A. Cowan & M. Hatherington (Eds.), *Family transitions* (pp. 273–301). Hillsdale, NJ: Lawrence Erlbaum Associates.

Field, T. (1994). The effects of mother's physical and emotional unavailability on emotion regulation. *Monographs of the Society for Research in Child Development, 59*(2–3), 208–227.

Field, T., Diego, M., & Hernandez-Reif, M. (2006). Prenatal depression effects on the fetus and newborn: A review. *Infant Behavior and Development, 29*(3), 445–455.

Garmezy, N. (1995). Development and adaptation: The contributions of the MacArthur Foundation and William Bevan. In F. Kessel (Ed.) (1994). *Psychology, science, and human affairs: Essays in honor of William Bevan* (pp. 109–124). Boulder, CO: Westview Press.

Ghosh-Ippen, C., Harris, W. W., Van Horn, P., & Lieberman, A. F. (2011). Traumatic and stressful events in early childhood: Can treatment help those at highest risk? *Child Abuse & Neglect, 35*(7), 504–513.

Greef, A. P., & Ritman, I. N. (2005). Individual characteristics associated with resilience in single-parent families. *Psychological Reports, 96*(1), 36–42.

Halverson, C. F. (2005). Personality in children. *Merrill-Palmer Quarterly, 51*(3), 254–257.

Hampson, R. B., & Beavers, W. R. (1996). Measuring family therapy outcome in a clinical setting: Families that do better or do worse in therapy. *Family Process, 35*(3), 347–361.

Hawley, D. R. (2013). The ramifications for clinical practice of a focus on family resilience. In D. S. Becvar (Ed.), *Handbook of family resilience* (pp. 31–49). New York: Springer.

Hawley, D. R., & DeHaan, L. (1996). Toward a definition of family resilience: Integrating life-span and family perspectives. *Family Process, 35*(3), 283–298.

Hill, R. (1949). *Families under stress*. Westport, CT: Greenwood.

Hill, R. (1971). *Families under stress*. Westport, CT: Greenwood. (Original work published in 1949).

Kaplan, H. B. (2002). Toward an understanding of resilience. In M. D. Glantz & J. L. Johnson (Eds.), *Resilience and development* (pp. 17–83). New York: Springer.

Karney, B. R., & Bradbury, T. N. (1995). Assessing longitudinal change in marriage: An introduction to the analysis of growth curves. *Journal of Marriage and the Family, 57*(4), 1091–1108.

Kumpfer, K. L. (2002). Factors and processes contributing to resilience. In M. D. Glantz & J. L. Johnson (Eds.), *Resilience and development* (pp. 179–224). New York: Springer.

Landau, J., & Saul, J. (2004). Facilitating family and community resilience in response to major disaster. In F. Walsh & M. McGoldrick (Eds.), *Living beyond loss* (pp. 285–309). New York: Norton.

Legge, K. (2013). *Parental self-compassion, attributions of child behaviour and sensitive responding*. Unpublished doctoral dissertation, University of Exeter.

Lester, B. M., Tronick, E. Z., LaGasse, L., Seifer, R., Bauer, C. R., Shankaran, S., et al. (2002). The maternal lifestyle study: Effects of substance exposure during pregnancy on neurodevelopmental outcome in 1-month-old infants. *Pediatrics, 110*, 1182–1192.

Lietz, C. A., & Strength, M. (2011). Stories of successful reunification: A narrative study of family resilience in child welfare. *Families in Society, 92*(2), 203–210.

Ludbrook, J. (2002). Statistical techniques for comparing measurers and methods of measurement: A critical review. *Clinical and Experimental Pharmacology and Physiology, 29*(7), 527–536.

Luthar, S. S. (2006). Resilience in development: A synthesis of research across five decades. In D. Cicchetti & D. J. Cohen (Eds.), *Developmental psychopathology, Vol 3: Risk, disorder, and adaptation* (2nd ed., pp. 739–795). Hoboken, NJ: Wiley.

Luthar, S. S., & Zelazo, L. B. (2003). Research on resilience: An integrative review. In S. Luthar (Ed.), *Resilience and vulnerability: Adaptation in the context of childhood adversities* (pp. 510–549). New York: Cambridge University Press.

Masten, A. S. (1994). Resilience in individual development: Successful adaptation despite risk and adversity. In M. C. Wang & E. W. Gordon (Eds.), *Educational resilience in inner-city America: Challenges and prospects* (pp. 3–25). Hillsdale, NJ: Lawrence Erlbaum Associates, Inc.

Masten, A. S. (2001). Ordinary magic: Resilience processes in development. *American Psychologist, 56*(3), 227–238.

Masten, A. S. (2011). Resilience in children threatened by extreme adversity: Frameworks for research, practice, and translational synergy. *Development and Psychopathology, 23*(2), 493–506.

Masten, A. S. (2013). Risk and resilience in development. *Oxford handbook of developmental psychology, 2*, 579–607.

Masten, A. S. A., Hubbard, J., Gest, S. D. S., Tellegen, A. A., Garmezy, N. N., & Ramirez, M. M. (1999). Competence in the context of adversity: Pathways to resilience and maladaptation from childhood to late adolescence. *Development and Psychopathology, 11*, 143–169.

Masten, A. S., & Coatsworth, J. D. (1998). The development of competence in favorable and unfavorable environments: Lessons from research on successful children. *American Psychologist, 53*(2), 205–220.

Masten, A. S., Best, K. M., & Garmezy, N. (1990). Resilience and development: Contributions from the study of children who overcome adversity. *Development and Psychopathology, 2*(4), 425–444.

McArdle, J. J., & Epstein, D. (1987). Latent growth curves within developmental structural equation models. *Child Development, 58*(1), 110–133.

McCubbin, H. I., & Patterson, J. (1983). The family stress process: The double ABCX model of adjustment and adaptation. In H. I. McCubbin, M. B. Sussman, & J. M. Patterson (Eds.), *Social stress and the family: Advances and developments in family's stress theory and research* (pp. 7–38). New York: Haworth.

McCubbin, H. I., McCubbin, M. A., Thompson, A. I., Sae-Young, H., & Allen, C. T. (1997). Families under stress: What makes them resilient. *Journal of Family and Consumer Sciences, 89*(3), 2–11.

McCubbin, M. A., & McCubbin, H. I. (1993). Families coping with illness: the resiliency model of family stress, adjustment, and adaptation. In C. B. Danielson, B. Hamel-Bissell, & P. Winstead-Fry. *Families, Health, and Illness*, (pp. 21–63). Maryland Heights, MO: Mosby Publishing.

Patterson, J. M. (1988). Families experiencing stress: I. The family adjustment and adaptation response model: II. Applying the FAAR Model to health-related issues for intervention and research. *Family Systems Medicine, 6*(2), 202–237.

Patterson, J. M. (2002). Integrating family resilience and family stress theory. *Journal of Marriage and Family, 64*(2), 349–360.

Peterson, S. M., & Yates, T. M. (2013). Early childhood relationships and the roots of resilience. *Resilience*, (pp. 11–17). In http://www.child-encyclopedia.com/

Rajendran, K. (2008). Impact of relationship with the caregiver and positive future expectations on behavioral and emotional resilience in adolescents in child welfare. Doctoral dissertation, State University of New York, Albany.

Rende, R., & Plomin, R. (1993). Families at risk for psychopathology: Who becomes affected and why? *Development and Psychopathology, 5*(04), 529–540.

Rodriguez, H., Trainor, J., & Quarantelli, E. L. (2006). Rising to the challenges of a catastrophe: The emergent and prosocial behavior following Hurricane Katrina. *The Annals of the American Academy of Political and Social Science, 604*(1), 82–101.

Rutter, M. (2012). Resilience as a dynamic concept. *Development and Psychopathology, 24*(02), 335–344.

Shonkoff, J. P., Garner, A. S., Siegel, B. S., Dobbins, M. I., Earls, M. F., McGuinn, L., ... & Wood, D. L. (2012). The lifelong effects of early childhood adversity and toxic stress. *Pediatrics, 129*(1), e232–e246.

Simon, J. B., Murphy, J. J., & Smith, S. M. (2005). Understanding and fostering family resilience. *The Family Journal, 13*(4), 427–436.

Stern, D. N. (2009). *The first relationship: Infant and mother*. Cambridge, MA: Harvard University Press.

Thompson, E. A., McCubbin, H. I., Thompson, A. I., & Elver, K. M. (1995). Vulnerability and resiliency in Native Hawaiian families under stress. *Resiliency in Ethnic Minority Families, 1*, 115–131.

Van Montfort, K., Oud, J. H. L., & Satorra, A. (2010). *Longitudinal research with latent variables*. Berlin: Springer.

Von Eye, A. (1990). *Introduction to configural frequency analysis: The search for types and antitypes in cross-classifications*. New York: Cambridge University Press.

Walsh, F. (2002). A family resilience framework: Innovative practice applications. *Family Relations, 51*(2), 130–137.

Walsh, F. (2003). Family resilience: A framework for clinical practice. *Family Process, 42*(1), 1–18.

Walsh, F. (2006). *Strengthening family resilience*. New York: Guilford Press.

Walsh, F. (2010). A family resilience framework for clinical practice: Integrating developmental theory and systemic perspectives. In W. Borden, W. (Ed.), (2010) *Reshaping theory in contemporary social work: Toward a critical pluralism in clinical practice* (pp. 146–176). New York, NY: Columbia University Press.

Walsh, F. (Ed.). (2011). *Normal family processes: Growing diversity and complexity*. New York, NY: Guilford Press.

Walsh, F. (2012). Facilitating family resilience: Relational resources for positive youth development in conditions of adversity. In M. Ungar (Ed.), *The social ecology of resilience* (pp. 173–185). New York: Springer.

Walsh, F. (2013). Community-based practice applications of a family resilience framework. In *Handbook of family resilience* (pp. 65–82). New York: Springer.

Werner, E. E. (2013). What can we learn about resilience from large-scale longitudinal studies? In D. S. Becvar (Ed.), *Handbook of resilience in children* (pp. 87–102). New York: Springer.

Werner, E. E., & Smith, R. S. (1992). *Overcoming the odds: High risk children from birth to adulthood*. Ithaca, NY: Cornell University Press.

Wu, L. L., & Thomson, E. (2001). Race differences in family experience and early sexual initiation: Dynamic models of family structure and family change. *Journal of Marriage and Family, 63*(3), 682–696.

Wyman, P. A., Cowen, E. L., Work, W. C., Raoof, A., Gribble, P. A., Parker, G. R., et al. (1992). Interviews with children who experienced major life stress: Family and child attributes that predict resilient outcomes. *Journal of the American Academy of Child & Adolescent Psychiatry, 31*(5), 904–910.

Chapter 8
Theoretical Bases of Intervention in Infant and Early Childhood Mental Health

Introduction

This chapter will present a number of intervention theories which recognize the importance of understanding patterns of adaptation throughout child development and include identifying factors that protect the individual against negative outcomes, as well as those factors which increase vulnerability. Child variables, family influences and the ecological contexts in which development occurs are all parts of the theoretical perspectives covered in this chapter.

In Chap. 1, in which the conceptualization of the field of infant mental health was discussed, it was stressed that clinicians in the field are engaged in different issues than those currently explored by researchers in clinical psychology and psychiatry. In the field of infant mental health, identification of the dynamic processes underlying development is studied, providing the theoretical bases for intervention. Since infant mental health is viewed from a developmental perspective, it is better to intervene sooner rather than later, and the strong theoretical foundations presented here affirm that early intervention is a way to decrease both the prevalence of problems and their severity.

From this perspective, the complex determinants of infant mental health focus on the issues of child temperament, attachment and emotional security, parental depression, and marital adjustment, as well as on the immediate environment, including ethnicity, culture and other demographic factors, all of which should be considered when establishing an intervention program (Shonkoff & Philips, 2000). In keeping with the themes of this book, considerable emphasis is placed on family process and the family/social context in order to understand and predict the onset, maintenance and developmental course of a young child's problems. What may be considered a problem in one community may be acceptable in another. Behavior that concerns families with unlimited resources might be overlooked by families struggling to meet basic needs, and parental fears and worries may also vary according to cultural context. To support this, research indicates that the views

C. Shulman, *Research and Practice in Infant and Early Childhood Mental Health*, Children's Well-Being: Indicators and Research 13,
DOI 10.1007/978-3-319-31181-4_8

adults hold regarding the appropriateness or inappropriateness of their children's behavior is a function of culture, both within and between countries (Ungar, 2008).

In order to intervene effectively, it is necessary to define the problems being addressed. In the field of infant mental health, these definitions occur on multiple levels, sometimes resulting in the fragmentation of intervention recommendations. The goal of this chapter is to present the general theoretical underpinnings which are at the base of intervention programs for young children and their families. The information gathered through the assessment process is interpreted and then becomes the cornerstone of the treatment program for the individual child. Each customized treatment program should be informed by research and theoretical perspectives. Academic research has targeted several prospective domains which are pertinent to research and intervention in infant mental health (Hoagwood & Olin, 2002; Raju, Higgins, Stark, & Leveno, 2006). For example, NIH recommends conducting research among high-risk populations and treating risk factors as an inherent focus of assessment and intervention in infant mental health studies. Secondly, in order to optimize research applicability, NIH suggests interdisciplinary research and stresses professional collaboration (Gone, 2004; United States Department of Health and Human Services, n.d.), both of which will be considered in the theoretical treatment models delineated below.

Psychodynamic Theory

The psychodynamic theory of mental health emphasizes the systematic study of psychological forces underlying human behavior, feelings and emotions and how these may relate to early childhood experience. Specifically, psychodynamic psychology refers to the psychological stream developed by Sigmund Freud (1955) which was the basis for intervention strategies based on his understanding of conscious and unconscious bases of human behavior. His daughter, Anna Freud, based her work with young children on the assumptions of psychodynamic theory with necessary adaptations for young children who cannot use some of the verbal techniques central to psychodynamic interventions with adults. Limited use of language and concrete thinking made the use of widespread techniques, such as free association, inappropriate for young children, although she was interested in accessing the same internal/implicit processes which reflected unresolved areas of conflict (Freud, 1988).

Dynamic interventions with children typically involve several goals. The therapist observes the child's play with representative objects and accompanies this play with a running commentary, enabling the child to put feelings into words. For example, if a 3-year-old plays with puppets and one puppet systematically hits another, the therapist can wonder aloud if the first puppet is mad at the second. The child's response to the therapist's clarification allows the therapist to understand if this interpretation was appropriate or not. If the therapist is able to correctly translate the child's actions into words and the child accepts this language, the child will shift to another level of play or to different content. If, however, the therapist misconstrues the meaning behind the child's play scenario, the feelings will remain unresolved or unidentified and the child will continue with similar play themes. An additional goal addresses unresolved core emotional conflicts and helps the child in settling these. For example, in a comparable situation where a young child has one doll hitting another and the second doll acts frightened, the therapist might infer that the child is occupied with the relationship between aggression and fear. If the child then makes the "frightened" doll leave the game, it might appear that the child sees withdrawal as the solution to the conflict. In this situation, the therapist might help the child solve the conflict by understanding other possible responses to aggression or fear.

Another core premise of psychodynamic theory is that parents often impart their own unresolved conflicts to their children. This intergenerational transmission is also a focal point for the therapist, who will try to assist the parents in supporting their child's mental health and refraining from undermining his or her social and emotional development. A clinician attempts to understand the parenting style in which the child is raised and may determine that the parents are too permissive or too strict, that they are abusive or neglectful, or that they unduly draw the child into their conflicts. Treatment goals would include helping the parents to change these behavior patterns. In addition to parenting styles, parental perceptions of their children were found to shape their relationships. Selma Fraiberg (1980, 1987) conceptualized these parental perceptions as stemming from their own early childhood experiences and formulated a therapeutic intervention called parent-infant psychotherapy. The goal was to help parents gain insight into the therapeutic process and to resolve their internal conflicts which prevented them from interacting with their child in a manner that fostered optimal development. This theory complements the attachment model and affects the manner in which the field of infant mental health is formulated today, although it does not take the infant's physiological and constitutional qualities into consideration nor the caregivers' perceptions of family dynamics.

Dynamic approaches, e.g. play and other expressive therapies, cannot reach children who are not yet sufficiently verbal, or who do not engage in symbolic play or in other methods of nonverbal communication of their inner states. Thus very young children, or older children with significant developmental or emotional challenges which interfere with age appropriate use of language and abstract thinking, will not be able to make use of the more traditional techniques integral to psychodynamic theory. Dynamic therapy focuses on the symbolic representation of feelings and conflicts and does not offer techniques for addressing lower developmental and functional levels. However, this may still be useful for parents striving to understand their child and the parent–child relationship.

The psychodynamic school addresses manifest problems in the child and/or the parent and views the therapeutic process as a response to the ever-changing interaction between the inner world of the individual and external demands. Although theoretically it should be possible to abstract intergenerational transmission of pathology and other processes which address risk factors in mental health, risk does not seem to be a focus of this intervention technique. The psychodynamic therapist undergoes intensive and strict training and continues to receive supervision while conducting therapy. Typically, part of the therapeutic process involves transference, the unconscious redirection of feelings from one person to another. In psychodynamic theory, transference is considered helpful to the therapist in understanding the patient's feelings. It is not a multidisciplinary, integrative or collaborative model of intervention, focusing instead on the importance of therapeutic intervention for the individual.

Attachment-Based Theory

Attachment-based therapies include a group of techniques which regard attachment theory as the base for understanding the presenting problems and for intervention. As presented in previous chapters, attachment theory was originally espoused by John Bowlby (1956, 1969, 1988) and has become a major scientific theory of social and emotional development and in infant and early childhood mental health. Attachment theory was an outgrowth of psychodynamic theory, in which the relationship between the therapist and the patient becomes an integral part of the therapeutic process. An additional level of therapeutic relationship involves the therapist who nurtures the parent so that he can in turn nurture his child. These parallel processes between therapist-parent and parent–child are part of the substance of relationships in the attachment model. Although the theory stands on its own, it has also been absorbed by several other theories, such as relational theory, described below. Bowlby was more interested in the clinical characterization of the quality of attachment and its implications than in converting the theory into intervention strategies. In addition, the term "attachment" as applied by practitioners is often used quite broadly and could be misleading as a model for intervention.

Attachment theory is based on the notion that the caregiver-infant relationship is the most important element in communicating to the young child what others expect of him and what he can expect of others. As a result, all intervention strategies based on attachment principles regard the fostering of relationships between infants, toddlers and young children and their caregivers as the primary goal of infant mental health interventions. Concomitantly, supporting nurturing relationships between young children and their caregivers has evolved into a primary focus of intervention as well as a means of intervention.

Infant mental health programs based on the attachment model posit that the most essential goal of intervention is to promote secure attachments between infants and their caregivers. Many studies suggest that early attachment experiences are important contributors to later child outcomes (Berlin, Appleyard, & Dodge, 2011; Sroufe, Carlson, Levy, & Egeland, 1999) and research has documented the benefits of attachment-oriented interventions. One of the most useful aspects of this line of research is to identify the parental variables which enhance the relationship. Specifically, it has been found that developing children need warm, supportive and responsive parents in order to establish a secureattachmentrelationship with their caregivers (Bowlby, 1988), including caregivers in child care settings (Rolfe, 2004).

Responsive parenting begins immediately after birth with the parents' ability to respond to their child's signals and soothing the infant, and continues as the parents establish a reciprocal interchange where responding becomes the stimulus to which the child reacts. This responsiveness on the part of the parent is likely to have a central impact on the quality of the parent–child relationship. When children are in need they seek out their caregivers, expecting them to attend to their needs. If the caregiver typically does not respond, the child may begin to perceive the social world as unsupportive, unsympathetic and insensitive, which may influence his subsequent relationships. The infant-caregiver relationship is perceived to be so powerful that it can shape the child's development of his self-concept (Stern & Elias, 2007), guide his behavior in other relationships throughout life (Berlin, Cassidy, & Appleyard, 2008) and determine his or her overall mental health (Lieberman & van Horn, 2011). Parent behaviors in the context of their interactions with their children have a major influence on child outcomes. For example, a balance of parental warmth and limit setting is strongly related to prosocial behavior (Hastings, McShane, Parker, & Ladha, 2007).

Edward Tronick's mutual regulation model and dyadic expansion of states of consciousness is an attachment-based theory which evolved from his extensive infant-parent research. Tronick developed the key concepts of mutual regulation and dyadically-expanded states of consciousness, where self- and interactive regulation operate optimally within open, dynamic systems. These dynamic systems function in the same way as any open biological system operates, where paradoxically, incorporating and integrating ever-increasing amounts of meaningful information allows the organism to reach more advanced coherent states (Tronick & Beeghly, 2011).

As more information is integrated, the system becomes more complex and more organized. Successful maturation of the differing states of arousal may be conceptualized as growth which allows more interpretation of information, which then increases and expands the complexity and coherence of the organization and the structure of these states of consciousness. Tronick proposed three principles which are involved in expanding the coherence, complexity and organization of the organism and which form the foundation of intervention strategies. Firstly, by interacting and communicating with people, the infant is exposed to progressively more and more complex stimulation in an ever growing reciprocal relationship requiring coherence predicated on organization. Secondly, as children grow and have more control over their motor functions and can cognitively understand how objects and people around them behave, they begin to act upon objects and understand the consequences of their actions. Finally, Tronick claimed that the young child will begin to engage with others only when his or her own sense of self begins to emerge. According to Tronick, the interaction of these factors involving relationships, development and sense of self is pivotal to the continued development of a healthy, open and self-organizing system.

Most intervention programs based on attachment theory strive to improve parenting behaviors and parent–child interactions, thus directly improving infant developmental and behavioral outcomes. Attachment-based infant and early childhood mental health interventions target the parent–child dyad in an attempt to facilitate more positive caregiver-infant interactions, strengthening the relationship overall, so that parents and caregivers can become more emotionally available, more contingently responsive and more nurturing to their children. With the support of the mental health practitioner, caregivers can increase the attention they give to the child in need and find effective ways of comforting the child during times of distress. In the attachment model of infant mental health, the effects of a secure attachment include better child outcomes and adaptive behaviors, with the securely attached child having richer language and more curiosity by first grade than the insecurely attached child. Thus the positive results of nurturing and supporting the parent can be perceived in domains of child development.

Intervention approaches based on attachment theory see the quality of relationship as a risk factor for mental health problems and as such they address aspects which can affect the parent–child relationship. Identifiable variables which have an impact on the quality of the dyadic relationship include child variables (e.g., temperament), parent variables (e.g., parental mental health status) and environmental variables (e.g., poverty, exposure to violence). In addition, there are several clinical applications based on attachment theory whose outcomes have been empirically investigated and which will be presented in Chap. 10.

Developmental Theories of Infant Mental Health

Several theories incorporate psychodynamic constructs and attachment theory, while broadening the context for understanding the variables to be considered in establishing an intervention program. By incorporating a developmental framework and including models of development as part of the foundation of infant mental health, it is possible to describe the process of development itself, including genetic and biological dispositions and environmental influences. These models describe individual differences in the ways that infants and children respond to sensory stimulation and plan motor activities, and include Sameroff's transactional model, Ayres' sensory motor integration model and Brazelton's emphasis on individual differences in behavior and development. These individuals and others were seminal in furthering developmentally-based treatment in the field of infant mental health. By adding the achievement of developmental milestones as part of the infant mental health paradigm, these theoreticians helped to shape the manner in which infant mental health is conceptualized today.

Sameroff: Transactional Model

As researchers search for the complexities in a multi-faceted model, a parallel process is occurring in the clinical arena, supported by clinical research examining causal factors leading to better or worse child outcomes. One developmental theory to arise from this movement is the transactional model (Sameroff, 1975, 2009, 2010), which provides a paradigm for child development across academic, research and clinical communities (Sameroff & Fiese, 2000). Arnold Sameroff's longitudinal research dismantles any remaining notion that a single individual or environmental factor has major consequences for developmental outcomes. His perspective maintains that no one factor is causal; rather, the accumulation of a variety of risk factors, independent of their specific qualities, determines influence (Sameroff, 2010). Sameroff's transactional model is now being applied in research endeavors that influence public health and policy (Halfon, 2014). This research perspective supports the need for clinical conceptual frameworks that can incorporate multiple variables for all team members to use as a common theoretical base, so that no single discipline will be the only lens through which a child's distress signals will be evaluated and understood. A premise of multiple causalities sets the stage for more complex clinical models.

The underlying assumptions in Sameroff's theory are necessary for the successful implementation of interventions that support child development and they reflect the interface between developmental and environmental factors without surrendering attention to the individual. According to Sameroff, child development has multiple contributors at multiple levels, and one goal of research should be to identify these contributors and to investigate the manner in which they are linked. Development occurs within a context and at each developmental level the child is capable of understanding and reflecting multiple processes, represented in family beliefs, thoughts, and culture. There is a consensus among researchers and clinicians regarding the assumptions that intervention processes must be targeted in relation to a particular problem for a particular child within a particular family within a particular culture.

A child's presenting behavioral and developmental problems are more likely than not to be the result of multiple variables. Usually, assessing across multiple functional domains requires a team effort rather than the isolated endeavors of a solo practitioner. Sameroff's transactional model reflects the assumptions of the neurorelational framework, which holds that multiple interconnected systems contribute to the complexities inherent in a child's and a family's behaviors. The neurorelational framework considers multiple domains in the context of multiple diagnostic categories, rather than narrowing the focus to a single causal domain.

Within the transactional model lies a complex process approach to child development, in which the child is viewed as a product of continuous, dynamic interactions between the child and the experience provided by the family and social contexts (Olson, Sameroff, Kerr, Lopez, & Wellman, 2005, p. 7). This description demonstrates the impact that the parent and child have on each other in real time and in the long term. The fact that there are multiple transactions occurring at any given time supports the premise that development is rarely the consequence of immediate causes or even previous experiences; rather, it is the result of the convergence of cumulative effects resulting from what a child brings, what a parent brings and the co-created dynamic between them.

Despite the mutual influence that the parent and the child exert on one another, a natural asymmetry exists in the proportion of the child's degree of need in relation to the parent's degree of need. It is obvious that a child needs considerably more assistance from a parent for healthy development to progress. Self- and other regulation are important vehicles through which development occurs. As development progresses, a balanced dynamic of self- and other regulation occurs through maturation, although these dynamics are subject to shifts at various points along the life cycle.

Greenspan: Developmental, Individual-Differences, Relationship-Based Model (DIR)

Stanley Greenspan's model incorporates a universal developmental perspective without compromising the individual profile, within a context which reflects the importance of the parent–child relationship. This model, sustaining multiple factors across various developmental domains while promoting an interdisciplinary perspective, brings a clinical interdisciplinary approach to older newborns and young children in infant mental health and early intervention settings. This clinical model provides a complex configuration for individual clinicians and practitioners as well as those who work in teams.

The DIR model assesses each infant or child across sensory, motor (movement and balance), affective (emotional) language and cognitive systems (Weider & Greenspan, 2005). Assessments are used to prioritize the functional aspects of a child's behavior, the parents' interpersonal style and the functional interactions between them. Treatment focuses on changing their existing interactions through coaching and modeling. Relational interpersonal development is assessed across functional emotional milestones that serve as the basis for Axis V in the Zero to Three diagnostic system (2005). This is a functional approach which does not rely solely on the set parameters provided by the test variables but allows evidence from multiple sources, specifically focusing on observable behaviors. This theoretical approach is another advanced and complex clinical model that bridges infant mental health (socioemotional) and early intervention (sensory motor, speech language and cognitive domains), and creates an integrated model of theoretical and intervention principles.

The DIR clinical perspective has a strong play-based component, and the emotional relationship between the child and the parent/s exhibited through naturalistic interactions is at the core of the assessment, diagnosis and intervention. Parents are always included in the process and are given as much information as they can assimilate in order to function as the healing agents for their child. DIR emerged from work with low-income families, but due to its inherent holistic approach it has attracted families whose children have developmental and learning delays. In fact DIR can be seen as applicable to all healthy and at-risk children.

Bagnato: Convergent Model

Coming from a psychoeducational perspective, Bagnato, Neisworth and Munson (1997) applied the interdisciplinary concept to assessment tools and instruments used in early intervention educational settings. Their convergent model links parents, teachers and discipline-specific professionals in the collection of information in authentic and natural ways. Bagnato and his associates critiqued and evaluated the standardized measurement tools used in infant mental health and early intervention circles corresponding to multiple factors (e.g., sensitivity, authenticity, equity and congruence). As there are multiple variables but no singular causation, input about the child is gathered from many settings, on numerous occasions, from several sources and by means of varied assessment instruments, and is used as the basis for establishing an appropriate individual, multidisciplinary intervention program in infant and early childhood mental health.

Als: Synactive Theory of Development

Als' synactive theory is a systems-oriented, relationship-based, integrative theory of development. It identifies the overlapping systemic forces that provide the basis for understanding observed behavior in vulnerable infants. Working specifically with preterm infants in hospital settings, Als developed a highly attuned and individualized bedside care protocol, based on applied theory from both development and risk models and integrating many disciplines and techniques. At its core, the approach is based on ongoing assessment (Als et al., 2004), by frequently tracking the infant's physiological, motor, attentional and regulation capacities. All interactions involving the infant – daily care activities, medical procedures or simple interaction – are entirely based on his or her need for rest or recovery after a stressful event.

Environmental demands, even mundane stimuli arising from lights and sounds, are carefully monitored, as are the individual's need for motor and physical support. Any support which could facilitate the infant's self-regulation is provided and parents are considered participants in the health care team. Als' integrative theory is one of the few which has undergone evidence-based outcome research. While the need for research continues, evaluations have found that preterm babies who were treated according to this protocol had less need for specific medical procedures, better behavioral outcomes at key stages, earlier initiation of oral feeding, better average daily weight gains, shorter hospital stays, more brain activity in the frontal lobe and a lower level of developmental disabilities than the comparison group (Als et al., 2003).

Ayres: Sensory Integration Theory of Development

Ayers (1972), an educational psychologist and occupational therapist, first proposed the term sensory integration dysfunction to describe large numbers of infants and toddlers who have sensory related disorders. Psychologists and other mental health practitioners also recognized that there were sensory components in the behavior problems which infants and toddlers exhibited, but they preferred to use the term regulatory disorder (Greenspan & Wieder, 2007). It is important to illuminate the differences between these two theoretical conceptualizations of early childhood in order to understand the developmental and functional implications of sensory disorders in young children. A more specific comprehension of the theory of sensory integration allows intervention and prevention strategies to be more effective.

Ayers postulated that sensory integration is the neurological process which allows the brain to function and make sense of the world. It has been used as the name of the theory and the intervention, and refers to a dynamic system which focuses on the critical influence that sensory processing has on human development and functioning and its contribution to social emotional development. Ayres proposed that dysfunction in sensory integration results in emotional and social distress for young children. Difficulties in sensory detection, or in the awareness or registration of incoming sensory signals, are seen in children who seek intensive levels of stimulation, including children who like to touch everything or lick objects, or those who do not seem to feel even highly intense sensations, such as not feeling pain when touching a hot surface. Difficulties in regulating the degree, intensity and nature of sensory input in a graded and adaptive manner impact negatively on the child's ability to achieve and maintain an optimal range of performance and adaptation to life challenges. Sensory integration problems can also be expressed in difficulty in perceiving specific characteristics of objects without seeing them, like feeling around in your pocket until you identify your keys among other objects in your pocket. Postural abnormalities and motor planning (i.e., dyspraxia) can also be symptoms of sensory integration issues (Ayres, Mailloux, & Wendler, 1987).

According to Ayres, difficulties in modulation are the most common behavioral profile in infants and very young children. While theoretical descriptions of children from birth to age 3 can be found in the literature (Schaaf & Miller, 2005; Williamson & Anzalone, 2001), there are few empirical studies validating this theoretical system. In infants and toddlers, sensory integration disorders often express themselves as sleeping or eating disorders or emotional outbursts after sensory input. The sensory integration model has been refined and differentiated over the years (Lane, Reynolds, & Dumenci, 2012) and the ecological model of sensory integration disorders is a hierarchal paradigm, beginning with sensory processing, during which the child receives and manages sensory information which results in appropriate responses moving up to emotion, which is the ability to accurately perceive emotional cues and to regulate affective and behavioral responses with the highest level encompassing attention, the ability to sustain performance and inhibit impulsivity for task completion and for effective interpersonal relationships.

This model explains child behaviors such as those of the child who cannot maintain friends and who fights with siblings and peers. This would be a child who does not participate in family routines and outings. This type of child would need specific conditions and instruction in order to complete a task, and making the surroundings appropriate to the child's level of arousal would be a very important step in improving the child's functional profile. Finally, the child with difficulties in sensory integration responds negatively to demands of the general culture and often misbehaves at birthday parties. The preferred method of intervention is derived from the theory and involves occupational therapy as sensory related problems are critically important in understanding, conceptualizing and treating early emotional and behavioral disorders. The intervention methods and tools pioneered by Ayres (1980) have continued to be investigated.

A growing number of theoreticians and practitioners are educated in sensory integration theory, assessment, and intervention techniques, and as such continue to strengthen and enhance Ayres' original body of work through research. The inclusion of sensory integration as one of the domains in infant mental health assessment and treatment is essential. Early identification of sensory related problems, the evaluation of related environmental and contextual areas and appropriate sensory based intervention can have dramatic and global effects on young children and their families.

Brazelton: Touchpoints Model

T. Berry Brazelton, a pediatrician, proposed a theory of child development based on the assumption that parents and families are the central and primary caregivers in ensuring the health and well-being of their children. Brazelton (1999) proposed that professionals and parents should partner in providing services for young children and developed an intervention based on this centrality of the supportive relationship between professionals and parents. Respecting parental strengths, promoting parent-infant attachment, nurturing the young child and enhancing the child's development potential are the underpinnings of the neurodevelopmental, neurorelational Touchpoints Model (Brazelton, O'Brien, & Brandt, 1997). Through the media including his syndicated column about child care, books and television appearances, Brazelton disseminated his belief that it is the professionals' responsibility to give parents knowledge regarding child development, and once the parents have such knowledge they would raise their children in a healthy manner, allowing the growing child to mature biologically and interactively.

Empirical findings have supported Brazelton's conviction that the assessment of the newborn can give relevant and significant information which predicts later infant-parent attachment patterns and subsequent infant development (Linn & Horowitz, 1983). Furthermore, research based on the assessment of the newborn during the first month of life revealed that the infants' ability to control their state is the most predictive of later functioning (Als & Brazelton, 1981), strengthening the fundamental importance of early state regulatory capacities for other more complex functions such as attention and social interactions.

Guralnick: Multidisciplinary Collaborative Team Work Model

Guralnick (1997), the main proponent of interdisciplinary team work in the field of infant and early childhood mental health, provides guidelines for setting up assessments which serve as the basis for intervention programs (Guralnick & Bricker, 1987). Specifically, he targets parents of children with special needs stemming from developmental delays or disabilities to come for a complete assessment, which becomes the basis upon which an intervention plan is established, using the recommendations of the assessment team. The teams members work together, employing a family systems approach in order to collect information from various disciplines in a coordinated manner. They identify areas where additional information is necessary and put forth a possible explanation of the child's difficulties based on developmental and interactional frameworks. One of the main purposes is to provide the parents with recommendations and suggested interventions based on a comprehensive understanding of the issues challenging the child and the family.

References

Als, H., & Brazelton, T. B. (1981). A new model of assessing the behavioral organization in preterm and fullterm infants: Two case studies. *Journal of the American Academy of Child Psychiatry, 20*(2), 239–263.

Als, H., Duffy, F. H., McAnulty, G. B., Rivkin, M. J., Vajapeyam, S., Mulkern, R. V., … & Eichenwald, E. C. (2004). Early experience alters brain function and structure. *Pediatrics, 113*(4), 846–857.

Als, H., Gilkerson, L., Duffy, F. H., Mcanulty, G. B., Buehler, D. M., Vandenberg, K., … & Jones, K. J. (2003). A three-center, randomized, controlled trial of individualized developmental care for very low birth weight preterm infants: medical, neurodevelopmental, parenting, and caregiving effects. *Journal of Developmental & Behavioral Pediatrics*, *24*(6), 399–408.

Ayres, A. J. (1980). *Southern California sensory integration tests-manual* (rev. ed.). Los Angeles, CA: Western Psychological Services.

Ayres, A. J. (1972). *Sensory integration and learning disorders*. Los Angeles, CA: Western Psychological Services.

Ayres, A. J., Mailloux, Z. K., & Wendler, C. L. W. (1987). Developmental dyspraxia: Is it a unitary function? *Occupational Therapy Journal of Research, 7*, 93–110.

Bagnato, S. J., Neisworth, J. T., & Munson, S. M. (1997). *LINKing assessment and early intervention: An authentic curriculum-based approach*. New York: Paul H Brookes Publishing.

Berlin, L. J., Appleyard, K., & Dodge, K. A. (2011). Intergenerational continuity in child maltreatment: Mediating mechanisms and implications for prevention. *Child Development, 82*(1), 162–176.

Berlin, L. J., Cassidy, J., & Appleyard, K. (2008). The influence of early attachments on other relationships. In J. Cassidy & P. R. Shaver (Eds.), *Handbook of attachment: Theory, research, and clinical applications* (2nd ed., pp. 333–347). New York: Guilford Press.

Bowlby, J. (1956). *The growth of independence in the young child.* Publisher not identified.

Bowlby, J. (1969). *Attachment and loss: Vol. 1. Attachment.* New York: Basic Books.

Bowlby, J. (1988). *A secure base: Clinical application of attachment theory.* London, UK: Routledge.

Brazelton, T. B. (1999). How to help parents of young children: The Touchpoints model. *Journal of Perinatology, 19*(6), S6–S7.

Brazelton, T. B., O'Brien, M., & Brandt, K. A. (1997). Combining relationships and development: Applying Touchpoints to individual and community practices. *Infants and Young Children, 10*(1), 74–84.

Fraiberg, S. (1980). *Clinical studies in infant mental health.* New York: Basic Books.

Fraiberg, S., Adelson, E., & Shapiro, V. (1987). Ghosts in the nursery: A psychoanalytic approach to the problems of impaired infant–mother relationships. In S. Fraiberg (Ed.), *Selected writings of Selma Fraiberg* (pp. 100–136). Columbus, OH: Ohio State University Press.

Freud, S. (1955). From the history of an infantile neurosis. In *The standard edition of the complete psychological works of Sigmund Freud, Volume XVII (1917–1919): An infantile neurosis and other works* (pp. 1–124).

Freud, A. (1988). The nursery school of the Hampstead child-therapy clinic. *Bulletin of the Anna Freud Centre, 11*(4), 265–269.

Gone, J. P. (2004). Mental health services for Native Americans in the 21st Century United States. *Professional Psychology: Research and Practice, 35*(1), 10–18.

Greenspan, S. I., & Wieder, S. (2007). *Infant and early childhood mental health: A comprehensive developmental approach to assessment and intervention.* Washington, DC: American Psychiatric Publications.

Guralnick, M. J. (1997). Effectiveness of early intervention for vulnerable children: A developmental perspective. *American Journal on Mental Retardation, 102*(4), 319–345.

Guralnick, M. J., & Bricker, D. (1987). *The effectiveness of early intervention for children with cognitive and general developmental delays.* Waltham, MA: Academic Press.

Halfon, N. (2014). Socioeconomic influences on child health: Building new ladders of social opportunity. *Journal of the American Medical Association, 311*(9), 915–917.

Hastings, P. D., McShane, K. E., Parker, R., & Ladha, F. (2007). Ready to make nice: Parental socialization of young sons' and daughters' prosocial behaviors with peers. *The Journal of Genetic Psychology, 168*(2), 177–200.

Hoagwood, K., & Olin, S. S. (2002). The NIMH blueprint for change report: Research priorities in child and adolescent mental health. *Journal of the American Academy of Child & Adolescent Psychiatry, 41*(7), 760–767.

Lane, S. J., Reynolds, S., & Dumenci, L. (2012). Sensory overresponsivity and anxiety in typically developing children and children with autism and attention deficit hyperactivity disorder: Cause or coexistence? *American Journal of Occupational Therapy, 66*(5), 595–603.

Lieberman, A. F., & Van Horn, P. (2011). *Psychotherapy with infants and young children: Repairing the effects of stress and trauma on early attachment.* New York: Guilford Press.

Linn, P. L., & Horowitz, F. D. (1983). The relationship between infant individual differences and mother-infant interaction during the neonatal period. *Infant Behavior and Development, 6*(4), 415–427.

Olson, S. L., Sameroff, A. J., Kerr, D. C., Lopez, N. L., & Wellman, H. M. (2005). Developmental foundations of externalizing problems in young children: The role of effortful control. *Development and Psychopathology, 17*(01), 25–45.

Raju, T. N., Higgins, R. D., Stark, A. R., & Leveno, K. J. (2006). Optimizing care and outcome for late-preterm (near-term) infants: A summary of the workshop sponsored by the National Institute of Child Health and Human Development. *Pediatrics, 118*(3), 1207–1214.

Rolfe, S. (2004). *Rethinking attachment for early childhood practice: Promoting security, autonomy and resilience in young children*. Melbourne, Australia: Allen & Unwin Publishers.

Sameroff, A. (1975). Transactional models in early social relations. *Human Development, 18*(1–2), 65–79.

Sameroff, A. (2009). *The transactional model*. Washington, DC: American Psychological Association.

Sameroff, A. (2010). A unified theory of development: A dialectic integration of nature and nurture. *Child Development, 81*(1), 6–22.

Sameroff, A. J., & Fiese, B. H. (2000). Transactional regulation: The developmental ecology of early intervention. In J. P. Shonkoff & S. J. Meisels (Eds.), *Handbook of early childhood intervention* (pp. 135–159). New York: Cambridge University Press.

Schaaf, R. C., & Miller, L. J. (2005). Occupational therapy using a sensory integrative approach for children with developmental disabilities. *Mental Retardation and Developmental Disabilities Research Reviews, 11*(2), 143–148.

Shonkoff, J., & Philips, D. (2000). *From neurons to neighborhoods: The science of early childhood development*. Washington, DC: National Academies Press.

Shonkoff, J. P., Garner, A. S., Siegel, B. S., Dobbins, M. I., Earls, M. F., McGuinn, L., … & Wood, D. L. (2012). The lifelong effects of early childhood adversity and toxic stress. *Pediatrics, 129*(1), e232–e246.

Sroufe, L., Carlson, E. A., Levy, A. K., & Egeland, B. (1999). Implications of attachment theory for developmental psychopathology. *Development and Psychopathology, 11*(1), 1–13.

Stern, R., & Elias, M. J. (2007). Emotionally intelligent parenting. In K. Maree & M. J. Elias (Eds.), *Educating people to be emotionally intelligent* (pp. 37–48). Westport, CT: Greenwood Publishing Group.

Tronick, E., & Beeghly, M. (2011). Infants' meaning-making and the development of mental health problems. *American Psychologist, 66*(2), 107–119.

Ungar, M. (2008). Resilience across cultures. *British Journal of Social Work, 38*(2), 218–235.

U.S. Department of Health and Human Services. (n.d.). H.H.S. Strategic Plan Goals and Objectives: FY 2007–2012 . Available: http://www.hhs.gov/strategic_plan/. Accessed 27 Mar 2015.

Weider, S., & Greenspan, S. (2005). Can children with autism master the core deficits and become empathic, creative and reflective? A ten to fifteen year follow-up of a subgroup of children with autism spectrum disorders (ASD) who received a comprehensive developmental, individual-difference, relationship-based (DIR) approach. *Journal of Developmental and Learning Disorder, 9*, 1–29.

Williamson, G. G., & Anzalone, M. E. (2001). *Sensory integration and self-regulation in infants and toddlers: helping very young children interact with their environment*. Zero to Three: National Center for Infants, Toddlers and Families, 2000 M Street, NW, Suite 200, - Washington, DC 20036–3307.

Zero to Three (Organization). DC, & 0-3R Revision Task Force. (2005). *DC: 0-3R: Diagnostic Classification of Mental Health and Developmental Disorders of Infancy and Early Childhood*. Zero to Three: National Center for Infants, Toddlers and Families, 2000 M Street, NW, Suite 200, Washington, DC 20036–3307.

Chapter 9
A Survey of Evidence-Based Interventions in Infant and Early Childhood Mental Health

Introduction

Knowledge about infant and early childhood mental health is increasing rapidly and research has generated data which have broadened that knowledge base in order to establish appropriate intervention programs. There are many models of intervention that try to tackle the pressing needs of infants, toddlers and young children and their families who are at risk for developing mental health problems, or those who have already been identified as needing services to deal with existing mental health issues, while the child is still young and the plasticity of the brain holds promise for lasting changes as a result of intervention (Fisher & Gunnar, 2010).

The challenge for the clinician is to assess the child's and family's needs and decide on the appropriate method of intervention. In order to do this, the clinician must understand the basic assumptions and principles of infant and early childhood mental health (presented in the first half of this volume) and the appropriate theoretical models upon which intervention at this age is based (see Chap. 8). Even when equipped with this knowledge, it can be quite challenging to treat very young children and their families. One of the main goals of this book is to provide knowledge regarding children's social and emotional development, the social context in which it occurs and the interplay between the two. An attempt to focus on the tensions which exist between developmental and social systems theories, between research findings and clinical presentations, between brain and behavior, and other dualities which have plagued this field since its inception is a complicated but essential mission.

Early childhood intervention is an imperative encompassing a spectrum from broad-based goals of health promotion and programs for prevention of non-optimal outcomes to specific intervention programs which target poverty, family violence and trauma, maternal depression and parental substance abuse. As the knowledge base has matured, the field of infant and early childhood intervention has evolved

C. Shulman, *Research and Practice in Infant and Early Childhood Mental Health*, Children's Well-Being: Indicators and Research 13,
DOI 10.1007/978-3-319-31181-4_9

from its original focus on children to a growing appreciation of the necessity of including parents and other family members, while also considering relational, community, societal and cultural factors. A natural extension of this advancement is recognition that individual programs are implemented in a multilayered context, and that their effects are always a result of wider influences in the social, economic and cultural milieu in which the services are provided.

All successful interventions are guided by theoretical models which specify the relationship between their stated goals and the strategies employed to attain them. The continuing growth of the field of infant and early childhood mental health has generated a broad array of intervention programs which have contributed to the knowledge base and have withstood rigorous scientific inquiry into the effectiveness of intervention. The commonalities across these programs serve as a base from which each develops. Early intervention programs are designed to affect children directly through the provision of explicit service delivery to them, or indirectly through their influence on the caregiving environment which theoretically produces changes in the child as a result of changes in the quality and content of child–adult caregiver interaction.

The ability of caregivers to meet their child's particular individual needs is a function of their own resources and the external circumstances of their lives. So the caregivers' emotional health, intelligence, level of education, and personal history, as well as their social networks, economic security and work status, and the family environment all contribute to the quality of relations established between the child and the adult caregiver. The cumulative effect of risk factors can compromise the interaction while the buffering effects of protective factors can enhance it. It is important to note that the relationship with primary caregivers is central in promoting sound mental health in children, particularly very young children. The most positive relationships are those which are warm, nurturing, individualized and reciprocal, and in which responses are sensitive and consistent (Feldman, 2012).

This chapter surveys various leading interventional strategies, including the theoretical basis of each, its intended goals and research which evaluates its effectiveness. The success of any intervention program is determined by the soundness of the strategy, its acceptability, and the quality of implementation (i.e., fidelity). Evaluation of effectiveness is dependent on defined outcome variables and the methodological analysis of the program. Some programs are longitudinal and effectiveness is determined by the associations between child variables at the onset of intervention and other identified outcomes after implementation. The determination of appropriate child and family outcomes and their assessment requires an appreciation of individual differences among children and their caregivers and awareness that caregivers can modify their behavior, which subsequently can change the nature of the child-caregiver relationship.

The evaluation of infant and early childhood mental health interventions is important on several levels. First, intervention studies can test theories about the importance of early experiences and the malleability of behavior in early childhood. Second, program evaluations enable policy makers to assess the outcome of their investment in a particular program. It is not enough to know that an intervention is effective; in addition, it is important to know which aspects of the program are having a significant effect, to what degree and under what circumstances; in short, what is working and why (Klein Velderman, Bakermans-Kranenburg, Juffer, & van IJzendoorn, 2006; Kraemer, Wilson, Fairburn, & Agras, 2002). Assessing programmatic influence is a research question and one of the main purposes of research in the field of infant and early childhood mental health is to evaluate interventions. Various research designs, whose goals are to assess the efficacy of intervention strategies, are presented below. Only when research methodology improves will evaluations of infant mental health interventions achieve more validity and lead to more significant research in the field of infant and early childhood mental health, resulting in more effective interventions.

Research Methodology and Designs Which Assess Intervention Effectiveness

In order to carry out an evaluation of an intervention protocol, it is important to plan what is being evaluated and, only after defining the variables to be assessed, decide on a measurement and analysis design which will address the issues to be evaluated. Asking meaningful questions will provide the answer to the most important question – whether the implementation of a particular intervention accomplishes what it set out to do and significantly improves the lives of young children and their families. After deciding on what is to be evaluated, it is necessary to decide on the focus of the evaluation. The focus in infant mental health interventions can be on variables having to do with child mental health, such as developmental and behavioral outcomes, which are central to the field. Another emphasis for evaluation research can be caregiver mental health variables such as depression, anxiety, disengagement, aggression and exposure to trauma. Strengthening the child-caregiver interaction is the central emphasis in many infant mental health interventions, and assessing variables dealing with, for example, consistency, sensitivity, synchrony, and reciprocity during play and everyday activities is often the initial step in evaluating intervention programs. Infant-caregiverrelationships are often at the center of implementation programs. Finally, mediational and moderating models of influence, risk and resilience factors must be included in the evaluation of infant mental health interventions in order to understand their effect on the implementation of a particular program addressing a certain risk factor.

Research into the outcomes of the Head Start program, which was originally meant to address risk from poverty for young children, for example, suffered from many limitations, including some which stemmed from not being able to define nuanced outcome variables. Longitudinal research assessing outcomes in this ambitious and important program revealed significant differences in readiness for school, learning behavior and academic performance between children who went through Head Start programs and children from similar backgrounds who did not participate in Head Start preschool programs as they entered first grade (Bierman, Nix, Greenberg, Blair, & Domitrovich, 2008), but surprisingly enough these differences seemed to disappear by fourth grade (Marcon, 2002). Only when a more nuanced approach was taken and longitudinal data was collected and analyzed as the children grew did significant differences emerge. More of the children who participated in Head Start completed high school and this is a very important finding, as a high school diploma has been found to be one variable which helps to break continuing cycles of poverty (Ludwig & Miller, 2005).

Once the variables to be evaluated are defined, they must be operationalized and quantified in order to study them. Performance measures enable a program to document the progress that participants are making according to stated goals of the intervention. There are various ways to measure different aspects of performance, and typically the ones used in evaluative research are those which indicate whether the work has made a difference in the life of the child and his or her family. These methodologies include assessment instruments such as intelligence tests, questionnaires regarding child behavior, and other measures of progress in child development and/or in the child-parent interaction. It is also possible to simply count the presence or absence of a targeted behavior in order to document that it has increased (e.g., using adaptive problem solving skills instead of physical aggression) or decreased (e.g., biting or other aggressive behaviors) according to the goals of the intervention strategy.

Data should be collected regularly, for without this constant review it is impossible to know how children and their families are progressing. Observations may be very helpful in order to examine how the intervention has worked. It is important to code these interactions in a systematic, reliable and valid manner; otherwise it is difficult to compare results. For example, the Emotional Availability scales (Biringen, 2000; Biringen et al., 1998) discussed in Chap. 6 have been used to assess intervention programs which help teach caregivers, specifically child care providers, how to be more sensitive and available to the multiple-risk children in their care (Biringen et al., 2012), and significant differences emerged in the emotional content in the child-caregiver relationship as a result of intervention. These and other evaluation techniques are used to document changes in child development or child-caregiver interactions as a result of participation in a particular program.

Evidence-Based Practice

Employing data collection and review processes in order to evaluate an intervention strategy is called evidence-based practice (EBP). In the field of children's mental health services research, the term "evidence-based practice" refers to a body of scientific knowledge about service practices or about the impact of clinical treatments or services on the mental health problems of children and adolescents. The knowledge base is created through the application of scientific methods that examine the impact of certain practices on outcomes for the child and his or her family. Evidence-based practice denotes the quality, robustness, or validity of scientific evidence as it is brought to bear on these issues. In infant and early childhood mental health, the term "evidence-based" is most often used to differentiate therapies that have been studied with varying degrees of scientific rigor from therapies that are used but have not been studied or have not been studied well.

There is a consensus regarding four criteria for defining evidence-based practice (Barth et al., 2011), which have been employed in evaluating infant mental health intervention programs. A therapeutic intervention should have a theory that links a hypothesized mechanism to a clinical problem, basic research to assess the validity of the hypothesized mechanism, preliminary outcome evidence to show that a therapeutic approach has an effect on the relevant outcomes, and process-outcome connections which display the relationships between process change and clinical outcomes. In essence, these criteria delineate a process for attaining a valid and substantiated theory about the impact of therapy (Hoagwood, Burns, Kiser, Ringeisen, & Schoenwald, 2014; Kazdin, 2015). According to these criteria, treatments are to be supported by either group design or single-subject experiments, and studies should clearly describe salient characteristics of the subjects. For a treatment to be considered "well established," two or more studies must show that it is superior to medication, placebo, or an alternative treatment or that it is equivalent to an already established treatment, or at least nine single-subject case studies must be conducted to establish its equivalence or superiority.

Evidence-based practice requires adaptation of empirical research methodology to practice-related constraints, as well as accommodation of practice settings to the incorporation of evidence-based practice. One reason that efficacy studies, which constitute a significant portion of the evidentiary basis in infant and early childhood mental health, have not been performed in service settings may be that the theory, methods, and models used to develop, refine, and test treatments do not mesh well with the reality of clinic-based or community-based care (Snell-Johns, Mendez, & Smith, 2004). It may be that treatments with proven high efficacy as tested in laboratory conditions will need to be adapted to clinics, homes, or other service settings. However, it may also be that service settings or the service practices themselves may have to adapt and find ways to deliver services which meet evidence-based practices.

Today it is not always clear that treatments which have been validated in efficacy studies can be effective when implemented under clinical conditions. For example, the use of treatment manuals, special training for clinicians, and continual clinical monitoring to ensure treatment fidelity are characteristics of many research-based interventions which few community-based treatment practices are able to implement, possibly because of the heterogeneous populations and high caseloads which are characteristic of clinical programs and are not features of most research-based studies. Thus, both evidence-based treatments and community centers are likely to need some modification in order to realize the potential benefits from evidence-based practice. In addition, the fidelity of practitioners' implementation of a particular intervention strategy and how it may influence the effectiveness of the intervention must also be assessed.

Fidelity dimensions refer to the ability to implement the intervention appropriately in a replicable manner and they address components of the intervention itself and include the clinical training, professional support, consultation, and monitoring of the practitioners who are using the intervention; the homogeneity or heterogeneity of the population being serviced; the setting and the types of services accessible to the child and/or family being serviced in addition to the intervention; the motivation, attitudes, and morale which characterize the service agency; and the overall service system, which includes referral and reimbursement mechanisms and interagency relations. The research base that constitutes evidence-based practice for infant and early childhood mental health interventions has not always attained a good match between research and practice. As the field of infant and early childhood mental health intervention research expands, there is an imperative to find the best match so that research can help identify the most effective aspects of interventions while taking into account the reality of practice settings in which the treatment is delivered.

Different statistical models are used to evaluate different types of programs and to address different hypotheses and outcome variables in evidence-based practice: it is not employing a specific statistical analysis, but rather the use of data to assess the effectiveness of an intervention program which makes it evidence-based. Most frequently randomized control trials are used in group models, and single-subject designs are used when focusing on changes in individual children or parents. Single-subject studies allow programs to document the relationship between teaching strategies and changes in child or caregiver behavior (Horner et al., 2005) and are well suited for intervention evaluation as they can be easily incorporated into existing routines. The assessment of fidelity is often accomplished through the single-subject design, by measuring intervention strategies and changes in behavior in order to establish that changes in the child's behavior were the result of the intervention. The infant and early childhood mental health programs surveyed below are all evidence-based and the research design chosen to assess its effectiveness is included in the description of each program.

Child Parent Psychotherapy (CPP: Lieberman & Van Horn)

Child parent psychotherapy (CPP) is a relationship-based approach to the treatment of mental health disorders in infancy and early childhood for young children who are experiencing mental health problems. Its focus is on enhancing the quality of the emotional relationship between the young child and the parents, giving prominence to a variety of factors that contribute to the child's clinical condition. These include the parent's unresolved psychological conflicts as these are reenacted in the relationship with the child (Basseches & Mascolo, 2009; Lebovici, 1999; Lieberman & Van Horn, 2011); the mutually reinforcing impact of reality-based stresses and psychological conflicts as obstacles to effective parenting (Lieberman & Pawl, 1993); the transactional nature of the parent-child contributions to the child's mental health problems (Lieberman, Silverman, & Pawl, 2000; Lieberman & Van Horn, 1998); and parental strengths as a scaffolding for building new parental competencies and alleviating maladaptive parenting practices (McDonough, 2000, 2004).

CPP is appropriate for infants, toddlers, and preschoolers who are experiencing mental health problems or whose relationship with their parents is negatively affected as a result of parental factors such as mental illness, child constitutional characteristics that interfere with the formation of a secure attachment, and/or discordant temperamental styles between the parent and child. It emphasizes the child's centrality as an active partner in the treatment by focusing on the child's emotional experience and embedding this experience in the child-parent relationship. The goal is to promote a psychological partnership in which the child's modulation and integration of affect are supported by the parent's increasing ability to provide concrete protection and developmentally appropriate responses. Using the format of joint parent-child sessions, CPP therapists rely on play, behavioral intervention, and psychosocial education to interpret the emotional experience of the child to the parent and to explain the parent's behavior to the child, in order to promote empathic understanding and encourage emotional reciprocity. Individual sessions with the parent and/or with the child may be added when clinically indicated as an adjunct to the joint child-parent sessions.

While the infant's, toddler's or preschooler's mental health is the ultimate goal, the primary therapy focus in child parent psychotherapy involves uncovering unconscious links between the parent's psychological conflicts and parenting practices that are not correctly attuned to the baby's needs and which disrupt the infant's development. Therefore, CPP emphasizes the growing child's autonomy during treatment, with a concomitant emphasis on helping parents reflect on their individual experience, including their own unresolved childhood conflicts. The therapeutic focus in CPP is on the child's subjective experience within the child-parent relationship, with the goal of enhancing the child's mental health by promoting reliance on the parents as sources of protection and safety, more accurate reality testing, and modulation and integration of positive and negative affect. CPP targets the child's maladaptive behaviors and perceptions of self and others, engaging the parent as an indispensable partner in this therapeutic process.

The assumptions of CPP include the conceptualization that mental health problems in infancy and early childhood need to be addressed in the context of the child's primary relationships, regardless of their etiology (Emde & Sameroff, 1989; Lieberman et al., 2000). Similarly, mental health risk factors in the first 3 years of life operate in the context of transactions between the child and his or her social environment, including family, neighborhood, community and larger society. The child's parents may live in circumstances that tax their resources, such as poverty, discrimination, low education, unemployment, violent neighborhoods, inadequate housing, transportation, and health services, substance abuse, and/or mental health problems. Such circumstances affect the child's development directly through the negative conditions they create and indirectly by impairing the parent's ability to provide adequate care. These negative circumstances have a cumulative effect on the child's development (Sameroff & Fiese, 2000).

Faced with such stressors, parents are often unable to support their children's development unless the intervention includes a concerted effort to help them improve their own circumstances and well-being. In addition, child rearing beliefs and parenting practices are imbued with deeply held and often unconscious cultural values about who is a worthy human being and which characteristics should be encouraged or discouraged in a child; therefore, CPP therapists must be particularly cognizant of the importance of learning about and incorporating culturally appropriate therapeutic practices in their work.

CPP is based on the premise that patterns of mental health and mental disturbance are transmitted from generation to generation. Transmission mechanisms include attachment perspectives and parental attribution (Dix & Grusec, 1985). These attributions are essential for the child's healthy development when they are flexible and predominantly positive; but when parental attributions are rigid, disconnected from the child's developmental stage and negative in emotional tone, they adversely affect the child's mental health.

CPP typically involves weekly sessions lasting between 60 and 90 min, with at least one parent and the child present. Other family members may be present if appropriate, depending on clinical considerations and practical need. The developing child is central in CPP and he or she is an active partner in the intervention. The child's behavior during the play session with the adult is the focus. It is intended for situations where the child is experiencing mental health problems or where the young child and the parent are negatively affected by the family's difficult circumstances, including parent depression or other mental illness, bereavement or chronic stress, exposure to trauma, child constitutional or developmental characteristics that interfere with the formation of a secure attachment and discrepancies in temperamental styles of the child and parent.

Five randomized studies have evaluated the effectiveness of CPP (Cicchetti, Rogosch, & Toth, 2006; Ghosh Ippen, Harris, Van Horn, & Lieberman, 2011; Lieberman, Van Horn, & Ghosh Ippen, 2005; Toth, Maughan, Manly, Spagnola, & Cicchetti, 2002). The comparison groups included young children and their caregivers who were found to be appropriate for CPP but were waitlisted. While they were waiting to begin their own therapy they participated as a control group for others who were already involved in therapy and continued to receive community intervention ("business as usual"). In order to assess whether the findings from the research are generalizable from university laboratory conditions to community settings, these studies all utilized broad samples including clinical community contexts. Data were collected before, during and after the intervention, in order to understand the change processes which are associated with this intervention technique. In addition, follow-up data were again collected 6 months after terminating therapy. Similar minimal attrition rates were reported for clinical and comparison groups. Although these studies were executed at different times, in different places, and with different populations, the results were analogous. Positive outcome variables consisted of more secure attachment, increases in children's intelligence scores and in parental responsivity and sensitivity, and decreases in child trauma symptoms and in adult symptoms of anxiety and depression.

The United States federal government funded a study evaluating the use of CPP with preschoolers who had witnessed domestic violence. For the 75 child-parent dyads, the children had witnessed physical abuse in the home (49 %) and in the community (46 %) and sexual abuse (14 %), and the mothers reported an average of 12 stressful events in their lives. The positive results for both children and mothers, as detailed above, were maintained for over 6 months (the follow-up period). These results are particularly robust as they were found at different sites (San Francisco and Rochester) and different instruments were used for evaluation. The training of the professionals was meticulous and for each site there was an average of 34 sessions which were spread over a 12 month period. As in the previous study, follow-up was 6 months after completion of treatment. The outcome variable coders who assessed the children's and mothers' behavior and the quality of the child-mother interaction were blind to group at all times of data collection. One particularly promising result was that the mothers continued to improve 6 months after terminating treatment.

Fidelity measures were developed in order to maintain treatment efficacy. A questionnaire was developed which therapists are given at the end of their year-long training, which they are asked to complete for each of two cases. The fidelity measures become part of the treatment plan. The therapist is asked to fill out the questionnaire directly after the initial assessment or first treatment session, identifying target goals, and to complete it again after a month in order to see what really happened. It is important to understand how the principles of CPP are embedded in each individual case. CPP has also incorporated a training program for trainers, which emphasizes the need for fidelity among all the trainers. This intervention is a good example of a treatment program based on theoretical principles, with a defined operational program, which has been evaluated for its effectiveness according to the targeted goals.

Incredible Years® (IY: Webster-Stratton, 2000, 2001, 2003, 2006)

Incredible Years® Parent Program is a parent training program designed to improve parenting practices which is intended to reduce behavioral problems and promote children's social and emotional competence. IY was developed because of the limitations of the programs which existed in the 1980s, which relied on verbal training or one-on-one therapy methods, none of which seemed effective in supporting parents who were trying to cope with disruptive behavior and emotional problems in their children. The IY Parent Program is based on cognitive social learning, self-efficacy and relationship-building theories, and uses video-based modeling techniques as the primary mode of intervention. Groups of parents of young children with behavioral or emotional problems participate in a training series which includes videos of actual parent-child interaction vignettes illustrating positive and less effective parenting behaviors. The group leaders show the vignettes and facilitate group discussion, peer support, self-reflection and problem solving, all of which results in collaborative learning. In addition, there are practice exercises which help operationalize techniques. Participants are encouraged to determine goals for themselves and their children, which are informed by their cultural beliefs. They take responsibility for accomplishing the assigned home activities, participate in values exercises regarding their short- and long-term goals, and work with group leaders to recognize and overcome their personal barriers. Since the 1980s, the Incredible Years® Training Series has been expanded to include three complementary curricula for parents, teachers, and children, all of which employ similar training methods and therapeutic processes. These programs are designed to reduce the multiple risk factors associated with poor parenting practices, early-onset conduct problems and emotional difficulties.

Incredible Years® has undergone extensive empirical evaluation and well-established evidence-based research supporting its intervention techniques for treating disruptive behavior disorders. The goals of the program are tailored specifically to a particular age group (infancy, toddlerhood, preschoolers through middle childhood) and a specific developmental stage, and include (1) promoting parent competencies and strengthening families by increasing positive parenting, parent-child attachment, and self-confidence about parenting; (2) increasing parents' ability to use child-directed play interactions to coach children's social-emotional, academic, verbal, and persistence skills; (3) reducing critical and physically violent discipline and increasing positive discipline strategies such as ignoring and redirecting, logical consequences, time-out, and problem-solving; (4) increasing family support networks; and (5) strengthening home-school bonding and parents' involvement in school-related activities.

Empirical evidence supporting the Incredible Years® programs reveals the efficacy of this parent treatment program for children, ages 2–8 years, diagnosed with ODD/CD. It has been demonstrated in 8 published randomized control group trials (RCTs) by the program developer and colleagues (Reid, Webster-Stratton, & Hammond, 2003, 2007; Webster-Stratton, 1990, 1998; Webster-Stratton, & Reid, 2004; Webster-Stratton, Reid, & Stoolmiller, 2008; Webster-Stratton, Rinaldi & Reid, 2011). Randomized controlled trial is an empirical method used to evaluate intervention programs and tests the efficacy of intervention techniques by assigning participants to a particular group randomly, which means that they have an equal probability of being assigned to any treatment group. Procedures are controlled to ensure that all participants in all treatment groups undergo the same conditions except for the factor that is unique to their group. When using RCT research to evaluate a treatment technique, the unique factor is the type of intervention they receive. The primary goal of conducting an RCT is to test whether an intervention works by comparing it to a control condition, usually either no intervention or an alternative intervention. The no intervention group is often a "waiting list" group, in order to avoid ethical problems associated with offering one group no treatment. Another alternative involves one group getting "treatment as usual", which is what they would receive in any event. Secondary goals of the RCT statistical analyses may include identifying factors that influence the effects of the intervention, including moderating variables, understanding the processes through which an intervention influences change, and specifying the change mechanisms that bring about the intervention effect.

In all of these studies, the results demonstrated that participation in the Incredible Years® program improved parental attitudes and parent-child interactions and reduced harsh discipline and child conduct problems, compared to wait-list comparison groups. Treatment component analyses indicated that the combination of group discussion, a trained facilitator, and video modeling produced the most lasting results, in comparison to treatment that involved only one of those three training components (Webster-Stratton, 1990, 1998). Perhaps most significantly, a recent 8- to 12-year follow-up of families treated because of their young children's conduct problems indicated that 75 % of the teenagers were typically adjusted, with minimal behavioral and emotional problems (Webster-Stratton, Reid & Stoolmiller, 2008). In addition, the Incredible Years® program has been replicated with treatment populations in five research projects by independent investigators in mental health clinics or doctor's offices with families of children diagnosed with conduct problems (Drugli & Larsson, 2006; Gardner, Burton, & Klimes, 2006; Lavigne et al., 2008).

Additional RCTs have been conducted with multiethnic, socioeconomically disadvantaged families (Reid, Webster-Stratton, & Beauchaine, 2001; Webster-Stratton, 1998; Reid, et al., 2007). Another six RCTs were conducted by independent investigators who studied prevention programs in high-risk populations and have found that the Incredible Years® parenting program increases parents' use of positive attention with their children (praise, coaching, descriptive commenting) and positive discipline strategies, and reduces harsh, critical, and coercive discipline strategies (see review by Webster-Stratton & Reid, 2010). These replications were executed in applied mental health settings, not in university research clinics, and the Incredible Years® group leaders were staff (nurses, social workers and psychologists) working at the centers or in doctor's offices. The program has also been found to be effective with diverse populations, including those representing Latino, Asian, African American, and Caucasian backgrounds in the United States (Reid et al., 2001), and in other countries such as the United Kingdom, Ireland, Norway, Sweden, Holland, New Zealand, Wales, and Russia (Gardner et al., 2006; Hutchings et al., 2007; Larsson et al., 2009; Raaijmakers et al., 2008; Scott et al., 2001, 2010).

Parent Child Interaction Therapy (PCIT: Eyberg)

Parental child interaction therapy was originally developed as a synthesis of different theories of child development. It is based on social learning theory (Patterson, 1982), which posits that children's behavior can be shaped by environmental responses; specifically, that those which are reinforced will appear more frequently in the future and those which are not reinforced will decrease. In addition Baumrind's (1967) theory of parenting styles which is based on the belief that parents have a particular style of interacting with their children and each style predicts certain child behavioral outcomes lies at the heart of this intervention. Finally, parent child interaction therapy is based on attachment theory, which predicts that children's behavior and development will reflect the security of the attachment bond which is established between the child and the parent (Bowlby, 1969).

Parent Child Interaction Therapy is conducted in weekly 1 h sessions, during which the therapist and parent discuss an interaction which occurred during the week between visits, have a play session and then have a feedback session. The goal is to improve the quality of parent-child interactions by reducing coercive cycles and increasing positive interactions, in an average of 25–28 weekly sessions which typically include the parent-child dyad. The first phase involves the therapist coaching the parent in five important skills in relating with the child, summarized in the acronym of PRIDE (**P**raising the child, **R**eflecting on the child's statements, **I**mitation of the child's play, **D**escribing the child's behavior, and bringing **E**nthusiasm into the interaction). After focusing on the elements directed at the child, the sessions move on to the next phase, where the parent becomes the focus. The parent is coached not just in how to respond and interact with the child, but also in how to direct and guide the child's behavior and use other behavioral techniques such as time-out. These give the parents tools to use when dealing with difficult behavior. At the end of each session the parents get "homework" assignments directing them to continue to use the techniques that they learned at home and to report about their experiences in the following sessions.

The effectiveness of this intervention has been studied in randomized controlled trials research with different populations. The first evidence-based study investigated the results of parent child interaction therapy with children with externalizing behavior problems, and it was found that parents were able to successfully generalize the use of the techniques they learned in the clinic to their homes and that they reported a decrease in family conflict. There was also a reduction in the children's externalizing behavior (Eyberg & Boggs, 1998). It has also been found effective with other child disorders such as depression (Lenze, Pautsch, & Luby, 2011) and aggression in young children (Nixon, Sweeney, Erickson, & Touyz, 2004). Research has also demonstrated that PCIT was successful when working with parental problems, such as with parents who were physically abusive to their young children (Chaffin et al., 2004; Eyberg & Robinson, 1983; Eyberg et. al.,

2001) and with parents who neglected their children (Eyberg & Matarazzo, 1980; Thomas & Zimmer-Gembeck, 2007).

PCIT was among the first intervention programs to be evaluated among diverse populations, including Mexican Americans (McCabe & Yeh, 2009) and Chinese (Leung, Tsang, Heung, & Yiu, 2008). For example, Hakman, Chaffin, Funderburk, and Silovsky (2009) conducted a randomized trial to test the efficacy of PCIT in preventing reports of physical abuse among abusive parents of 4- to 12-year-olds. Results indicated that participants in PCIT were less likely to have a subsequent report for abuse at follow-up (after an average period of 2 years). It is interesting to note that participants in a PCIT treatment group who also received individualized services targeting parental depression, substance abuse, and marital dysfunction did not have more favorable outcomes than those receiving only PCIT. These studies have suggested that long-term interventions targeting improvement in the quality of the parent-child relationship may modify the early developmental trajectory of maltreated children. This continues to be a highly regarded, researched intervention technique which has proven its effectiveness among different cultures and populations, with different problems exhibited by children with various parenting disruptions.

Interaction Guidance (IG: Susan C. McDonough, 2000, 2004)

Interaction guidance is an intervention aimed at promoting and nurturing the caregiving relationship. The interaction guidance therapeutic treatment model incorporates principles of a family system theory into a multigenerational transactional preventative intervention. The resulting therapeutic approach focuses on the infant-caregiver relationship rather than on either the infant or the caregiver alone. Interactions between the infant, toddler or preschooler and the caregiver are observed and serve as the focus of the therapeutic relationship. Caregiver interactions with the infant are understood both as a reflection of the family structure and caregiving nurturance style, and as a reflection of the caregiver's and child's representational world. To facilitate the parents' understanding of their child's growth and development, they are treated as active participants in observing both their behaviors and those of their infant; while trying to make meaning of the behaviors they are also involved in understanding their own style of interaction when relating to their child. The use of videotapes in treatment allows for immediate feedback to the parents or family regarding their own behavior and its effect on the infant's behavior, as well as the effect of the infant's behavior on their own. Through viewing samples of parent-child play interaction, the family members participating in the interaction guidance intervention program become more aware of salient interactive behaviors that are positive and need to be reinforced, elaborated, and extended, and those interactions that were less enjoyable or inappropriate and require redirection, alteration or sometimes elimination. The use of videotape also provides parents with the opportunity to listen more carefully to the things that they say to their child and the manner in which they say them.

This approach was created specifically to meet the needs of infants and their families who previously were not successfully engaged in mental health treatment or who refused treatment referral. Many of these families could be described as being overburdened by multiple risk conditions, such as inadequate housing, poverty, poor education, family mental illness, substance abuse, large family size, lack of a parenting partner and inadequate social support. In an effort to reach such overburdened families, the therapists invite each family to take an active role in the creation and evaluation of their family's treatment program. The goal is to develop a therapeutic approach that involves the family members in deciding what is important to them and how they can feel that they are coming away with something helpful to them in their unique circumstances. In this way interaction guidance is an approach which is sensitive to each family's strengths and vulnerabilities.

Interaction guidance addresses the unique needs of each family by involving extended family or household members in the treatment plan when appropriate or necessary, offering supplementary help when such assistance is asked for or deemed critical to treatment success, providing the option of follow-up services at the conclusion of treatment and including the family in the evaluation of treatment progress (McDonough, 2000, 2004). This is done by encouraging family members to define the problem or issue of concern as they see it, emphasizing a family's strengths while recognizing its vulnerabilities and limitations, and embracing a nonjudgmental stance in work with families while conveying societal norms for the family's caregiving behavior. Specifically, interaction guidance therapists' work is characterized by certain therapeutic practices that interaction guidance therapists use to facilitate family system change, which include:

1. asking rather than assuming that the family believes that you will be helpful to them. This allows the family to understand that the ultimate decision to participate in treatment rests with them. Asking for their opinion also reinforces the role of the parents as the decision makers in the family and responsible agents in guaranteeing their child's welfare. Deferring to their expertise as the individuals who know their child best affords the parents legitimate power in making or influencing decisions about what is best for their child;
2. embracing a culturally sensitive, nonjudgmental approach in coming to know the family. Every family has its own unique story to share with people outside its immediate circle, and listening to family stories can reveal culturally specific patterns of family interaction and communication that can be acknowledged and sensitively explored. Information gathered through these discussions can provide the therapist with essential knowledge that will guide the therapist's family-specific, culturally sensitive practice;
3. taking a cooperative stance when identifying problems and generating potential solutions for treatment. Nearly all parents want to play a meaningful role in their child's life. Often the strategies that overburdened families use do not fulfill this

parental desire. Asking them what they have discovered about what works best and not so well for their own family invites an open discussion between the therapist and the family;

4. emphasizing family strengths while recognizing family vulnerabilities. The majority of families that participate in interaction guidance interventions are doing the best they can in caring for their children and themselves. By emphasizing the phrase "the best they know how to do now", a therapist can communicate the belief that parents can acquire new ways of thinking, coping, behaving, and feeling. It also conveys acceptance and respect of the parents without assuming that it is all that they are capable of achieving. Building on strengths can instill the confidence that they are able to make and maintain personal and family changes to adequately protect and nurture their young children.

Therapists who practice interaction guidance begin by establishing a positive working alliance, as the families with whom they work often have a history of unproductive contacts with social service professionals. Clearly many overburdened families have spent years struggling to resolve complex life problems. It is suggested that during the initial meeting the therapist should offer some concrete assistance, which may involve something as practical as arranging a scheduled appointment at the family's convenience rather than during regular clinic hours. The message to be conveyed is that the therapist intends to work hard towards making this experience a productive one for the family. The therapist should clarify with the parents what it is that they believe to be the problem or issue of concern. While meeting with the parents it is important to take note of parental attitudes and behaviors which are of critical importance.

Often overburdened families are confronted with a plethora of problems and issues of concern. For these families everyday life challenges preoccupy much of their psychic and physical energies. Providing instrumental help, advice and guidance on how to address a pressing family concern may provide some relief, albeit temporary, for the caregivers. Demonstrating a willingness to work with family members at addressing what they believe to be of critical importance provides concrete evidence of the therapist's commitment to forming an active working alliance with the family. Many worrisome family issues or inadequate problem solving techniques are rooted in longstanding family pathology.

There are no randomized controlled trials evaluating the efficacy of this intervention technique; rather, it has been assessed using more traditional research designs. The authors have analyzed changes in the quality of child-parent interactions through videotapes which revealed changes in interactional patters as detailed above. In addition, more qualitative data was analyzed from the family exit interviews, which revealed that parents discussed relocating their limited resources to better meet the infant's needs and restructuring the family so that the infant received more consistent quality care from one family member, and reported that participating in interaction guidance helped them identify and treat their own mental health issues. It is particularly difficult to define relevant outcome measures for evidence-based research which would be appropriate for the multi-problem, multi-risk families that participate in Interaction Guidance intervention. More effort is needed to define outcome measures and design appropriate research methodologies which can address the efficacy of this intervention for behavior problems in young children living in complex families.

Since its inception, Interaction Guidance has been monitoring the fidelity of implementation. All therapists are trained by an accredited trainer and criteria have been developed which must be met before attaining certification. The Interaction Guidance Adherence Scales were developed (McDonough, 2004) and have become an ongoing part of the training. Group leaders are required to continue using the scale periodically to decrease drifting away from the original methods of Interaction Guidance. Efficacy studies and translations of the manual, and international trainings which are now underway, will add more evidence-based findings and help to assess the transportability of this significant intervention in the field of infant and early childhood mental health.

Home Visiting Intervention

Several models of intervention which are based on professionals visiting at risk families in their home to observe and interact with the families in their natural settings exist (Olds, 2006, 2007). Moss et al. (2011) assessed the effectiveness of an adaptation of home visiting programs. This intervention was based on shortening the amount of time the home visits continued. The target population was families in which maltreatment of the children was identified are maltreated. Maltreatment has been identified as having deleterious long term effects on children's social, emotional, and cognitive development. Maltreated children are at high risk for developing both externalizing and internalizing behavior problems.

This intervention program was based on the attachment model and focused on enhancing maternal sensitivity to child emotional and behavioral signals in order to promote greater child security. Sensitivity was defined as responding to child distress signals with comfort and appropriate structuring, and promoting and supporting active child exploration when the child is not distressed. All intervention sessions were primarily focused on reinforcing sensitive parental behavior by means of personalized parent-child interaction, video feedback, and discussion of themes related to attachment/emotion regulation (e.g. child negative emotion, discipline, and separation anxieties).

The program consisted of 8 home visits of approximately 90 min which followed this sequence: (1) 20 min during which the parent and therapist discussed a theme which the parent chose and which could involve child related questions and issues and thinking about problematic interactions for which the parents would like alternative responses; (2) 10–15 min of a videotaped interactive session with toys provided by the therapist. The activities were chosen by the therapist as a function of child age and dyadic needs, in order to build reciprocity or child proximity seeking and to encourage the parent to follow the child's lead; (3) 20 min during which feedback was given to the parent after watching the videotape of the preceding play session. The discussion about the child-parent interaction revolved around the parent's feelings and observations of self and child during the interaction, while the therapist focused on positive sequences and provided feedback that reinforced parental sensitive behavior towards the child and its impact on child behavior; finally (4) 10–15 min were dedicated to wrapping up the session. Progress was highlighted and the parent was encouraged to continue similar activities with the child during the coming week.

Results revealed significant intervention effects for the intervention group in parental sensitivity and child attachment security when pre- and post-intervention scores were compared between groups. Fidelity of the intervention was maintained through carefully choosing the therapists from a pool of experts in the field of infant and early childhood mental health and a rigorous training session. The therapists received a detailed manual and were observed by the researchers.

Efficacy was tested in this randomized controlled trials study by examining the effects of the intervention on maternal sensitivity and child attachment style, using separate univariate analyses of covariance (ANCOVAs). These analyses were used to examine group differences at post-test, with initial scores (pretest) on each variable being entered as a covariate. In addition, family SES risk index and parental age were also included as covariates for analyses on parental sensitivity. The use of the ANCOVA is recommended when testing treatment efficacy (Gliner, Morgan, & Harmon, 2003) and it has been employed in comparable studies assessing the efficacy of interventions. Furthermore, hierarchical linear regression analyses revealed that parents in the intervention group exhibited higher levels of sensitivity following intervention than those in the control group and children in the intervention groups exhibited more secure attachment than those who were not in the intervention group. This research demonstrated the effectiveness of a short-term, attachment-based intervention in enhancing parental sensitivity and young children's attachment security.

References

Barth, R. P., Lee, B. R., Lindsey, M. A., Collins, K. S., Strieder, F., Chorpita, B. F., … & Sparks, J. A. (2011). Evidence-based practice at a crossroads: The emergence of common elements and factors. *Research on Social Work Practice*, *22*(1), 108–119.

Basseches, M., & Mascolo, M. F. (2009). *Psychotherapy as a developmental process*. New York, NY: Routledge.

Baumrind, D. (1967). Child care practices anteceding three patterns of preschool behavior. *Genetic Psychology Monographs*, *75*, 43–88.

Bierman, K. L., Nix, R. L., Greenberg, M. T., Blair, C., & Domitrovich, C. E. (2008). Executive functions and school readiness intervention: Impact, moderation, and mediation in the head start REDI program. *Development and Psychopathology*, *20*(03), 821–843.

Biringen, Z. (2000). Emotional availability: Conceptualization and research findings. *American Journal of Orthopsychiatry*, *70*(1), 104–114.

Biringen, Z., Robinson, J., & Emde, R. (1998). *Emotional availability scales* (3rd ed.). Unpublished manuscript. Retrieved from http://www.emotionalavailability.com

Biringen, Z., Altenhofen, S., Aberle, J., Baker, M., Brosal, A., Bennett, S., ... & Swaim, R. (2012). Emotional availability, attachment, and intervention in center-based child care for infants and toddlers. *Development and Psychopathology, 24*(01), 23–34.

Bowlby, J. (1969). *Attachment and loss: Vol. 1. Attachment*. New York, NY: Basic Books.

Chaffin, M., Silovsky, J. F., Funderburk, B., Valle, L. A., Brestan, E. V., Balachova, T., ... & Bonner, B. L. (2004). Parent-child interaction therapy with physically abusive parents: efficacy for reducing future abuse reports. *Journal of Consulting and Clinical Psychology, 72*(3), 500–510.

Cicchetti, D., Rogosch, F. A., & Toth, S. L. (2006). Fostering secure attachment in infants in maltreating families through preventive interventions. *Development and Psychopathology, 18*, 623–650.

Dix, T. H., & Grusec, J. E. (1985). Parent attribution processes in the socialization of children. In J. J. Goodnow, I. E., Sigel, A. V., & McGillicuddy-DeLis (Eds.), *Parental belief systems: The psychological consequences for children* (pp. 201–233). Mahwah, NJ: Lawrence Elbaum Associates.

Drugli, M. B., & Larsson, B. (2006). Children aged 4–8 years treated with parent training and child therapy because of conduct problems: Generalisation effects to day-care and school settings. *European Child & Adolescent Psychiatry, 15*(7), 392–399.

Emde, R. N., & Sameroff, A. J. (1989). Understanding early relationship disturbances. In A. J. Sameroff & R. N. Sameroff (Eds.), *Relationship disturbances in early childhood* (pp. 3–14). New York, NY: Basic Books.

Eyberg, S. M., & Boggs, S. R. (1998). Parent-child interaction therapy for oppositional preschoolers. In C. E. Schaefer & J. M. Briesmeister (Eds.), *Handbook of parent training: Parents as co-therapists for children's behavior problems* (2nd ed., pp. 61–97). New York, NY: Wiley.

Eyberg, S. M., Funderburk, B. W., Hembree-Kigin, T. L., McNeil, C. B., Querido, J. G., & Hood, K. (2001). Parent-child interaction therapy with behavior problem children: One and two year maintenance of treatment effects in the family. *Child and Family Behavior Therapy, 23*, 1–20.

Eyberg, S. M., & Matarazzo, R. G. (1980). Training parents as therapists: A comparison between individual parent-child interaction training and parent group didactic training. *Journal of Clinical Psychology, 36*, 492–499.

Eyberg, S. M., & Robinson, E. A. (1983). Conduct problem behavior: Standardization of a behavioral rating scale with adolescents. *Journal of Clinical Child Psychology, 12*, 347–357.

Feldman, R. (2012). Oxytocin and social affiliation in humans. *Hormones and Behavior, 61*(3), 380–391.

Fisher, P. A., & Gunnar, M. R. (2010). Early life stress as a risk factor for disease in adulthood. In R. A. Lanius, E. Vermetten, & C. Pain (Eds.), *The impact of early life trauma on health and disease: The hidden epidemic* (pp. 133–141). New York, NY: Cambridge University Press.

Gardner, F., Burton, J., & Klimes, I. (2006). Randomised controlled trial of a parenting intervention in the voluntary sector for reducing child conduct problems: Outcomes and mechanisms of change. *Journal of Child Psychology and Psychiatry, 47*(11), 1123–1132.

Ghosh Ippen, C., Harris, W. W., Van Horn, P., & Lieberman, A. F. (2011). Traumatic and stressful events in early childhood: Can treatment help those at highest risk? *Child Abuse & Neglect, 35*(7), 504–513.

Gliner, J. A., Morgan, G. A., & Harmon, R. J. (2003). Pretest-posttest comparison group designs: Analysis and interpretation. *Journal of the American Academy of Child & Adolescent Psychiatry, 42*, 500–503.

Hakman, M., Chaffin, M., Funderburk, B., & Silovsky, J. F. (2009). Change trajectories for parent-child interaction sequences during parent-child interaction therapy for child physical abuse. *Child Abuse & Neglect, 33*(7), 461–470.

Hoagwood, K., Burns, B. J., Kiser, L., Ringeisen, H., & Schoenwald, S. K. (2014). Evidence-based practice in child and adolescent mental health services. *Psychiatric Services, 52*(9), 1179–1189.

Horner, R. H., Carr, E. G., Halle, J., McGee, G., Odom, S., & Wolery, M. (2005). The use of single-subject research to identify evidence-based practice in special education. *Exceptional Children, 71*(2), 165–179.

Hutchings, J., Bywater, T., Daley, D., Gardner, F., Whitaker, C., Jones, K., . . . & Edwards, R. T. (2007). Parenting intervention in Sure Start services for children at risk of developing conduct disorder: pragmatic randomised controlled trial. *BMJ, 334*(7595), 678–685.

Kazdin, A. E. (2015). Clinical dysfunction and psychosocial interventions: The interplay of research, methods, and conceptualization of challenges. *Annual Review of Clinical Psychology, 11*, 1–2.28.

Klein Velderman, M., Bakermans-Kranenburg, M. J., Juffer, F., & van IJzendoorn, M. H. (2006). Effects of attachment-based interventions on maternal sensitivity and infant attachment: Differential susceptibility of highly reactive infants. *Journal of Family Psychology, 20*(2), 266–274.

Kraemer, H. C., Wilson, G. T., Fairburn, C. G., & Agras, W. S. (2002). Mediators and moderators of treatment effects in randomized clinical trials. *Archives of General Psychiatry, 59*(10), 877–883.

Larsson, B., Fossum, S., Clifford, G., Drugli, M. B., Handegård, B. H., & Mørch, W. T. (2009). Treatment of oppositional defiant and conduct problems in young Norwegian children. *European Child & Adolescent Psychiatry, 18*(1), 42–52.

Lavigne, J. V., LeBailly, S. A., Gouze, K. R., Cicchetti, C., Pochyly, J., Arend, R., . . . & Binns, H. J. (2008). Treating oppositional defiant disorder in primary care: a comparison of three models. *Journal of Pediatric Psychology, 33*(5), 449–461.

Lebovici, S. (1999). The genesis of mental representations. In P. Fonagy, A. M. Cooper, & R. S. Wallerstein (Eds.), *Psychoanalysis on the move: The work of Joseph Sandler* (pp. 75–86). New York, NY: Routledge.

Lenze, S. N., Pautsch, J., & Luby, J. (2011). Parent-child interaction therapy emotion development: A novel treatment for depression in preschool children. *Depression and Anxiety, 28*(2), 153–159.

Leung, C., Tsang, S., Heung, K., & Yiu, I. (2008). Effectiveness of parent-child interaction therapy (PCIT) among Chinese families. *Research on Social Work Practice, 19*(3), 304–313.

Lieberman, A. F., & Pawl, J. H. (1993). Infant–parent psychotherapy. In C. H. Zeanah Jr. (Ed.), *Handbook of infant mental health* (pp. 427–442). New York, NY: Guilford Press.

Lieberman, A. F., Silverman, R., & Pawl, J. H. (2000). Infant-parent psychotherapy: Core concepts and current approaches. In C. Zeanah (Ed.), *Handbook of infant mental health* (2nd ed., pp. 472–484). New York, NY: Basic Books.

Lieberman, A. F., & Van Horn, P. (1998). Attachment, trauma, and domestic violence: Implications for child custody. *Child and Adolescent Psychiatric Clinics of North America, 7*(2), 423–443.

Lieberman, A. F., & Van Horn, P. (2011). *Psychotherapy with infants and young children: Repairing the effects of stress and trauma on early attachment*. New York, NY: Guilford Press.

Lieberman, A. F., Van Horn, P., & Ghosh Ippen, C. (2005). Toward evidence-based treatment: Child-parent psychotherapy with preschoolers exposed to marital violence. *Journal of the American Academy of Child & Adolescent Psychiatry, 44*(12), 1241–1248.

Ludwig, J., & Miller, D. L. (2005). Does Head Start improve children's life chances? Evidence from a regression discontinuity design. *The Quarterly Journal of Economics, 122*(1), 159–208.

Marcon, R. A. (2002). Moving up the grades: Relationship between preschool model and later school success. *Early Childhood Research and Practice, 4*(1), 2–22.

McCabe, K., & Yeh, M. (2009). Parent-child interaction therapy for Mexican Americans: A randomized clinical trial. *Journal of Clinical Child & Adolescent Psychology, 38*(5), 753–759.

McDonough, S. (2004). Interaction guidance. In A. J. Sameroff, S. C. McDonough, & K. Rosenblum (Eds.), *Treating parent-infant relationship problems: Strategies for intervention* (pp. 79–86). New York, NY: Guilford Press.

McDonough, S. C. (2000). Interaction guidance: An approach for difficult-to-engage families. In C. R. Zeanah (Ed.), *Handbook of infant mental health* (2nd ed., pp. 485–493). New York, NY: Basic Books.

Moss, E., Dubois-Comtois, K., Cyr, C., Tarabulsy, G. M., St-Laurent, D., & Bernier, A. (2011). Efficacy of a home-visiting intervention aimed at improving maternal sensitivity, child attachment, and behavioral outcomes for maltreated children: A randomized control trial. *Development and Psychopathology, 23*(01), 195–210.

Nixon, R. D., Sweeney, L., Erickson, D. B., & Touyz, S. W. (2004). Parent-child interaction therapy: One-and two-year follow-up of standard and abbreviated treatments for oppositional preschoolers. *Journal of Abnormal Child Psychology, 32*(3), 263–271.

Olds, D. L. (2006). The nurse-family partnership: An evidence-based preventive intervention. *Infant Mental Health Journal, 27*(1), 5–25.

Olds, D. L. (2007). Programs for parents of infants and toddlers: Recent evidence from randomized trials. *Journal of Child Psychology and Psychiatry, 48*, 355–391.

Patterson, G. R. (1982). *Coercive family process* (Vol. 3). Kouvola, Finland: Castalia Publishing Company.

Raaijmakers, M. A., Smidts, D. P., Sergeant, J. A., Maassen, G. H., Posthumus, J. A., Van Engeland, H., & Matthys, W. (2008). Executive functions in preschool children with aggressive behavior: impairments in inhibitory control. *Journal of Abnormal Child Psychology, 36* (7), 1097–1107.

Reid, M. J., Webster-Stratton, C., & Beauchaine, T. P. (2001). Parent training in Head Start: A comparison of program response among African American, Asian American, Caucasian, and Hispanic mothers. *Prevention Science, 2*(4), 209–227.

Reid, M. J., Webster-Stratton, C., & Hammond, M. (2003). Follow-up of children who received the Incredible Years intervention for oppositional-defiant disorder: Maintenance and prediction of 2-year outcome. *Behavior Therapy, 34*(4), 471–491.

Reid, M. J., Webster-Stratton, C., & Hammond, M. (2007). Enhancing a classroom social competence and problem-solving curriculum by offering parent training to families of moderate-to high-risk elementary school children. *Journal of Clinical Child and Adolescent Psychology, 36*(4), 605–620.

Sameroff, A. J., & Fiese, B. H. (2000). Transactional regulation: The developmental ecology of early intervention. In J. P. Shonkoff & S. J. Meisels (Eds.), *Handbook of early childhood intervention* (pp. 135–159). New York, NY: Cambridge University Press.

Scott, S., Sylva, K., Doolan, M., Price, J., Jacobs, B., Crook, C., & Landau, S. (2010). Randomised controlled trial of parent groups for child antisocial behaviour targeting multiple risk factors: the SPOKES project. *Journal of Child Psychology and Psychiatry, 51*(1), 48–57.

Scott, S., Webster-Stratton, C., Spender, Q., Doolan, M., Jacobs, B., & Aspland, H. (2001). Multicentre controlled trial of parenting groups for childhood antisocial behaviour in clinical practice: Commentary: Nipping conduct problems in the bud. *British Medical Journal, 323* (7306), 194–200.

Snell-Johns, J., Mendez, J., & Smith, B. (2004). Evidence-based solutions for overcoming access barriers, decreasing attrition, and promoting change with underserved families. *Journal of Family Psychology, 18*, 19–35.

Thomas, R., & Zimmer-Gembeck, M. J. (2007). Behavioral outcomes of parent-child interaction therapy and triple P – Positive parenting program: A review and meta-analysis. *Journal of Abnormal Child Psychology, 35*(3), 475–495.

Toth, S. L., Maughan, A., Manly, J. T., Spagnola, M., & Cicchetti, D. (2002). The relative efficacy of two interventions in altering maltreated preschool children's representation models: Implications for attachment theory. *Development and Psychopathology, 14*, 877–908.

Webster-Stratton, C. (2003). The Incredible Years: parent, teacher, and child training series (IYS). In *Preventing violence and related health-risking social behaviors in adolescents: An NIH State-of-the-science conference* (pp. 73–77). https://consensus.nih.gov/2004/2004youthviolencepreventionsos023program.pdf#page=77

Webster-Stratton, C. (2006). The incredible years: A trouble-shooting guide for parents of children aged 2–8 years. *Incredible Years.*

Webster-Stratton, C. (1990). Long-term follow-up of families with young conduct problem children: From preschool to grade school. *Journal of Clinical Child Psychology, 19*, 144–149.

Webster-Stratton, C. (1998). Preventing conduct problems in head start children: Strengthening parent competencies. *Journal of Consulting and Clinical Psychology, 66*(5), 715–730.

Webster-Stratton, C. (2000). *The incredible years training series.* Washington, DC: US Department of Justice, Office of Justice Programs, Office of Juvenile Justice and Delinquency Prevention.

Webster-Stratton, C., & Mihalic, S. F. (2001). *The incredible years: Parent, teacher and child training series.* Boulder, CO: Center for the Study and Prevention of Violence, Institute of Behavioral Science, University of Colorado at Boulder.

Webster-Stratton, C., & Reid, M. J. (2004). Strengthening social and emotional competence in young children and the foundation for early school readiness and success: Incredible years classroom social skills and problem-solving curriculum. *Infants & Young Children, 17*(2), 96–113.

Webster-Stratton, C., & Reid, M. (2010). Adapting the Incredible Years, an evidence-based parenting programme, for families involved in the child welfare system. *Journal of Children's Services, 5*(1), 25–42.

Webster-Stratton, C., Reid, J. M., & Stoolmiller, M. (2008). Preventing conduct problems and improving school readiness: Evaluation of the Incredible Years teacher and child training programs in high-risk schools. *Journal of Child Psychology and Psychiatry, 49*(5), 471–488.

Webster-Stratton, C., Rinaldi, J., & Reid, J. M. (2011). Long-term outcomes of Incredible Years Parenting Program: Predictors of adolescent adjustment. *Child and Adolescent Mental Health, 16*(1), 38–46.

Chapter 10
Early Childhood Mental Health Consultation

Introduction

Manyinfants and young children spend numerous hours daily in child care facilities, where they are cared for by adults other than their parents. The backgrounds and knowledge bases of care providers in these facilities are varied and often the programs are unsupervised. Some care providers hold graduate degrees in early childhood studies or in child development, while others have no formal training in the field. Similarly, some providers have acquired years of experience, while others are at the outset of their professional development. Caregivers are responsible for all the children in their care, and provide for their developmental, emotional and social needs as well as basic nurturance. Invariably, the group of children will include a number of children at risk for adverse social emotional outcomes resulting from exposure to socio-emotional stressors (see chapter 5), while some children may already have received a diagnosis of some developmental disorder or have been identified as having special needs. As a result, daycare providers are expected to cope with potentially disruptive and challenging behaviors, which are occurring more frequently and at a younger age than previously (e.g., Fox, Henderson, Marshall, Nichols, & Ghera, 2005), developmental problems requiring individual care and familial conditions (including parental mental illness or incarceration), as well as poverty and exposure to violence or trauma.

Even caregivers with academic training or many years of experience may feel ill-equipped to address such complex issues. The level and intensity of some of these concerns, specifically the disruptive behavior problems encountered in the classroom, are often the basis for expulsion, even of very young children. According to Gilliam (2005), the best way to reduce expulsion is to ensure that daycare providers have access to a mental health consultant with expertise in the social emotional development of the young child.

C. Shulman, *Research and Practice in Infant and Early Childhood Mental Health*, Children's Well-Being: Indicators and Research 13,
DOI 10.1007/978-3-319-31181-4_10

Issues to be Considered in Mental Health Consultation in Early Childhood

Mental health consultation in early childhood settings is a problem-solving and capacity-building intervention implemented through a collaborative relationship between a professional consultant with mental health expertise and one or more individuals directly involved with the child. These people may be staff members at a child care center, other service providers and/or family members, each having his or her expertise and knowledge of the child and of child development. Early childhood mental health consultation emphasizes the importance of the quality of the young child's social and emotional environments as well as addressing the needs of the individual child. The goals of early childhood mental health consultation include strengthening the capacity of child care staff, families and systems to promote positive social and emotional development as well as to "prevent, identify, treat, and reduce the impact of mental health problems among children from birth to 6 years of age and their families" (Kaufmann, Perry, Hepburn, & Duran, 2012, p. 6).

The role of the consultant is not to assume total responsibility for particular problems, but rather to support the child care staff in their daily challenges. The consultant can fulfill this function by helping the staff to understand the mental health perspective and incorporate it into their work. The consultant can apply assorted techniques, such as fostering optimal development in each child, observing the day care center or home climate, examining relationships in the classroom and assessing the appropriateness of activities for each child, and thus promoting learning and social emotional development. By building relationships with the child care staff and with the parents, consultants recognize the importance of the environmental systems within which the infant or child develops and functions.

Early childhood mental health consultants enter the field from a variety of professional backgrounds. In addition to the unique needs of the setting and the population, the consultant's discipline (e.g., social work, psychology, psychiatry, special education or counselling), orientation, training, professional and life experience all contribute to the ways in which the consultant will define and prioritize his or her work (Steier, 2013). For example, a child or developmental psychologist who focuses on children's strengths and weaknesses will request a developmental evaluation to understand a particular child's unique developmental profile in order to guide intervention decisions. A mental health consultant with a background in family therapy, however, may spend more time on parent education and training. Although there is no one accepted method of consultation in early childhood, a consensus regarding the consultative model does exist and will be presented in this chapter. Discussion of the consultative setting, the consultative relationship, consultative skills and the importance of reflective practice, problem-solving and capacity-building in early childhood consultation will follow. Lastly, research findings supporting this model, as well as ethical issues and challenges to the implementation of the consultative model in early childhood, will be considered.

Early childhood mental health consultation has not yet been formally incorporated into the early childhood care system, although it is part of the Head Start program, as this program's performance standards require programs to incorporate the services of mental health professionals in order to enable the timely and effective identification of and intervention in family and staff concerns about a child's mental health (Head Start Performance Standards and Other Regulations, 45 CFR Part 1304.24.2). Aside from the Head Start programs, only a few states, including Maryland, Connecticut, and Michigan, have statewide consultation programs. In the Unites States, consultation programs serve limited geographic areas or service specific targeted populations, at best (Gilliam & Shahar, 2006; Johnston & Brinamen, 2006).

The issues which can be addressed through early childhood mental health consultation include promoting nurturing interactions and promoting interventions which are needed in order to help teachers manage challenging behaviors in appropriate ways (Brinamen, Taranta, & Johnston, 2012). Approximately 20 % of preschoolers have some type of emotional or behavioral problem, some of which will recede without intervention as the child matures. Approximately half of these children, however, will carry persistent problems into later childhood or adolescence (Campbell, 1995; Lavigne et al., 2008). Less experienced teachers and teachers who cope with more psychosocial stressors tended to be less effective in their behavior management strategies (Li Grining et al., 2010). Children in their classrooms exhibited poorer quality social interactions. The challenge that these behaviors pose for teachers is illuminated by the number of young children who are expelled from their educational placement. Gilliam (2005) reported that in almost 4000 state-funded classes randomly selected across the nation, 10.4 % of preschool teachers reported at least one expulsion in their classroom over the past 12 months. In a follow-up study (Gilliam, 2008) it appears that the rates are considerably higher in the less-regulated private frameworks than in state-supported preschool programs.

Because early childhood mental health consultation is not clearly defined, there is great variety in existing early childhood mental health consultation programs, including differences in the array of services offered, the background and abilities of the consultants and the roles they fulfill. It is not clear who receives consultative service or how long the consultation should be. Duran et al. (2009) surveyed several states and conducted a cross-site analysis of effectiveness of early childhood mental health consultation programs, delineating the variations in practice. There is a need to explore the mechanisms of early childhood mental health consultation programs, to identify the effects of specific components of early childhood mental health consultation programs on teachers and child outcomes, and to understand how much consultation is needed to produce good outcomes.

Virmani, Masyn, Thompson, Conners-Burrow, and Whiteside Mansell (2013) used data collected in an evaluation of early childhood mental health consultation programs in Head Start and state funded pre-kindergarten programs to examine the relationship between the consist nature of (e.g. regularity) and the frequency of consultation, as well as the approach to consultation and changes in teacher-child interactions. Outcome measures were defined as changes in teacher-child interactions, measured using the Caregiver Interaction Scale (CIS: Arnett, 1989), and results suggested that the regularity with which teachers and consultants met in order to discuss children, their families, and teacher issues was associated with gains in quality of teacher-child interaction. They also investigated the operationalization of the consultative approach at each site and found that improvements in interactions were more likely when consultants offered teachers information about age-appropriate abilities, needs and feelings related to the child's behavior and information about resources and services for children.

Green, Everhart, Gordon, and Gettment (2006) surveyed 655 Head Start directors, staff members and mental health consultants in an effort to determine what makes consultation effective from the perspective of the recipient. Results suggested that the ability of a mental health consultant to build positive collaborative relationships with early childhood staff members was seen as the most important factor leading to the success of early childhood mental health consultation. In addition, responders reported that consultants who provided more frequent services tended to have more positive relationships with early childhood staff members, suggesting that both the frequency with which the consultant appeared at the program and the skills of the consultant in developing relationships are at the foundation of early childhood mental health consultation success. From these research findings it seems that there is a consensus that frequent meetings between the consultant and the care provider are central to success, but the consultative model is still not clearly defined and the differences between sites often make it seem as if there is no real model of early childhood mental health consultation. Yet there is a model of early childhood mental health consultation which is being implemented and evaluated (Johnston & Brinamen, 2006; Virmani et al., 2013).

The Consultative Model and Its Principles

The consultative model is based on providing support to young children through consultation with the adults who are responsible for their care, thereby promoting the children's social and emotional wellbeing. Most of the principles of a consultative model are consistent across settings but can vary on the basis of factors such as the population served, the type of setting or agency, the vision or mission of each program, and the extent to which the consultant will be available. These principles are formulated for early childhood settings but they can be applied in other programs, as they would be consistent with such programs as home visiting programs, primary care agencies and homeless shelters, where the consultative model is particularly suitable for enabling adults to support young children.

Optimally, a consultant will begin his or her relationship with a program by clarifying the philosophy of the program and the purpose of the consultation, preferably with the involvement of the principal or director of the program. This clarification can result in a review of the scope of expected services. Next, the consultant may spend time with the families, children and staff members so as to get acquainted with the community where the program operates. After the orientation phase, it is important to negotiate and establish mutual expectations regarding duration, intensity and frequency of consultation, and to define specific areas of responsibility, methodology and focus. Practical considerations, such as meeting schedules, information transfer and methods of prioritizing crises or new concerns also need to be addressed. Afterwards, observation in the classroom and other settings can begin, followed by one-on-one consultations with various colleagues, family members and community representatives, when appropriate. After mapping the situation, the consultant can identify and prioritize immediate needs and determine how to reduce the identified pressing issues.

When using systematic instruments for data collection to identify problems and understand contextual influences, it is important to focus on the strengths of the child, the staff and the program. By beginning with short-term problem-solving, the consultant can model collaboration with and respect for parents and staff and launch a long-term partnership with the goal of selecting culturally competent, effective and feasible strategies. It is imperative at this stage to define operational goals and to enumerate the steps to attain them and, in parallel, to identify informal and formal indicators of success.

A variety of factors contribute to choosing the best intervention for addressing a particular issue. These include the specific goals of mental health consultation, the nature of the issues and concerns, the setting, the availability of mental health practitioners and other experts, the time frame and the cost. In addition, placing these goals and steps within a time line makes the intervention plan more attainable. Implementation will begin with distinctly defined activities, notification of the program director and discussion about the implementation. During the implementation stage, it is imperative to model effective strategies and to provide supplementary materials. After assessing the recommended strategies, the consultant will provide support and coaching, monitor progress and give consistent and frequent feedback. Both professionals and family members are vital to this stage, which assesses whether the intervention is meeting the stated needs and evaluates the proposed outcomes and indicators for examining success.

To strengthen the collaborative relationship, it will be important to identify further sources of support outside the specific educational program which may be able to address the mental health needs of the child, family and staff. If necessary, the consultant may make a referral for further consultation or complementary services for the child or his family. The program should be revisited regularly and all members of the team who will consider new strategies and intervention plans must be updated often. Complete documentation and frequent meetings can assist in these evaluative processes, which can address changes not only in the child or program but also in the consultative relationship. Periodic review is integral to the process of identifying the necessary supports for maintaining behavioral changes in staff, child, program or family and is also part of the ongoing review of strengths, and needs to be addressed through the consultative model (Dougherty, 2013; Duran et al., 2009).

The Consultation Setting

Early childhood mental health consultation is now expanding into new settings with new models that serve infants, young children and their families. Traditionally, consultation was performed in day care facilities and focused on the child or on the program and was implemented according to various models. Today these models of intervention are often combined. It is also possible to apply the principles of early childhood mental health consultation in the home setting and in other early childhood care systems such as child welfare, although these applications can be challenging.

Child-centered consultation focuses on the needs of a specific child in the classroom. This is the classic form of early childhood mental health consultation, where staff members are concerned, alarmed or frustrated about a particular child's behavior and request help from the mental health consultant. The primary goal of this type of consultation is to develop a plan to address the factors contributing to the child's difficulties in functioning well in his or her child care setting and to include the family in the intervention plan. Case consultation about individual children who exhibit difficult behaviors is not always sufficient to solve behavioral or emotional problems. Additional services for caregivers, such as therapeutic groups which help professionals to cope with the challenges of caring for children with behavior problems, may complement the consultation (Watson & Gatti, 2012). Another option entails weekly consultations with parents and staff to enhance parental understanding and build collaborations, which can also be generalized to the day care staff. When necessary, it might be appropriate to refer some parents to other community-based mental health support services (Gilkerson, 2004).

The goal of child-centered early childhood consultation is twofold: to reduce the impact of challenging classroom behavior by a particular child and to facilitate staff engagement with that child in ways that will improve his or her behavior. By collaborating with the child, the teacher and caregiver and other staff members, the consultant helps to develop techniques and strategies which will support the child's positive behavior, promote his or her development and support staff engagement (Green et al., 2006).

Consultation may include assessment or referral in addition to working with on-site staff. In order to understand the child's presenting behaviors and determine intervention strategies which will best support his or her development, the consultant will need to observe the child in the classroom and gather information from a variety of sources, including parents, welfare workers, and other therapists involved in the child's care. The consultant will need to partner with the teachers and parents to design and implement an intervention program, possibly including a behavior management component. Consultants may recommend additional strategies beyond those offered in the day care center and may refer the child to a specialist, such as a speech and language pathologist or a community mental health professional, to address identified issues or issues which still need to be clarified. Clearly, parental consent must be obtained before embarking on consultation with an individual child. Often, consultation regarding a particular child promotes the healthy emotional development of other children in the program, as interventions applied to one child may be generalizable to others and may affect the program as a whole.

Program-centeredconsultation focuses on the program as a self-contained entity and is therefore broader in scope than child-centered consultation. In this context, the consultant aims to determine how program-specific factors affect the social and emotional development of participating children and how the overall quality of the program can be improved. The consultant may be asked to assist with specific concerns about social interactions with a particular teacher or group of children, with time management, with staging of activities and its effect on children's behavior and with approaches to the physical environment which can nurture overall mental health goals in early childhood. The primary goal is to improve the overall quality of the program (Alkon, Ramler, & McLennan, 2003) by assisting the staff to develop the ability to cope with problematic behavior through programmatic change (Green et al., 2006). Consultation to programs is often based on a preventative model which addresses problems by improving overall quality of care, advancing staff development strategies, enhancing children's social and emotional development and supporting optimal family functioning.

In programmatic consultation, facilitation of the program's success is aimed at developing a mental health approach in strengthening the quality of the program, by means such as establishing a staff development plan. In addition, opportunities for discussion of staff concerns are incorporated into the program in order to address possible work-related stress and work or workplace conflict, thus providing the staff with options for identifying and examining their relationships toward the children with whom they work and their families. Most early childhood mental health consultation programs use a combination of child- and program- centered approaches, including models in which the consultant observes the child in the center and focuses on the specific issues that the staff have raised, as well as incorporating some programmatic changes from which all the children in the program will benefit.

The Adult Client

Although the consultant is contacted regarding a child's problematic behavior or a programmatic difficulty, the consultation is usually conducted with the child's adult care providers who have diverse characteristics, various needs, diverse and distinct motivations and unique life experiences. In order to establish the consultative relationship between the consultant and the caregiver who requested the consultation, it is imperative that the consultant shows respect and empathizes with the caregiver, yet at the same time attempts to motivate him or her to improve the level or type of social emotional support offered to the child.

Increasing the caregiver's comprehension of children and of effective ways of facilitating healthy emotional development improves the overall level of childcare in a program, as well as the caregiver's feeling of competence in fulfilling his or her role (Alkon et al., 2003). Consultation should therefore focus on recognizing the caregiver's existing skills and on increasing his or her knowledge, on addressing teacher needs and on providing support in managing the challenging behavior of specific children. The kinds of skills and knowledge that caregivers have can vary greatly in a field comprised of novice and veteran caregivers, and consisting of staff members with graduate degrees alongside those lacking any degree. At best, the consultant discovers each person's needs and aspirations through attentive observation and discussion about private concerns and experiences. Capacities that need to be boosted may include successful management of classroom transitions, the impact of tone of voice on children's behavior and modeling intervention techniques.

The Consultant

Professionals from many disciplines may become consultants, although most frequently they come from child psychiatry, clinical psychology, clinical social work, marriage and family counseling and psychiatric nursing. Regardless of the consultant's original profession, his or her area of expertise must be rooted in a comprehensive knowledge of child development milestones and the underlying concepts of the young child's social emotional development and behavior, including the centrality of attachment theory (Rolfe, 2004) and the significance of relationships for the developing infant.

The consultant should have highly-honed observation, listening, interviewing and assessment skills, familiarity with the principles of adult learning and the competence to work with adults. Because of the diversity in the population of young children needing mental health consultation services and the environments in which they live, the consultant must be sensitive to the community's strengths and attitudes, including possible resistance to mental health services. Sometimes the consultant will need to employ alternative intervention strategies which might include short-term behavioral intervention. At other times, in-depth work in developing the relationship between the child and the caregivers and/or parents is the central emphasis of the consultation.

The child's relationship with his or her parents and with the caregivers in the educational program can be assessed by observing the child's response to separation from primary caregivers at morning drop-off at the child care program and to whom the child turns for comfort if necessary as the parents or primary caregivers leave. Likewise, observing how the child and home caregivers reunite at the end of the day provides keys to understanding the nature and quality of their interactions. The importance of relationships for the developing infant is at the forefront of early child mental health, and one of the important areas of the consultant's work is to help the staff and parents to understand the myriad of ways in which relationships shape development. This is only one example of the significance of mental health concepts, philosophy and activities which must be integrated into group settings.

In some situations, it will be necessary to distinguish between resistance to consultation and culturally appropriate behavior, as many immigrant cultures do not subscribe to Western culture's philosophy regarding psychological assistance. For example, many Hispanic immigrants in the United States will turn to their extended family for both support and guidance rather than follow through on a referral for consultation (Vega & Lopez, 2001). In addition, an understanding of family systems and the dynamics of the particular child care facility is vital. By recognizing family and staff differences and smoothing the communication between diverse perspectives, the consultant can enable all involved parties to feel validated and understood.

The consultant must also have specialized knowledge and experience regarding specific topics of concern to the staff and family members (e.g., developmental or mental health disorders, failure to thrive and low-weight infants and aggressive behavior), the ability to work with varied sub-groups (e.g., fathers who are less involved, adolescent mothers, cohabiting unmarried parents, parents with less than a high school education, joint custody parents), and states of emotional health (e.g., postpartum depression, bereavement and trauma), as well as social issues of substance abuse, violence and poverty. These areas are often stressors in the life of the child, the family or the community where the program is functioning and are often identified as a top priority to be addressed. Sometimes the caregiver is also experiencing similar stressors in her life, particularly if she lives in the same community or comes from a similar culture. This list is not exhaustive, but points to the necessity of possessing appropriate professional skills.

The consultation process is only productive in bringing about change when the staff believes that the consultant appreciates the problem, perceives the need for action and provides support for carrying out the proposed changes. The effective consultant not only has to have expertise in a particular content area but will also have the interpersonal skills to motivate staff to take action. When the consultant is interpersonally warm and sensitive, the staff member and the family feel attended to and believe that the consultant is committed and caring. This is the first step toward establishing the collaborative relationship which is the foundation of the consultative model. The consultant's ability to be empathic and to understand the staff member's subjective experience allows the staff or family member to trust the consultant and believe that their message has been conveyed and heard. The ability to suspend judgment and to communicate to the staff member that he or she is valued stems from a respectful stance which avoids the position of the expert and instead stresses the mutuality of endeavor (Steier, 2013).

The integration of these areas allows early childhood mental health consultants to build on an existing foundation, incorporating a position of alignment with promotion, prevention and intervention with young children and their caregivers. The consultant's aim is to transform the manner in which early care providers think and feel about the children they care for and how they think about themselves as professionals. The consultant can actively encourage staff to consider the role they play in the lives of the children in their care, especially how their actions contribute to the development of the children's social competence and emotional regulation (Cohen & Kaufmann, 2000). The importance of the consultant being familiar with practical aspects of group care and its impact on children's development and being able to make a clear distinction between consultation and treatment is crucial to success in the early childhood consultative model.

A mental health consultant can be an invaluable resource for supporting caregivers in an educational setting in developing and maintaining classroom environments that promote social and emotional development. This is critical, as preschool children who develop social skills and good emotional regulation are more prepared for elementary school and more likely to succeed throughout their early school years (Bowman, Donovan, & Bums, 2000; Domitrovich, Moore, & Greenberg, 2012; Shonkoff & Philips, 2000). Moreover, social and emotional competence have been associated with more positive peer and teacher relationships (LaFreniere & Sroufe, 1985) and less aggressive behavior (Denham et al., 2002; Lemerise & Arsenio, 2000). Having access to early childhood mental health consultation helps early childhood educators identify problems sooner and develop suitable skills prior to the occurrence of serious problems or expulsion (Gilliam, 2005).

The Consultative Relationship

The ways that consultants approach their work can transcend the setting to provide caregivers with a sense of direction and a mechanism they can trust and through which services can be delivered. Consultants must not underestimate the importance of relationship-building with the caregivers and families with whom they work, as the consultant's relationship with center staff can be seen as a catalyst for changes which may occur (Duran et al., 2009). In order to establish a collaborative relationship it must be clear that the consultant and the early childhood care provider are each skillful in their distinct fields and that the consultant has no authority over the staff members, who are free to accept the consultant's suggestions or not. It is important, yet albeit time consuming, to establish a productive working relationship. Trust and mutual respect lie at the core of the consultative model, enabling two professionals to discuss issues despite differences of opinion and varying perspectives. Once a level of comfort, trust and mutual respect has been achieved, caregivers can safely acknowledge areas in need of improvement, while identifying ways to continually adjust their own program and pursue their own professional growth. Accordingly, by forming and modeling a non-judgmental relationship and a partnership with caregivers, teachers and families it is hoped that all those parties will in turn form positive relationships between themselves.

Virmani et al. (2013) focus on several areas of competence which support the consultative relationship. The "magical moment of connection" (Goodson, Mackrain, Perry, O'Brien, & Gwaltney, 2013) may occur between the consultant and a child, care provider, family member or other member of the team, with the understanding that additional levels of relationship are an outgrowth of the initial connection. Consensus has been attained regarding the ten key elements of the consultative stance, which set the stage for collaborative relationship-based work between the consultant and the caregiver professional.

The ten elements of the collaborative consultative relationship which are the source of viable change are: (1) establishing mutuality of endeavor; (2) emphasizing centrality of relationships; (3) understanding parallel process as an organizing principle; (4) being patient; (5) accepting consideration of all levels of influence; (6) having awareness of all voices (especially the child's) and being able to represent each; (7) avoiding the position of expert; (8) wondering instead of knowing; (9) feeling empathy towards another's subjective experience; and (10) holding out hope. Adults need to feel understood, be respected and be able to understand and anticipate the needs of children in their care. These domains of competence are at the heart of the reciprocity which characterizes the childcare and consultative relationship.

As stated above, central to establishing a consultative relationship is avoidance of the expert or teacher mode, and operating instead in a collaborative mode with staff members whenever looking for creative solutions. The consultant strives to become a partner who brings expertise in infant mental health to the relationship, while being open to and respectful of the existing staff's expertise. By the time the consultant enters a child care program or is invited to address difficulties, an entrenched history has developed among the staff, possibly based on misinterpretation and false assumptions. The consultant must address these issues within the relationship, and begin by working out misinterpretations of staff actions.

In order to address these issues and to build a collaborative relationship, the consultant encourages open, empathic communication, based on active and supportive listening. It may be helpful to set aside time for fixed forums of communication, such as staff meetings, during which it is important to have amicable interactions despite the reality that issues are typically brought up only after they have become critical. The consultant can help the facility's director to understand that the more the staff feels understood, the more willing they will be to embrace the organization's philosophy.

As staff members begin to respond to the budding relationship with the consultant, the relationship will develop. This relationship-based work (Bertacchi & Norman-Murch, 1999) reinforces respect for the individual, including positive regard towards all people, recognizing both their strengths and vulnerabilities. Respect involves an awareness that people do not always agree and that differences of opinion may move those involved to discover a new solution to the problem. In addition respect brings with it an appreciation of different cultures, perspectives and areas of expertise. Developing respect for the other is a priority in building the consultative relationship, because respect, among other things, is based on being sensitive to the specific context in which the consultation occurs. The staff member and the consultant must understand each other as both influencing and being influenced by their environment. For example, if caregivers are frightened to come to work because their center is located in a violent neighborhood, the consultant must be able to respect the feelings which accompany the caregiver each morning and afternoon as she comes to and leaves work, and to be part of the process of clarifying with the caregiver her feelings for the children in her charge who experience the violence in their community.

The consultant and the caregiver develop a relationship in tandem, which is committed to evolving growth and change. The consultant is committed to promoting the mental health development of young children concurrently with the development and growth of caregivers, families and staff. The relationships of the consultant and staff members are rooted in shared goals for families, children and the program and the on-going process of sharing and communicating goals transpires throughout the consultation, as an outgrowth of this mutuality.

To initiate a productive working relationship, the consultant and staff members discuss the roles that they will take during the consultation. This step ensures that the consultant and the staff members will each have an opportunity to express their preferences and that both understand and agree on the basic parameters of the consultation. At this initial juncture, it is critical for both parties to recognize the importance of a coordinated, non-hierarchical relationship for achieving the mutually agreed-upon goals. When staff members feel that they have something to contribute they are less likely to be passive in developing a solution, to feel threatened or to be reluctant to express disagreement when problem-solving begins.

Heller et al.'s (2011) research revealed that, on the whole, daycare providers reported positive and growthful relationships with consultants, while Green et al. (2006) reported that a positive relationship with a consultant is correlated to positive child outcome variables, as detailed above. The consultants' stance ("way of being"; Johnston & Brinamen, 2006, p. 15) engenders positive relationships and supports the caregiver's ability to perceive the child and his or her behavior patterns, the caregiver's own role in the interaction and the influence of the day care setting.

Consultative Skills

Reflective Practice

The theoretical model of consultation in early childhood is based on the principles of infant mental health and relationship-based practice, which incorporates the capacity for thoughtful consideration of multiple perspectives. Reflective practice is an essential tool for supporting and sustaining the consultative process. Shahmoon-Shanok (2006) defined reflective supervision as "a collaborative relationship for professional growth that improves practice by cherishing strengths and partnering around vulnerabilities to generate growth" (p.8).

In early childhood mental health consultation, reflective supervision aims to create a relational climate between the consultant and supervisor, director and other staff members as well as with the specific caregivers with whom he or she is working. Only when all levels of this relationship are realized will the overall goal of optimizing the effectiveness of the child care program through consultation be accomplished. Fenichel (1992) characterized reflective supervision as a partnership in which the person receiving consultation does not feel alone, is not overwhelmed by uncertainty, and feels safe enough to express his or her thoughts, feelings and reactions. To achieve these goals, three crucial components of reflective supervision must be incorporated into the consultative stance. These are reflection, collaboration and regularity, each of which allows both the professional caregiver and the consultant to learn more about each other as participants in the consultative relationship and about the overall aim of consultative work. This stance helps to build competencies in a nurturing and supportive framework while enhancing the caregiver's ability to meet the needs of the young children, their parents and families with whom he or she is working.

Reflective supervision supports the consultant's ability to develop positive relationships with childcare providers through parallel processes. The consultant listens empathically, communicates with authenticity and builds collaborative relationships, resulting in the care providers responding to the children in their care with increased empathy, warmth and understanding. Reflective practice affords an opportunity for the caregivers to learn new skills. Typically, caregivers have limited opportunities to reflect on their work or to consider their own emotional response to it. Through the reflective relationship, the daycare caregiver learns new social and emotional skills which will help in the development of more meaningful relationships with children, coworkers and families. Thus, through the consultative process, the caregivers become increasingly more reflective and less reactive when coping with the challenges of their profession.

Reflective practice provides a unique opportunity for considering the varying perspectives of all involved parties. The child caregiver becomes aware that he or she has a uniquely informed perspective based on experience, education and personal background. Together, the consultant and the caregiver take the opportunity to reflect on how these perspectives affect the situation and how this enhanced understanding can be used to support positive change. Through reflection, the providers can deconstruct a problematic situation and move forward with deliberation. The key to reflection is slowing down and thinking about specific issues, perspectives and difficulties faced on a daily basis in early childhood settings. It is important to encourage a climate in which it is possible to find time to discuss and elaborate on specific issues. Once a framework for reflection becomes the norm, it becomes possible to address specific problems and attempt to solve them.

Problem-Solving

The collaborative relationship which develops between the consultant and the person working with infants and very young children in day care facilities allows for problem-solving and capacity-building within a specific time period and around particular issues. As stated above, the primary role of the early childhood mental health consultation is to assist staff in addressing concerns and solving problems regarding specific children and/or families or certain elements of the care program. The underlying goal of the consultation is to help staff members to develop enabling attitudes and skills which will help them function more effectively with specific children's issues and respond adeptly to similar issues if they arise in the future. Effective problem-solving involves assessment of the issue, selection of the optimal intervention strategies and implementation of the developed plan. During and after implementation, it is important for the consultant and the day care practitioner to assess the strategy and learn what was accomplished and how to continue to understand problem solving options.

The consultant needs to be flexible in the use of problem-solving strategies and must adapt to the specific features of the case. By flexibly negotiating between programmatic obstacles and child-focused concerns, the consultant begins by receiving permission to observe the child and to initiate the process of information-gathering. In order to observe the child in the day care setting, the consultant must prepare the care providers for his or her presence. In addition, it is important to gather information from different sources, specifically from parents and from providers, and to acknowledge that adults will have varied perspectives about a child. One of the first problems to be solved is that of sharing different views of the child as neutrally as possible, helping the adults unite around the common cause of understanding the child and resolving how to best promote social and emotional development.

To identify the various elements which can help with problem-solving, the consultant can observe the child's way of relating to children and adults in naturally occurring interactions, and likewise observe and interpret the adults' responses to the child's interactional efforts. Identifying helpful and less effective responses to the child can be one way of enhancing the quality of the day care provider-child relationship. Similarly, the consultant can observe the program itself, acknowledging routines, activities, practices and goals as they manifest themselves throughout the day.

After observation, the consultant should reflect on what he or she has observed, since such information only becomes useful when providers incorporate it into their developing understanding of the child and apply it to problem-solving. The consultant can verify that what was observed is typical behavior and determine that enough information has been collected in order to begin problem-solving about issues and possible responses. As the consultant does not possess the caregivers' or teachers' breadth of interaction with the child, his or her knowledge is based on intermittent and anecdotal information and therefore further information will need to be collected from the care providers, who possess a more comprehensive perspective of the child's behavior. The consultant must recognize the need to respond to the caregivers' subjective experience of the child. Helping the caregivers express their concerns and questions in a clear fashion is often a preliminary step to problem-solving about presenting issues. The consultant wants to elicit the provider's current thoughts about the child's behavior and the reasons for that view because the provider's response to behavior is determined by the meaning ascribed to it. To place the child's behavior in context, it is imperative to include his parents in the process and to impart to them that the child's behavior can only be considered meaningfully if it relates to other aspects of the child's experience. Therefore, it is also necessary to gather information from the parents regarding the child's developmental history, relational history, constitutional peculiarities and current functioning outside of the child care setting.

Once equipped with this information, the consultant can begin to problem-solve regarding the identified difficulties of the child or program. Since there will be discrepancies regarding both the existence and the interpretation of behaviors, the consultant must understand that differences in meaning can be attributed to differing adult perceptions of the child and the behavior. The consultant can empathize equally with the parent's and the provider's experiences, and by presenting each group's perception to the other, can begin to problem solve around misperceptions and misinterpretation. This establishes a commonality of purpose and an ability to hold multiple views of the child and the child's behavior throughout the problem-solving phase.

Capacity Building

Early childhood mental health consultation is primarily geared toward capacity building for care providers and teachers. Targeted capacities in early childhood mental health consultation include improving the skills of the staff who work in the program and improving the context and educational strategies which are employed in the program. Programs can be improved through structural issues such as teacher education, lower teacher-child ratios and larger allotment of physical space (Mashburn & Pianta, 2006), each of which influences the emotional climate in the program and the caregivers' and teachers' abilities to build nurturing relationships. In order to build these capacities in the classroom, the early childhood mental health consultant is involved in observations, one-on-one meetings with teachers or supervisors, team meetings, formal and informal exchanges of information, mentoring and coaching. Furthermore, the consultant helps the caregivers develop the ability to operationalize the issues which cause them concern about specific children, and how to observe those children and interpret those observations. These skills will hopefully be applied whenever the caregivers need to observe a problem behavior in the future.

Research Findings

Early childhood mental health consultation has been the subject of research studies in order to assess its treatment efficacy. Policymakers and program managers require empirical studies of the outcomes of early childhood mental health consultation intervention techniques in order to investigate its efficacy and incorporate funding on a statewide level. Evaluation of early childhood mental health consultation intervention is quite complex, and in order to research program effectiveness it is necessary to decide on outcome measures and the method to be used in evaluating the results of early childhood mental health consultation programs.

This complex process is dependent on the relationships established between different people coping with differing issues. Although it is valuable to understand the pathways through which change occurs and what is expected to change, it is not easy to identify and operationalize the variables to be assessed in outcome research. Three review articles (Brennan, Bradley, Allen, & Perry, 2008; Hepburn, Perry, Shivers, & Gilliam, 2013; Perry, Allen, Brennan, & Bradley, 2010) summarize the results of empirical research examining outcomes of the early childhood mental health consultation model.

Evaluative research of the consultation model has focused on assessing the achievement of the early childhood mental health consultation goals and on measured changes in the child, in teacher behavior, and in the classroom environment. In regard to the child in the educational framework, outcome measures encompass decreases in challenging behaviors and increases in prosocial behaviors and positive cognitive growth. Perry, Dunne, McFadden, and Campbell (2008) evaluated a program offering individualized (child-specific) consultation, where pre- and post-tests of children indicated that social skills had improved, problem behavior had decreased and more than 75 % of the 200 children at risk for expulsion were able to remain in their current child care placements. Gilliam (2007) found, in a randomized trial of short-term early childhood mental health consultation, that early childhood mental health consultation had a positive effect on child behaviors expressed within the early childhood classroom setting. General long-term outcome variables focus on enhanced child functioning.

As for the care providers, the target behaviors and personal characteristics which can be modified include attitudes and beliefs, self-efficacy, stress and competence. In addition, the quality of adult-child interactions and the quality of care and emotional climate in the program are other aspects that are being evaluated. Williford and Shelton (2008) found that children whose teachers received individually-based consultation which imparted methods for reducing problem behavior showed a greater reduction in externalizing behaviors post-intervention than did a control group. Teachers in the intervention group also increased their use of appropriate teacher strategies to address problematic behaviors. Raver et al. (2008) found that early childhood mental health consultation led to higher levels of positive classroom climate, teacher sensitivity and behavior management while gender, race, ethnicity and exposure to poverty were moderating factors with regard to the effectiveness of the consultation. Alkon et al. (2003) found that early childhood centers which received mental health consultation services for more than 1 year demonstrated improvements in environmental rating scale scores as well as in teacher self-report self-efficacy and competence. Conners-Burrow, Whiteside-Mansell, McKelvey, Amini-Vermani, and Sockwell (2012) reported that teachers receiving consultation services exhibited greater decreases in permissiveness and detachment as measured by research assistant ratings on the caregiver interaction scale (CIS: Arnett, 1989) as compared to teachers not receiving consultation.

In addition to positive outcomes for the children and for the caregivers, early childhood mental health consultation has been shown to have a positive effect on the program itself. Since the quality of care which the children in a particular day care facility receive has been shown to have an impact on particular children, on intervention techniques and on the emotional climate in the program, effects of early childhood mental health consultation on the framework were also investigated. Mashburn and Pianta (2006) found that among the 2439 4-year-olds enrolled in 617 prekindergarten classrooms, the children who developed better social skills, including prosocial overtures to their peers, the ability to wait for their turn and sharing abilities were those who had higher-quality emotional interactions with their caregivers in the educational setting. In fact, the quality of these interactions was a better predictor of social skills development than were many other factors, including the caregivers' level of education and/or field of study, class size and child-teacher ratio.

In addition, changes in the emotional climate of the preschool program as measured by the use of classroom management strategies which support the healthy social and emotional development of young children also showed improvement in programs in which early childhood mental health consultation was employed. Raver et al. (2008) found more teacher responsiveness and less harshness in early childhood programs which integrated early childhood mental health consultation with other programs such as Incredible Years parent and teacher training series (Webster-Stratton, 2000, 2003, 2006). Cumulative research results are presented in Table 10.1 below.

While mental health consultation has been suggested as an approach which helps teachers develop nurturing relationships with children and manage challenging behaviors, there is still minimal empirical research to support that claim. A meta-analysis of research between 1985 and 2008 (Brennan et al., 2008) revealed that early childhood consultation was significantly related to reduced staff turnover.

Research in early childhood mental health consultation is promising but still in its early stages. The complexity of the model makes it difficult to understand what aspects of the model are the core skills, and it is necessary to continue to search for a way to assess the parceling of effects of the various components of the model. Reports from the field make it clear that the success of the early childhood mental health consultation model is dependent on the establishment of good relationships between the consultant and the staff, and between the child's family and the program. Just as in early childhood itself, relationships provide the basis for development in the context of a supportive, respectful and nurturing environment.

Table 10.1 Impact of early childhood mental health consultation

Impact on child	Impact on caregiver	Impact on program
Decrease in expulsion or risk for expulsion	Increase in self-efficacy	Increase in positive interactions
Decrease in externalizing and internalizing behaviors	Increase in sense of competence	Decrease in negative interactions
Increase in prosocial behaviors and social skills	Decrease in job-related stress	Increase in teacher sensitivity
	Reduction in staff turnover	Increase in teacher classroom management skills

Virmani et al. (2013)

One of the most important roles of the consultant is to be a catalyst, supporter and participant in the ongoing, dynamic process of finding the best in every adult who cares for children and the best in every child to whom providers give their time, energy and considerable care. It is essential to develop better research designs that align with common frameworks and measurement approaches, which would lead to a more unified and efficient manner of assessing the evidence base for implementing early childhood mental health consultation models. With further collaboration among research partners and more rigorous research practice, efficacy can be enhanced and long-term sustainability can be established.

Challenges in Early Childhood Mental Health Consultation

Early childhood mental health consultation has been proven to positively affect children, caregivers and caregiver-child relationships, but there has been less research in the area of early childhood mental health consultation with parents. It must be noted that working with young children, particularly those whose behavior is quite challenging, may evoke complex emotions among staff and parents. These emotions are at the foundation of some of the difficulties in the ways that adults respond to challenging behavior of young children. Finding those ways which support the child and the relationship between the child and the caregiver is one of the main challenges in the early mental health consultative model (Johnston & Brinamen, 2006).

Despite the benefits, many challenges arise when implementing early childhood mental health consultation. For example, confusion regarding the specifics of what a consultant does often leads to problems in defining areas of responsibility (Duran et. al., 2009). Caregivers and teachers are unsure about the role of the consultant and presume that he or she will provide traditional direct therapeutic services to children and families, rather than offering more broad-based support and guidance. On the other hand, a consultant may arrive imagining he or she will address a particular issue only to find that other issues need to be addressed first in order to establish a relationship with the caregiver, teacher, director or parent. In hierarchical care systems, open communication may not be fostered and it may be difficult to achieve understanding between administrators, supervisors, consultants and direct care providers. In order to enhance mental health consultation in early childhood more resources need to be allocated and areas of responsibility and goals need to be clarified. Consultants must focus on supporting caregivers and teachers as they implement new practices and guide them as they assist children in adapting to these changes. Change is often a process that occurs over time and requires skill and patience to initiate and maintain, but once changes have been implemented it is important that the consultant help caregivers, teachers and parents to note the small but significant changes that occur over the course of the consultative relationship.

References

Alkon, A., Ramler, M., & MacLennan, K. (2003). Evaluation of mental health consultation in child care centers. *Early Childhood Education Journal, 31*(2), 91–99.

Arnett, J. (1989). Caregivers in day-care centers: Does training matter? *Journal of Applied Developmental Psychology, 10*(4), 541–552.

Bertacchi, J., & Norman-Murch, T. (1999). Implementing reflective supervision in non-clinical settings: Challenges to practice. *Zero to Three, 20*(1), 18–23.

Bowman, S., Donovan, D., & Bums, M. (2000). *Eager to learn: Educating our preschoolers.* Washington, DC: National Academy Press.

Brennan, E. M., Bradley, J. R., Allen, M. D., & Perry, D. F. (2008). The evidence base for mental health consultation in early childhood settings: Research synthesis addressing staff and program outcomes. *Early Education and Development, 19*(6), 982–1022.

Brinamen, C. F., Taranta, A. N., & Johnston, K. (2012). Expanding early childhood mental health consultation to new venues: Serving infants and young children in domestic violence and homeless shelters. *Infant Mental Health Journal, 33*(3), 283–293.

Campbell, S. B. (1995). Behavior problems in preschool children: A review of recent research. *Journal of Child Psychology and Psychiatry, 36*(1), 113–149.

Cohen, E., & Kaufmann, R. K. (2000). *Early childhood mental health consultation.* Center for Mental Health Services, Substance Abuse and Mental Health Services Administration, US Department of Health and Human Services.

Conners-Burrow, N. A., Whiteside-Mansell, L., Mckelvey, L., Virmani, E. A., & Sockwell, L. (2012). Improved classroom quality and child behavior in an Arkansas early childhood mental health consultation pilot project. *Infant Mental Health Journal, 33*(3), 256–264.

Denham, S. A., Caverly, S., Schmidt, M., Blair, K., DeMulder, E., Caal, S., … & Mason, T. (2002). Preschool understanding of emotions: Contributions to classroom anger and aggression. *Journal of Child Psychology and Psychiatry*, *43*(7), 901–916.

Domitrovich, C. E., Moore, J. E., & Greenberg, M. T. (2012). Maximizing the effectiveness of social-emotional interventions for young children through high-quality implementation of evidence-based interventions. In B. Kelly & D. F. Perkins (Eds.), *Handbook of implementation science for psychology in education* (pp. 207–209). New York, NY: Cambridge University Press.

Dougherty, A. (2013). *Psychological consultation and collaboration in school and community settings.* Stamford, CT: Cengage Learning.

Duran, F., Hepburn, K., Irvine, M., Kaufmann, R., Anthony, B., & Horen, N. (2009). *What works? A study of effective childhood mental health consultation programs: Executive summary.* Georgetown University Center for Child and Human Development. www.gucchd.georgetown.edu/78358.html

Fenichel, E. (1992). *Learning through supervision and mentorship to support the development of infants, toddlers and their families: A source book.* Zero to Three/National Center for Clinical Infant Programs, 2000 14th Street North, Suite 380, Arlington, VA 22201-2500.

Fox, N. A., Henderson, H. A., Marshall, P. J., Nichols, K. E., & Ghera, M. M. (2005). Behavioral inhibition: Linking biology and behavior within a developmental framework. *Annual Reviews of Psychology, 56*, 235–262.

Gilkerson, L. (2004). Irving B. Harris distinguished lecture: Reflective supervision in infant-family programs: Adding clinical process to nonclinical settings. *Infant Mental Health Journal, 25*(5), 424–439.

Gilliam, W. S. (2007). *Early childhood consultation partnership: Results of a random-controlled evaluation* (Final report and executive summary). New Haven, CT: Child Study Center, Yale University School of Medicine.

Gilliam, W. S. (2008). Implementing policies to reduce the likelihood of preschool expulsion. *Foundation for Child Development Policy Brief, 7*, 2–10. Retrieved from http://medicine.yale.edu/childstudy/zigler/Images/PreKExpulsionBrief2_tcm350-34772.pdf

Gilliam, W. S. (2005). *Prekindergarteners left behind: Expulsion rates in state prekindergarten systems.* New York, NY: Foundation for Child Development.

Gilliam, W. S., & Shahar, G. (2006). Preschool and child care expulsion and suspension: Rates and predictors in one state. *Infants & Young Children, 19*(3), 228–245.

Goodson, B. D., Mackrain, M., Perry, D. F., O'Brien, K., & Gwaltney, M. K. (2013). Enhancing home visiting with mental health consultation. *Pediatrics, 132*(Suppl 2), S180–S190.

Green, B. L., Everhart, M., Gordon, L., & Gettman, M. G. (2006). Characteristics of effective mental health consultation in early childhood settings: Multilevel analysis of a national survey. *Topics in Early Childhood Special Education, 26*(3), 142–152.

Heller, S. S., Boothe, A., Keyes, A., Nagle, G., Sidell, M., & Rice, J. (2011). Implementation of a mental health consultation model and its impact on early childhood teachers' efficacy and competence. *Infant Mental Health Journal, 32*(2), 143–164.

Hepburn, K. S., Perry, D. F., Shivers, E. M., & Gilliam, W. S. (2013). Early childhood mental health consultation as an evidence-based practice. *Zero to Three, 33*(5), 10–19.

Johnston, K., & Brinamen, C. (2006). *Mental health consultation in child care: Transforming relationships among directors, staff, and families.* Washington, DC: Zero to Three Press.

Kaufmann, R. K., Perry, D. F., Hepburn, K., & Duran, F. (2012). Assessing fidelity for early childhood mental health consultation: Lessons from the field and next steps. *Infant Mental Health Journal, 33*(3), 274–282.

LaFreniere, P. J., & Sroufe, L. A. (1985). Profiles of peer competence in the preschool: Interrelations between measures, influence of social ecology, and relation to attachment history. *Developmental Psychology, 21*(1), 56–69.

Lavigne, J. V., LeBailly, S. A., Gouze, K. R., Cicchetti, C., Pochyly, J., Arend, R., . . . & Binns, H. J. (2008). Treating oppositional defiant disorder in primary care: A comparison of three models. *Journal of Pediatric Psychology, 33*(5), 449–461.

Lemerise, E. A., & Arsenio, W. F. (2000). An integrated model of emotion processes and cognition in social information processing. *Child Development, 71*(1), 107–118.

Li Grining, C., Raver, C. C., Champion, K., Sardin, L., Metzger, M., & Jones, S. M. (2010). Understanding and improving classroom emotional climate and behavior management in the "real world": The role of Head Start teachers' psychosocial stressors. *Early Education and Development, 21*(1), 65–94.

Mashburn, A. J., & Pianta, R. C. (2006). Social relationships and school readiness. *Early Education and Development, 17*(1), 151–176.

Perry, D. F., Allen, M. D., Brennan, E. M., & Bradley, J. R. (2010). The evidence base for mental health consultation in early childhood settings: A research synthesis addressing children's behavioral outcomes. *Early Education and Development, 21*(6), 795–824.

Perry, D. F., Dunne, M. C., McFadden, L., & Campbell, D. (2008). Reducing the risk for preschool expulsion: Mental health consultation for young children with challenging behaviors. *Journal of Child and Family Studies, 17*(1), 44–54.

Raver, C. C., Jones, S. M., Li-Grining, C. P., Metzger, M., Champion, K. M., & Sardin, L. (2008). Improving preschool classroom processes: Preliminary findings from a randomized trial implemented in Head Start settings. *Early Childhood Research Quarterly, 23*, 10–26.

Rolfe, S. (2004). *Rethinking attachment for early childhood practice: Promoting security, autonomy and resilience in young children*. Melbourne, Australia: Allen & Unwin Publishers.

Shahmoon-Shanok, R. (2006). Reflective supervision: A method of implementation. In G. M. Foley & J. D. Hochman (Eds.), *Mental health in early intervention: Achieving unity in principles and practice*. Baltimore, MD: Paul H. Brookes.

Shonkoff, J., & Philips, D. (2000). *From neurons to neighborhoods: The science of early childhood development*. Washington, DC: National Academies Press.

Steier, A. (2013). *Smart Support at southwest human development: Arizona's system of early childhood mental health consultation*. media.education@umn.edu.

Vega, W. A., & Lopez, S. R. (2001). Priority issues in Latino mental health services research. *Mental Health Services Research, 3*(4), 189–200.

Virmani, E. A., Masyn, K. E., Thompson, R. A., Conners-Burrow, N. A., & Whiteside Mansell, L. (2013). Early childhood mental health consultation: Promoting change in the quality of teacher–child interactions. *Infant Mental Health Journal, 34*(2), 156–172.

Watson, C., & Gatti, S. N. (2012). Professional development through reflective consultation in early intervention. *Infants & Young Children, 25*(2), 109–121.

Webster-Stratton, C. (2000). *The incredible years training series*. US Department of Justice, Office of Justice Programs, Office of Juvenile Justice and Delinquency Prevention.

Webster-Stratton, C. (2003). The Incredible years: Parent, teacher, and child training series (IYS). In *Preventing violence and related health-risking social behaviors in adolescents: An NIH state-of-the-science conference* (pp. 73–77). https://consensus.nih.gov/2004/2004youthviolencepreventionsos023program.pdf#page=77

Webster-Stratton, C. (2006). The incredible years: A trouble-shooting guide for parents of children aged 2–8 years. *Incredible Years*.

Williford, A. P., & Shelton, T. L. (2008). Using mental health consultation to decrease disruptive behaviors in preschoolers: Adapting an empirically-supported intervention. *Journal of Child Psychology and Psychiatry, 49*(2), 191–200.

Chapter 11
Applications of Infant and Early Childhood Mental Health Research in Policy and Practice

Introduction

Research into the interrelatedness of neurobiology, genetics, neuroendocrinology and environmental factors is quite complex, but with appropriate research designs and statistical analyses which are suitable for the types of questions being asked, major advances have been made. Zeanah (2009) in the Handbook of Infant Mental Health, third edition, states that "infant mental health has a much more visible profile than when previous versions of this handbook were published" (p. 531). The United States government put infant and early childhood development on the national agenda by establishing a multidisciplinary committee whose responsibility was to integrate the current scientific knowledge regarding early childhood development, a formidable but important task. The result was a book published by the National Research Council and Institute of Medicine, edited by Jack Shonkoff and Deborah Phillips (2000), called "From Neurons to Neighborhoods", which reflects the necessity of synthesizing information garnered from different fields. Indeed, this book reflects the need for understanding child development contextually.

One of the core concepts upon which development is predicated, according to Shonkoff and Phillips, is that "human relationships, and the effects of relationships on relationships, are the building blocks of healthy development" (p. 27). One of the basic assumptions in the field of infant and early childhood mental health is that caring relationships are the main mediators of successful human developmental and behavioral adaptation, resulting in optimal outcomes. Developmental or behavioral disturbances in infants and toddlers are embedded in disturbances in the infant-caregiver relationship (Ainsworth et al., 1978; Bowlby 1969; Sameroff & Fiese, 2000). It is practically impossible to consider problems in infancy as independent of the infants' relationships with their primary caregivers, as the infant cannot survive without the caregiver. Through a relationship with a sensitive and warm adult caregiver, the infant learns to trust the world and with growing confidence explores

C. Shulman, *Research and Practice in Infant and Early Childhood Mental Health*,
Children's Well-Being: Indicators and Research 13,
DOI 10.1007/978-3-319-31181-4_11

the environment and learns about objects, people and him- or herself. Therefore, the primary goal of intervention programs is to strengthen the foundational relationship between caregiver and infant, helping both the child and the caregiver learn to adapt more successfully to each other.

These assumptions regarding the centrality of relationships, particularly those in the earliest stages of development, are the benchmarks of infant and early childhood mental health; they are seen as formative and constitute the basic structure within which all meaningful development unfolds. The nonprofit organization Zero to Three was founded in 1977 to communicate the message that in order for all infants and toddlers to get a strong start in life, it is critical to gather information about the importance of nurturing the developing infant in order to maximize developmental potential.

Parents, professionals and policymakers are the intended audience, as Zero to Three deals with key issues affecting young children and their families including child care, development, early intervention, and the impact of culture on early childhood development, all of which are basic to the field of infant and early childhood mental health. Zero to Three integrates perspectives of infant and child development from various fields and is rooted in the empirical study of development, with the aim of promoting a child's overall physical and mental health and emotional well-being in the context of his family and culture. This is eminently clear from the title of the January 2015 issue of the organization's journal - Connecting Science, Policy, and Practice - which highlights the integrative philosophy of the organization. Topics discussed included the science of epigenetics and the inequities faced by many young children today who experience racial and ethnic disparities in health outcomes, educational achievement, and well-being.

This chapter is likewise integrative, reviewing the implications of our knowledge in the field of infant and early childhood mental health which can foster policies and professional standards. It will highlight several important policy areas that can support the social and emotional development of very young children, with some suggestions for a policy agenda to promote infant and early childhood mental health. In addition, it will present the components of training programs for professionals who want to work in the field of infant mental health or are already working and want to deepen their professional knowledge, strategies and techniques. Finally, it will survey what has been accomplished and what challenges remain for prevention programs in infant and early childhood mental health, with some recommendations about possible next steps.

Policy Agenda: Promoting Infant and Early Childhood Mental Health

Public policies that promote optimal social– emotional development in the early years can help to establish the foundation needed for successful adaptation in later years. Therefore it is important to identify the conditions which promote social and emotional development and those conditions which present threats to optimal mental health. With limited funding to funnel into programs and resources in the field of infant and early childhood mental health, it is important to identify interventions which evidence-based research has found to be effective, in order to prioritize which programs should be funded (Zigler & Gilliam, 2009). There is a need to educate policymakers regarding the nature of mental health, the mental health needs of infants and toddlers and possible causes of early mental health problems. As the field of infant and early childhood mental health continues to mature, parents, professionals and policymakers will have to collaborate in order to advance a policy agenda that meets the social and emotional needs of very young children.

Policy Agenda: Creating Mental Health Informed Systems

Because of limited resources and pressing needs in other fields, infant mental health programs have not been supported to the extent necessary to provide support for the social– emotional development of infants and toddlers (Knitzer & Cohen, 2007). Policymakers rarely have the background or even the interest to interpret and translate empirical findings into practical policies. Infant mental health reflects a complex, overlapping system of confluent components which may be different for each individual child, making policy decisions difficult. In general, policymakers do not support comprehensive, integrated strategies that address parents, their children, and the family situation together. Coordinated attention to children's social– emotional development across a broad set of policies affecting physical and mental health, social services, and family support is required in order to achieve positive mental health outcomes (Huang et al., 2005; Lally, Lurie-Hurvitz, & Cohen, 2006).

There are many ways this can be accomplished. Infant and early childhood mental health services can be brought to child care facilities, incorporated into home visiting models and practiced in family support settings, such as community clinics. A core set of mental health services should be available to families with young children. Policymakers will decide whether these services should be offered to all families, allowing those who feel that they want help or support the opportunity to receive services, or whether the services should be available only to families who are at risk and may take less initiative in turning to service providers for help. There is also an approach which believes that infant and early childhood mental health services should be accessible only for those with an identified mental health disorder. At whatever level it is decided to offer these services, they should be enmeshed in the primary care system, as the families and children with problems and challenges are generally first identified there. These services need to be expanded through policy changes.

Addressing risk factors such as mental illness or poverty, which have deleterious effects on developmental and behavioral outcomes, should be a high priority (Lally et al., 2006; Nelson & Mann, 2011). Early identification of children in need of services is an important step in beginning intervention as early as possible. In order to realize that goal, a policy of screening should be instituted to detect social–emotional problems, such as relationship disorders, depression, and self-regulation problems, in infants and toddlers. Screening for family risk factors that might affect children's social–emotional development. For example, looking for poverty, pre- and postnatal parental depression, family isolation, parental mental illness, or parental substance abuse should also be an integral part of the screening process. If a question about a child's mental health status arises during screening, it is possible to refer the child for a full evaluation or to begin a targeted mental health intervention.

In addition to targeted mental health interventions, some of which were surveyed in Chap. 8, it is possible to infuse early services and child care frameworks with the principles of infant mental health. A public health approach to infant mental health would incorporate mental health supports into community services with which young children have contact, in order to support their social emotional development. Applying infant mental health principles in normative frameworks has two clear advantages. The first one is that all children, not just those identified as needing support, will be the recipients of a richer program with an emphasis on social and emotional goals. A programmatic decision to include infant mental health content in child care and preschool settings must be made on a policy level. For example, if a child has experienced trauma and is not in a targeted intervention program like child parent psychotherapy, it is possible that the staff of the childcare center or preschool where the child spends his or her daytime hours can offer support. If the staff has knowledge regarding trauma and its effects on children and has a sense of the child's vulnerabilities, it will be possible to help the child.

Understanding that trauma is akin to terror and that the child has experienced trauma, abuse or neglect, and may exhibit affect dysregulation and/or hyper-arousal makes it easier to be empathic to the child, even when his or her behavior is challenging. Traumatized children are overwhelmed by feelings of unpredictability, terror and helplessness, which upset their ability to cope. Such children have a distorted sense of danger and may feel unmitigated terror in situations which would not evoke those feelings in other children who have not experienced trauma. They may be isolated and angry. If the caregiver understands the trauma experience and identifies possible vicarious trauma in staff members, it will be possible to help staff members change their attitude towards such children and respond more empathically. Reflection replaces reactivity; curiosity replaces depersonalization; care replaces anger; and the staff feels important and supportive of the child who is clearly suffering. Epstein, Seron, Oglensky, and Saute (2014) describes such a system for child care professionals, and emphasizes the need for supervision from a professional specializing in trauma.

Similarly, care for abused and neglected infants and young children can be delivered in regular educational frameworks which adopt a mental health perspective, with appropriate considerations systematically incorporated into policies and decisions affecting children and their families. Children from birth to 5 years of age have disproportionately high rates of maltreatment, with long-term consequences for their mental and physical health. It is crucial to incorporate systemic change in the agencies which provide services by integrating infant and early childhood mental health principles into existing systems of care for young children and their families. The recommended approach is to attempt to integrate components of mental health, particularly those focused on relationship building, into existing key service systems, such as primary health care offices or clinics, child care facilities, community centers and other places where children and their families congregate. A number of programs successfully incorporate core infant and early childhood principles into their program strategy and several of these will be surveyed below.

Support Programs for Families at Risk

Keys to Caregiving, a home visiting program developed in Australia, is grounded in relationship-building principles of infant mental health and was begun by Barnard, Morisset, and Spieker (1993) as an alternative for families for whom the traditional 3-month nurse home visiting program was ineffectual. The mothers in these families were characterized as solitary, with little support and many problems. Research assessing the efficacy of this program contrasted the Keys for Caregiving program, in which the home visiting nurses stressed relationship building, with a program in which the home visiting nurses provided educational and resource information, and found significantly more behavioral changes in the children (e.g., "less fussy", more talkative) and more positive emotional changes in the mothers (lessening of depressive symptoms, happier) in the Keys to Caregiving group than in those enrolled in the comparison program.

Parent Service Program (1980), which was developed and researched in northern California, is a nonprofit organization dedicated to integrating family support systems into early childhood programs and family-serving organizations. The purpose is to strengthen partnerships between educators and service providers who work with families in supporting the well-being of children, families, and communities. This is accomplished by adding activities which bring parents together and having them make decisions regarding the activity opportunities which they think will be most meaningful for them (Link, Beggs, & Seiderman, 1997). Although this program has no formal infant mental health components, when compared with a matched group of parents who did not participate in the Parent Service Program, the parents from the Parent Service Program reported significantly less isolation and maternal depression as a result of participation in the program. The program has been replicated at over 500 sites throughout 12 states nationally, reaching an estimated 40,000 families in the United States, and although it is necessary to continue to evaluate mental health outcomes for the parents and young children, it is clear that the support provided in Parent Service Program has been helpful for many families.

The Learning to Live Together (Rosenthal & Gatt, 2010) program was developed in Israel for caregivers working in child care facilities in which toddlers and preschoolers spend many hours of their day. The program was developed to deal with the negative responses that caregiversreport when faced with young children's challenging behavior. The goals of the program are to help toddlers and preschoolers learn empathy, play together and resolve conflicts, while helping the caregivers to understand the behavior of the child. Incorporating relational principles from early childhood mental health, this program attempts to point out how behaviors are maintained and how they can be changed within a meaningful relationship. The program uses videotapes in order to train caregivers to comprehend the complexities of their interactions. These interactions are interpreted together with the Learning to Live Together consultant, who provides empirical knowledge regarding social and emotional development and relationship development.

The program also involves teaching specific intervention skills that support social and emotional development. The program clarifies explicit and implicit attitudes and beliefs that adults in the child's life hold concerning children's social and emotional development and concerning their own role in promoting this development. The training consists of 12 workshop meetings guided by an early childhood mental health expert, which are followed by four small-group consultation meetings which deal with understanding and responding to challenging behaviors and interactions with children.

Caregivers who interact with children around their feelings and intentions and those of others, and help children express their own feelings and understand the emotions, intentions and social behavior of others (Denham et al., 2002; Dunn, 2000; Ruffman & Perner, 2005), infuse principles of infant mental health into their programs. For example, the Learning to Live Together program encourages caregivers to coach a shy or withdrawn child to communicate his or her interests more clearly, as well as helping him or her to understand the interests and intentions of others. Caregivers also use various playful interventions to support a child with difficulties in self-regulation in finding appropriate and acceptable regulatory behaviors. This is done in a non-judgmental manner, and caregivers are encouraged to recognize their own difficulties in regulating emotions when they become stressed as well as the reciprocal nature of regulation.

Research has evaluated the results of this intervention on two levels. Firstly, pre- and post-test measures revealed that the caregivers expressed more warmth towards the children, listened more attentively, enjoyed them more and expressed less hostility during routine care after participating in the program. Secondly, caregivers who participated in Learning to Live Together were compared with matched caregivers who did not participate, and empirical findings demonstrated that by the end of the year caregivers in the comparison group who did not receive the training engaged significantly more frequently in offensive and punitive interactions with the children, offered less frequent positive interactions and less support during emotional arousal, and promoted children's social skills less frequently. The children's behavior also changed as a result of participation in the program, showing greater social competence, less aggression and less social withdrawal (Beer, 2007).

Incorporating Mental Health Perspectives in Policy Decisions

In addition to incorporating mental health principles into existing programs and establishing complementary programs in the community, other policy decisions can inculcate infant mental health principles into community services. The addition of a clinical mental health professional, who can help parent and professional tolerate the stress inherent in dealing with mental health issues, has been demonstrated to be effective. Hawaii Healthy Start is an innovative infant mental health program which was originally set up to address families with young children in which there was documented child abuse and/or neglect. Paraprofessionals were trained to go into the homes of these families and provide support (Wallach & Lister, 1995). A subgroup of mothers who had experienced so much grief, trauma or depression that the program was not effective for them was identified by the home visitors as problematic. The solution was found by providing a mental health professional consultant who was hired to support the staff. Empirical results showed less absenteeism for the staff on sites where professional supervision was available.

At this point in time, Head Start and Early Head Start are the only federally funded projects that require early childhood programs to include mental health professionals on their staffs. Early Head Start is the component of Head Start that serves the nation's most impoverished pregnant women, infants, and toddlers, a population in which a high level of mental health issues might be anticipated (Center on the Developing Child at Harvard University, 2007). Congress increased the funding allocated for Early Head Start services in the 2007 reauthorization of Head Start and provided additional funds in the American Recovery and Reinvestment Act of 2009, and yet the program currently serves fewer than 4 % of eligible infants and toddlers nationally. Early Head Start provides a model for integrating mental health services into child development programs.

All Early Head Start programs are required to screen children for developmental and/or behavioral concerns. Programs must employ or contract with mental health professionals to consult with program staff and to provide family-centered mental health services (U.S. Department of Health and Human Services & Administration for Children & Families, 2005). A national evaluation of Early Head Start produced positive findings with implications for social–emotional development. At 3 years of age, Early Head Start children had more positive interactions with their parents than control group children and displayed less aggressive behavior (Love et al., 2005). Increasing numbers of Early Head Start parents use the mental health services provided, including treatment for depression, crisis intervention, child abuse and neglect services, substance abuse prevention and treatment, and domestic violence services, suggesting that these services are an important resource (Hoffman & Ewen, 2007).

In addition to direct access to mental health services, mental health consultation in early child care and education programs is a promising strategy to increase infant mental health resources in the community (Gilliam, 2008; Perry, Allen, Brennan, & Bradley, 2010). Early childhood mental health consultation refers to mental health professionals collaborating with professionals in other fields to prevent or address early childhood mental health problems (Johnston & Brinamen, 2006; Perry et al., 2010). Early childhood mental health consultants have knowledge of child development and parenting and understand the dynamics of early childhood settings. Consultation can be focused on program staff or on specific children or families, with the intention of strengthening the capacity of programs to recognize and address social– emotional issues (Brennan, Bradley, Allen, & Perry, 2008). Gilliam (2008) identified a growing need for mental health consultation in early care and education settings when he found a high rate of expulsion from preschool programs for behavior issues among 3- and 4-year-olds. Programs participating in his study that had access to early childhood mental health consultation were less likely to exclude children for behavior issues.

Policy Agenda: Establishing Prevention Programs

Head Start is anexample of a policy decision taken to support populations who are at risk for non-optimal development by establishing a prevention intervention program. Prevention work is a challenge for researchers as it is very difficult to isolate variables when studying the effects of prevention intervention, but it is an important societal venue for change in the field of infant and early childhood mental health.

Prevention has been conceptualized as having three tiers (Mrazek & Haggerty, 1994). Universal prevention, like putting fluoride in water to help prevent tooth decay, is a procedure which is considered to be beneficial for every individual in a particular population; selective prevention is appropriate for individuals in the population who have a high risk level for a particular problem; while indicated prevention targets those who manifest sub-threshold but detectable symptoms that may become a diagnosable disorder. Societies place different values on different services in general and in the field of prevention intervention specifically. Universal prevention, in which something is seen as important for all infants and all families, is only universal to the eligible population. Decisions are made according to the degree to which members of the population believe that government can be involved in certain areas and how they believe this involvement should occur. In the United States, where individuality is highly valued, the government often supports services but is not the implementer. In more socialist countries, where the government is more involved in the daily lives of the citizens, universal prevention includes more services provided by the government.

Universal prevention programs establish programs for health promotion or prevention of the onset of problems. In the field of infant and early childhood mental health, this can be translated as programs to enhance social and emotional development or to avert the onset of disorders. These include education programs regarding infant and child development and healthy parenting skills, and access to available services when needed. These services are provided on the individual, family, group or community level, depending on the service. Quality child care has been identified as a universal value and has been operationalized as providing warm, supportive interactions in a safe and stimulating environment (Scarr, 1998). Although the quality of child care has been found to be related to cognitive and linguistic outcomes (NICHD Early Child Care Research Network, 2005), more importantly perhaps, the quality of the parent-child relationship was a better predictor of child outcomes than any combination of child care variables.

Selective interventions are those which are provided to families of young children who are at risk for poor social and emotional outcomes, based on particular dimensions. Although some may be functioning well, with no outward signs that their risk will manifest in poorer outcomes, others may show difficulties and challenging behavior. Interventions are designed to address the risks of a particular population and certain measures are defined as the outcome variables to be monitored. Olds, Sadler, and Knitzman (2007) studied the Nurse-Family Partnership program which was designed to combat abuse and neglect in young, first-time mothers, in which nurse practitioners visited the home before the 28th week of pregnancy and continued through the child's second birthday.

The program was based on attachment theory, social learning theory and human ecology theory and was supported by the public health professional community. The basis of the program was the understanding that the period encompassing pregnancy and the early years of the child's life is the earliest opportunity to intervene and possibly prevent adverse maternal, child, and family outcomes. The program was designed for low-income mothers who had had no previous live births and its goals of improving pregnancy outcomes; improving children's health and development by helping parents provide more sensitive and competent care of the child; and improving parental life course by helping parents plan future pregnancies, complete their education, and find work were evaluated in three separate large-scale, randomized controlled trials with different populations living in different contexts.

The research findings from these studies indicate that the program has been successful in achieving many of its main goals. There were fewer child injuries that could be associated with child abuse and neglect and better infant emotional and language development, and the mothers had fewer subsequent pregnancies and found work to a greater degree than mothers who did not go through the program.

Indicated approaches to prevention intervention are employed when sub-threshold syndromatic problems are already evident in young children. These interventions are aimed at ameliorating the effect of the early manifestations of abnormality. Insecure and disordered attachment styles have been identified as a risk factor for adaptive functioning. Because sensitive and responsive parenting has been demonstrated to be associated with secure attachment, many indicated intervention approaches which have been developed as prevention programs are grounded in attachment-based strategies. For example, Juffer, Bakermans and van IJzendoorn (2012) developed an attachment based intervention based on results from several previous techniques (e.g., Rolfe, 2004). Their technique, called video-based intervention to promote positive parenting, is targeted at dyads at risk for the adverse consequences of insecure attachment, and this intervention strategy has been shown to reduce externalizing problems in young children.

Prevention interventions in infant and early childhood mental health are challenging for several reasons. To establish the validity of these programs it is important to work with the families of young children in the planning and implementation of the prevention programs. It is likewise important to recognize personal, familial, cultural and organizational values which have an influence on intervention. Without understanding these diverse systems, it is difficult to match the prevention program to the population. Ongoing research into prevention programs is vital. By identifying the components of the targeted recipients, the content of the methods and the elements of implementation, such as frequency, intensity and length of services, it will be possible to link the outcomes from research in a meaningful manner. Clinicians and researchers need to work together in order to establish a continuum of services and policies which will ensure that families have access to individualized services as early as possible.

Policy Agenda: Training Professionals

In addition to instituting infant and early childhood consultation in care systems, it is equally important to have programs which train professionals who will be working in infant and early childhood mental health programs. Many practitioners who potentially could provide mental health services come from disciplines which are not mental health professions. The education and training of many professionals who work with young children do not include developmental components or treatment strategies which are appropriate for children with mental health problems and their families. Didactic courses, practicums, and internships in infant and early childhood mental health should become integral components of undergraduate and graduate curricula in psychology, education, social work, nursing, occupational therapy and speech and language therapy in order to build capacity to achieve this goal. Professionals in these fields are in a position to guide and support the parent-child relationship, but although they are expected to work within the relational context to promote infant mental health, their training has not prepared them to do so.

A program for training professionals to work in the field of infant and early childhood mental health should include a core set of principles pertaining to the understanding of infant development in context. These core principles must be delineated and transmitted in a clear and coherent framework, which includes imparting information from development theory, the family systems approach, human ecology and relational psychology. The training experiences should be supervised by multidisciplinary infant mental health professionals, in order to provide specific training that differentially develops knowledge and skills appropriate to the degree to which professionals will be involved with the infants and their families. This is dependent on the professional discipline of origin and will be different for psychologists, occupational therapists, social workers, speech and language pathologists, nurses, and other professionals. The supervision should also promote professional development in the context of a supportive relationship. The nature of that relationship may be a model for the one that the trainee will establish with the parents in the families of young children with whom he or she will be working. Because of the multidisciplinary nature of infant and early childhood mental health, it is also important at the training stage to emphasize professional boundaries. Professionals in the field of infant mental health cannot all provide the same services. By defining the boundaries of professional strengths of each of the various disciplines from which professionals come to the infant mental health field, it is possible to maximize the abilities of each professional.

Training in infant and early childhood mental health occurs on many levels, for many different people, for many different reasons. Some people working in the field want to specialize, while others need the continuing education to remain in their place of work. Some programs award degrees while others are certificate programs. In 2011, the Hebrew University of Jerusalem established an advanced degree program to train professionals to specialize in infant mental health. The students, after completing the 2 year program of study, return to the field, to their practice with young children in need and their families, bringing with them the knowledge and skills obtained during their studies. The program is a specialization track in the interdisciplinary program in early childhood graduate studies which is associated with the Schools of Social Work and Education.

Policy Agenda: Incorporating Diversity-Informed Tenets

It is extremely important for professionals in the field of infant mental health to be sensitive to and respectful of diversity. The Irving Harris Foundation, which supports infant and early childhood programs on all levels (Glink, 2012), has published a manifesto on the subject of diversity-informed practice (Ghosh Ippen, Norona, & Thomas, 2012), which emphasizes the following themes: Professionals must reflect on their own culture, personal values and beliefs and on the impact that racism, classism, sexism, able-ism, homophobia, xenophobia, and other systems of oppression have had on their lives in order to provide diversity-informed, culturally attuned services on behalf of infants, toddlers, and their families.

Diversity-informed infant mental health practice recognizes non-dominant ways of knowing bodies of knowledge, sources of strength and routes to healing within diverse families and communities. Families define who comprises them and how they are structured; no particular family constellation or organization is inherently optimal compared to any other. Diversity-informed infant mental health practice recognizes and strives to counter the historical bias towards idealizing (and conversely blaming) biological mothers as primary caregivers while overlooking the critical child rearing contributions of other parents and caregivers including fathers, second mothers, foster parents, kin, and felt family, early care and educational providers and others.

Diversity and inclusion must be considered proactively in undertaking any piece of infant mental health work. Such consideration requires the allocation of resources such as time and money for this purpose and is best ensured when opportunities for reflection with colleagues and mentors, as well as ongoing training and consultation, are embedded in agencies, institutions and systems of care. Infant mental health workforces will be most dynamic and effective when culturally diverse individuals have access to a wide range of roles, disciplines and modes of practice and influence. Diversity-informed infant mental health practitioners, regardless of professional affiliation, seek to understand the impact of social policies and programs on diverse infants and toddlers and to advance a just policy agenda for and with families.

Conclusions and Recommendations for Policymakers, Researchers and Practitioners

Research in neurobiological, behavioral and social sciences has led to major advances in understanding the conditions that influence whether children begin life on a pathway toward optimal development or not. Consensus has been reached regarding the importance of early experience. Intervention that begins early has the potential to shape the future of the infant, the family and the community in which the child grows up. The effects of interactions between genetics and environment on the development of the brain and the unfolding of behavior are complex and multi-directional. It is important to understand that child characteristics and environmental variables are at play in a particular context for a particular child and family, in order to individualize the intervention program to the specific needs and circumstances of adversity. Within this dynamic system of child and environment, of biology and ecology, of genes and context, of nature and nurture, it is necessary to acknowledge the central role of early relationships as a source of adaptation or of risk.

The challenges which remain to be addressed by policymakers include the high levels of economic hardship among families with young children despite increases in maternal education, increased rates of parent employment, and a strong economy; increasing cultural diversity; and the persistence of significant racial and ethnic disparities in health and developmental outcomes. There are high levels of serious family problems and adverse community conditions which are detrimental for children, and their cumulative effect must be addressed through services, collaborations between agencies, and training in the field of infant mental health, which should be accompanied both by research to add to our knowledge base and by translational research to develop appropriate intervention techniques. Evaluation research can also assess the effectiveness of existing treatment programs and serve as the basis for the development of additional complementary programs. Scientists, policymakers, community leaders, practitioners, and parents must all work together to identify and sustain policies that are effective and consider new approaches.

It is in the best interest of policymakers, practitioners, children and families to understand the dynamic processes in child development, the centrality of relationships and the effects of environmental risk factors. Based on what is known today there are important directions for continuing research which can only be realized with support from policymakers. More resources, like those invested in reading and arithmetic, need to be allocated to translating the knowledge base regarding children's emotional regulatory and social development into effective strategies for fostering the development of the healthy self in the child, which is manifested in curiosity, self-direction and persistence in learning in order to continue growing and developing. School readiness initiatives should not simply be about skill achievement and performance, but should also address emotional and social development and the ability to make friends, be cooperative and solve problems adaptively. Similarly, it is important to set reducing the disparities among children from different backgrounds as a social policy goal.

There is more consensus among researchers and practitioners today than there was even 10 years ago and hopefully this important trend will continue. The points upon which agreement has been achieved are the foundational points from which the field of infant and early childhood mental health will progress during the twenty-first century. These points include the understanding that helping parents of young children is by far the most long-lasting and effective way to help young children and that the relationship which is forged between the practitioner and parents should be based on respect and understanding. By recognizing that parents have needs and wishes and listening to them, it is possible to understand more about the child and the environment in which he or she is developing. It is imperative that we not only reach those children diagnosed with behavior and/or emotional problems and their families but also address the needs of those children who are at risk for non-optimal social and emotional development and their families.

These assumptions support a strength-based approach which recognizes the need for all interested parties to work together and which provides opportunities to share knowledge and experience across contexts. The staff members who work with young children with social and emotional problems also need to acknowledge their own feelings about the violence or abuse that the children they care for are experiencing. Engaging in collaborative problem solving can build bridges between parents and professionals, scientists and practitioners, and clinicians and policymakers. It is imperative that connections across systems be maintained and that knowledge from the field of infant and early childhood mental health be combined with child care resources in order to cope effectively with the challenges of young children growing up in a complex, diverse world. In order to effectively address young children's mental health needs, resources must be allocated for effective screening, early detection, treatment, and ultimately prevention of serious childhood mental health problems.

This agenda requires cooperation between the early childhood community and the mental health community with a shared focus on the treatment and prevention of severe behavioral disorders. In order to achieve this, policymakers must provide the fiscal support needed to develop and support multi-disciplinary programs for very young children and their families. It is my hope that this book will contribute to achieving a fruitful relationship between research and practice and assist practitioners and policy makers in dealing with the tension between intervention strategies and prevention perspectives, while never losing sight of the multidisciplinary approach that is at the foundation of work in the field of infant and early childhood mental health.

References

Ainsworth, M. D. S., Blehar, M. C., Waters, E., & Wall, S. (1978). *Patterns of attachment: A psychological study of the strange situation*. Mawah, NJ: Lawrence Erlbaum Associates.

Barnard, K. E., Morisset, C. E., & Spieker, S. (1993). Preventive interventions: Enhancing parent-infant relationships. In C. R. Zeanah (Ed.), *Handbook of infant mental health* (pp. 386–401). New York, NY: Guilford Press.

Beer, T. (2007). *Developing caregivers' competencies in the preschool classroom*. Unpublished doctoral dissertation. Hebrew University.

Bowlby, J. (1969). *Attachment and loss: Vol. 1. Attachment*. New York, NY: Basic Books.

Brennan, E. M., Bradley, J. R., Allen, M. D., & Perry, D. F. (2008). The evidence base for mental health consultation in early childhood settings: Research synthesis addressing staff and program outcomes. *Early Education and Development, 19*(6), 982–1022.

Center on the Developing Child at Harvard University. (2007). *The timing and quality of early experience combine to shape brain architecture* (Working paper #5). Retrieved February 23, 2015, from http://developingchild.harvard.edu/index.php/library/reports_and_working_

Denham, S. A., Caverly, S., Schmidt, M., Blair, K., DeMulder, E., Caal, S., . . . & Mason, T. (2002). Preschool understanding of emotions: contributions to classroom anger and aggression. *Journal of Child Psychology and Psychiatry, 43*(7), 901–916

Dunn, J. (2000). Mind-reading, emotion understanding, and relationships. *International Journal of Behavioral Development, 24*(2), 142–144.

Epstein, C. F., Seron, C., Oglensky, B., & Saute, R. (2014). *The part-time paradox: Time norms, professional life, family and gender*. New York, NY: Routledge.

Ghosh Ippen, C., Norona, C. R., & Thomas, K. (2012). From tenet to practice: Putting diversity-informed services into action. *Zero to Three, 33*(2), 23–28.

Gilliam, W. S. (2008). Implementing policies to reduce the likelihood of preschool expulsion. *Foundation for Child Development Policy Brief, 7*, 2–10. Retrieved from http://medicine.yale.edu/childstudy/zigler/Images/PreKExpulsionBrief2_tcm350-34772.pdf

Glink, P. (2012). The Irving Harris Foundation's investment in the professional development network. *Zero to Three (J), 33*(2), 5–8.

Hoffman, E., & Ewen, D. (2007). *Supporting families, nurturing young children: Early Head Start programs in 2006* (CLASP policy brief No. 9).

Huang, L., Stroul, B., Friedman, R., Mrazek, P., Friesen, B., Pires, S., et al. (2005). Transforming mental health care for children and their families. *American Psychologist, 60*(6), 615–627.

Johnston, K., & Brinamen, C. (2006). *Mental health consultation in child care: Transforming relationships among directors, staff, and families*. Washington, DC: Zero to Three Press.

Juffer, F., Bakermans-Kranenburg, M. J., & van IJzendoorn, M. H. (Eds.). (2012). *Promoting positive parenting: An attachment-based intervention*. London: Routledge.

Knitzer, J., & Cohen, E. P. (2007). Promoting resilience in young children and families at the highest risk: The challenge for early childhood mental health. In D. F. Perry, R. K. Kaufmann, & J. Knitzer (Eds.), *Social and emotional health in early childhood: Building bridges between services and systems* (pp. 335–359). Baltimore, MD: Paul H Brookes Publishing.

Lally, R., Lurie-Hurvitz, E., & Cohen, J. (2006). Good health, strong families, and positive early learning experiences: Promoting better public policies for America's infants and toddlers. *Zero to Three Journal, 26*(6), 6–9.

Link, G., Beggs, M., & Seiderman, E. (1997). Serving families. Retrieved February 2015, http://eric.ed.gov/?id=ED414067

Love, J. M., Kisker, E. E., Ross, C., Raikes, H., Constantine, J., Boller, K., ... & Vogel, C. (2005). The effectiveness of early Head Start for 3-year-old children and their parents: Lessons for policy and programs. *Developmental Psychology, 41*(6), 885–901.

Mrazek, P. J., & Haggerty, R. J. (Eds.). (1994). *Reducing risks for mental disorders: Frontiers for preventive intervention research*. Washington, DC: National Academies Press.

Nelson, F., & Mann, T. (2011). Opportunities in public policy to support infant and early childhood mental health: The role of psychologists and policymakers. *American Psychologist, 66*(2), 129–139.

NICHD Early Child Care Research Network. (2005). *Child care and child development: Results from the NICHD study of early child care and youth development*. New York, NY: Guilford Press.

Olds, D. L., Sadler, L., & Knitzman, H. (2007). Programs for parents of infants and toddlers: Recent evidence from randomized trials. *Journal of Child Psychology and Psychiatry, 48*, 355–391.

Perry, D. F., Allen, M. D., Brennan, E. M., & Bradley, J. R. (2010). The evidence base for mental health consultation in early childhood settings: A research synthesis addressing children's behavioral outcomes. *Early Education and Development, 21*(6), 795–824.

Rolfe, S. (2004). *Rethinking attachment for early childhood practice: Promoting security, autonomy and resilience in young children*. Melbourne, Australia: Allen & Unwin Publishers.

Rosenthal, M. K., & Gatt, L. (2010). 'Learning to live together': Training early childhood educators to promote socio-emotional competence of toddlers and pre-school children. *European Early Childhood Education Research Journal, 18*(3), 373–390.

Ruffman, T., & Perner, J. (2005). Do infants really understand false belief? *Trends in Cognitive Sciences, 9*(10), 462–463.

Sameroff, A. J., & Fiese, B. H. (2000). Transactional regulation: The developmental ecology of early intervention. In J. P. Shonkoff & S. J. Meisels (Eds.), *Handbook of early childhood intervention* (pp. 135–159). New York, NY: Cambridge University Press.

Scarr, S. (1998). American child care today. *American Psychologist, 53*(2), 95–108.

Shonkoff, J., & Philips, D. (2000). *From neurons to neighborhoods: The science of early childhood development*. Washington, DC: National Academies Press.

U.S. Department of Health and Human Services, Administration for Children & Families. (2005). *Child maltreatment 2003*. Washington, DC: U.S. Government Printing Office. Retrieved from http://www.acf.hhs.gov/programs/cb/stats_research/index.htm#can

Wallach, V. A., & Lister, L. (1995). Stages in the delivery of home-based services to parents at risk of child abuse: A healthy start experience. *Research and Theory for Nursing Practice, 9*(2), 159–173.

Zeanah, C. (Ed.). (2009). *Handbook of infant mental health* (3rd ed.). New York, NY: Guilford Press.

Zigler, E. F., & Gilliam, W. S. (2009). Science and policy: Connecting what we know to what we do. *Zero to Three, 30*(2), 40–46.

Index

A
Abuse, 30, 73, 108, 130, 167, 171, 206, 209, 211, 215
Adaptation, 26, 45, 81, 83, 105, 117, 125–129, 131, 132, 136, 145, 146, 154, 163, 174, 203, 204, 214
Additive risk model, 88, 127
Adolescent motherhood, 189
Adoption studies, 107
Adverse childhood experience, 96
Adversity, 73, 91, 117, 125–130, 137–140, 214
Aggression, 27, 44, 107, 147, 161, 170, 209
Anxiety, 38, 59, 84, 94, 95, 107, 108, 112, 117, 161, 167
Assessment
  caregiver report measures, 107
  infant toddler social and emotional screening (ITSEA), 55
Attachment
  ambivalent, 58, 85
  anxious, 85
  attachment relationship, 111
  attachment styles, 5, 6, 58, 59, 94, 108, 110, 111, 175, 211
  avoidant, 3, 58, 59
  brain development, 102
  definition, 7
  developmental context, 27
  disorganized, 58, 86, 108, 211
  early experiences, 14, 102
  figures, 85, 108, 111
  foster care, 147, 148
  insecure, 211, 212
  maternal depression, 94, 136
  overview, 58–59
  parenting, 6, 25, 166, 168
  secure, 6, 14, 26, 58–60, 94, 110, 148, 150, 165–167, 175, 212
  social development, 54, 74
  strange situation paradigm, 58, 106
  theory, 2, 106, 148–150, 170, 211
Attunement, 3, 6, 117–118

B
Beck Depression Inventory (BDI), 55
Behavior
  foster care, 57, 76, 128, 147, 214, 215
  maternal depression, 86, 94, 136, 159
  regulation, 15, 95
Behavioral genetics
  intervention strategies based on behavioral genetic, 72
  research findings from behavioral genetics, 71–72
  research methods for studying behavioral genetics, 70–71
Bonding, 7, 29–30, 50, 114, 115, 117, 118, 168
Brain and behavior in early development, 26–29

C. Shulman, *Research and Practice in Infant and Early Childhood Mental Health*, Children's Well-Being: Indicators and Research 13,
DOI 10.1007/978-3-319-31181-4

C
Caregiver, 2–8, 11, 12, 14–16, 26, 29, 31, 32, 34, 44, 47–51, 59, 60, 68, 73, 85, 86, 101–106, 109, 111–113, 115–118, 128, 148–150, 155, 160, 161, 164, 166, 171, 173, 181, 184, 186–195, 197–199, 203, 204, 206, 208, 214
Case conceptualization, 10
Case management, 186
Child Behavior Checklist (CBCL), 55
Child care
  access to mental health in, 181, 209
  consultation in, 181–199
  mental health considerations in, 9, 10, 92, 109, 182, 188–191, 195, 196, 204–207, 212, 215
Child-centered consultation model, 186, 187
Child characteristics in the relational context, 112
Child factors
  temperament, 31
  family functioning and, 84, 139, 187
Child-parent psychotherapy (CPP)
  empirical support for, 84
  developmental context, 165
  intervention modalities, 166, 167
  theoretical bases of, 147
Child rearing, 10, 43, 49, 52, 54, 56–57, 109–111, 166, 214
Child resilience, 12
Child risk factors, 94–96
  prematurity, 94–96
Cognitive development, 26–27, 174
Collaboration, 8, 139, 146, 185, 186, 193, 198, 215
Colorado Adoption Project (CAP), 70
  analysis of data, 71
  description, 70
  findings, 71
Community based interventions, 163
Conceptualizing early development, 24–26
Configural STATS, 134
Consultation relationship, 182, 187, 190
Cortisol, 58, 59, 94
Creation of meaning, 102
Critical period, 5, 14
Cross-cultural diversity, 56, 110, 111
Cultural differences in attachment behavior, 58–60
Cultural differences in childrearing, 56–57
Culturally determined "ideal child, 55–56
Cultural sensitivity
  cultural competence, 57
  cultural ecological model, 154
  multicultural perspective, 43
  intervention, 46, 54
  observation, 45, 46, 52, 54, 55
  social development, 54
  sociocultural context, 111
  theoretical models for culture, 56

D
Defining infant mental health, 7–10
Developing countries
  infant and early childhood mental health in, 96–97
Developmental change, 2, 13–15, 25, 26, 29, 31, 34, 67, 71, 76
Developmental context of infant mental health
  attachment and, 145
  brain development and, 26–27
  child care and, 191
  CPP and, 164–167
  emotional development, 23–38
  foster care and, 88
  language development, 23, 28, 29
  neural plasticity, 11, 37
  socioeconomic status social development, 88, 91
Developmental context of social and emotional functioning in the early years, 29–31
Developmental stages and social and emotional growth, 34–35
Developmental task, 2, 15, 28–29, 34, 36
Developmental theories of infant mental health, 150
Development in the earliest years, 12–13
Diagnostic Classification, 103
  0-3 (DC:0-3R):overview, 103
Diagnostic Statistical Manual of mental Disorders (DSM)
  attachment and, 103
Diathesis stress model, 72–74, 88
Differential susceptibility theory, 74
Divergent validity, 25
Diversity
  awareness model, 54
  tenets, 213–214
Divorce, 86, 127
Domestic violence, 167
Dopamine, 72–74, 117

Double ABCX model
family coping with adversity, 130
Dyadic relationship, 4, 45, 107, 132, 150

E

Early childhood mental health consultation
adult client, 187–188
capacity building, 195
challenges in early childhood mental health consultation, 198–199
collaborative relationship, 182, 185, 193
consultant, 188–190, 192, 195, 197, 199
consultation setting, 186–187
consultative model and principles, 184–185
consultative practice, consultation relationship, 182, 187, 190–192
consultative skills, 192–195
issues in, 182–184
overview, 181
principles of, 181, 184–185
training in, 182
Early Head Start, 209
Early intervention, 72, 145, 152, 153, 160, 204
Ecological models
ecosystem model, 154
Bronfenbrenner, 101
Emotion, 3–5, 8–9, 14, 15, 27, 28, 32, 34–36, 47, 51, 86, 94, 95, 102, 106, 107, 111–114, 116, 139, 146, 154, 174, 198, 208
Emotional availability (EA), 105–109
scales, 197–201
Emotional development
assessment, 37
depression and, 108, 145, 189, 206
overview, 23
poverty and, 90
theoretical models of, 159, 160
Emotion regulation
bi-directional dynamic, 4, 81, 117
models of, 4
parenting and, 109
synchronization, 4
Empathic responding, 117
Empathy, 23, 37, 49, 191, 193, 208
development of concern for others, 37
Environmental risk factors
exposure to violence, 84, 150
infant caregiver relationship and, 90–96
neuroscience and, 7, 69
parental substance abuse, 86, 159
parenting, prenatal substance exposure, 84
poverty, 60, 90–93
Evidence-Based Interventions in Infant and Early Childhood Mental Health, 159–175
a survey of, 159–175
Evidence-based practice, 162–164
Executive functioning, 27
Experience-dependent development, 11
Experience-expectant development, 11

F

Face to face paradigm, 126
still face paradigm, 31, 113, 114
Family factors
aggression, 27, 44, 107, 147, 161, 162, 170, 209
models, 130
overview, 133
structure, 87, 171
Family resilience, 125–140
Family strengths model, 130
Fathers, 9, 25, 26, 52, 95, 189, 214
cultural factors, 54
Fetal development
brain development, 96, 102, 113
maternal depression, 86, 94, 96, 136, 159, 207
maternal stress, 54, 107
neural plasticity, 76, 159
neurobiology, 203
overview, 94
substance abuse of parents, 60, 86, 117, 165, 171, 172, 189, 209
Fight/flight response, 82, 155
Foster care
brain and development, 26–29
insightfulness and, 52
intervention and, 9, 10, 147, 148
models of, 10–12
policy and, 204
Foundation for the concern for others, 36–37

G

Gaze behavior, 47–48
Gene-environment interaction mode, 76, 88
Gene-environment interplay, 72–75
General models of the nature-nurture controversy, 75–76

Genetic factors
emotional development and, 13
fetal development and, 94
maternal depression and, 86, 94, 96, 136, 159, 207
parental substance abuse and, 159, 206
resilience and, 127
stress in infancy and, 70, 71
temperament and, 6, 7, 12, 16, 27, 31–34, 37, 48, 49, 60, 71, 74, 84, 85, 88, 89, 91, 101, 125, 145, 150, 165, 166
Goodness of fit model, 89
Greenspan's Developmental, Individual-Differences, Relationship-Based Model (DIR), 152
Growth curve modeling, 90
Guralnick, M.J., 23
Multidisciplinary Collaborative Team Work, 156

H
Harsh parenting, 74
Head Start, 9, 69, 161, 162, 183, 184, 209, 210
Heritability, 94
Hierarchal linear modeling (HLM), 90
History of infant and early childhood mental health, 2–7
Home Measurement of Environment (HOME), 55
Home visiting programs, 184
evidence based intervention, 174–175

I
Implications of early development for later development, 14–15
Implicit and explicit socialization, 49–50
Incredible Years® (IY), 167–169
Individual differences
analysis of variance (standard error), 70
attachment relationships and, 85, 111, 148
emotional development in, 31–37
family functioning and, 84, 87, 132, 137, 139, 187
foster care and, 10, 88
maternal depression and, 86, 93, 94, 96, 136, 159, 207
stress in infancy and, 69–72
Infant and early childhood mental health interventions, 149, 160, 164
Infant caregiver relationship
assessment, 161
emotional availability scales, 106, 162
Infant development
brain and, 26–29
neural plasticity, 159
poverty and, 90–93
prevention interventions, 210–212
temperament and, 12
Infant mental health
definition, 2
emotional development and, 23–38
empirical foundations of, 36, 37
mental health consultation, 181–199, 210
social development, 8, 30, 36, 54, 84, 101, 215
training, 213
Infant-parent attachment relationship, 155
Infant Toddler Social and Emotional Assessment (ITSE), 55
Insecure attachment, 94
Interaction guidance (IG), 171–174
International Classification of Diseases (ICD)
Interrelational context, 112–117
Intersubjectivity, 3, 35, 114, 117
Intervention effectiveness, 295–297
research methodology and designs, 161–162
Intervention in infant and early childhood mental health, 267–285
theoretical bases of, 145–156
Interventions, 165
child parent psychotherapy, 164–167
home visits, 205, 207, 209
Incredible Years, 167–169, 197
parent child interaction therapy (PCIT), 170–171
social and cultural context, 43–60, 139

J
Jealousy, 112–114

L
Language development, 12, 211
Life course patterns, 211
Limit setting, 273
cultural differences, 149
Longitudinal research designs
adoption, 107
families, 133, 134
general, 84–86
resilience, 135–137
temperament, 135, 136
Longitudinal Resilience Research Statistics, 133–135

Louisiana Twin Study
analysis of data, 71
findings, 71

M
Marital relationship of parents
competence, 128
fathers and, 109
violence, 55
Mediation models in research, 89, 92, 135, 136
Mental health informed systems, 205–210
Mental representation, 26, 35, 108
Mindfulness and reflective thinking, 6–7
mentalizing, 6
Models of care
child centered, 186, 187
foster care, 88
program centered, 187
Moderator models in research, 87, 89
Mother-infant interaction, 3, 60, 110
Multicultural perspective
overview, 43
theoretical models, 10–12

N
Nature *vs.* nurture controversy, 67–76, 101
Neural plasticity, 159
Neurobiology of infant development, relational context, stress, temperament, 203
Non-optimal developmental outcomes, 82, 159
Nurse-family partnership, 211

O
Observational methods, 46
Overcoming adversity, 137, 138
Oxytocin, 117

P
Parental attribution, 166
Parental awareness, 51–52
Parental characteristics and risk, 60, 86
Parental mental health, 150
Parental risk factors, 30, 86
depression, 93–94
Parent child interaction therapy (PCIT), 170–171
Parent education, 182
Parenting, 6, 7, 10, 25, 27, 29, 30, 51–55, 57, 59, 60, 72, 74, 84, 92, 94, 96, 102, 108–111, 117, 126–129, 131, 136, 147, 149, 165–172, 210–212
across cultures, 108–111
dysfunctional parenting, 6
models, 10
stress, 57
styles, 16, 25, 27, 52–54, 109, 111, 147, 170
Parent report measures
considerations, 82
limitations, 52
overview, 107
recommendation, 156
selecting an instrument, 46
Parent staff relationship, 185, 186, 188
Pediatric health care providers, 162, 182, 187, 190, 192, 193
Play
pretend, 16, 47, 51
symbolic, 147
Policy, 7, 8, 53, 151, 160, 196, 203–216
Policy agenda
creating mental health informed systems, 205–207
establish prevention programs, 210–212
incorporate mental health perspectives in policy decisions, 209–210
incorporating diversity-informed tenets, 213–214
policymakers, 8, 196, 204, 205, 214–216
promoting infant and early childhood mental health, 204
support programs for families at risk, 207–209
training professional, 212–213
Poverty, 60, 69, 84, 86, 90–93, 96, 127, 139, 150, 159, 161, 162, 165, 172, 181, 189, 196, 205, 206
Prematurity, 127
Prevention
challenges in, 204
continuum of services model, 212
early experiences and, 11–12
levels of, 210–212
primary health care settings, 207
programs, 204, 210–212
successful programs for, 210–212
Primary care providers
challenges and future directions, 205
prevention and, 212
role of, 205
treatment and intervention model, 205

Problem-solving, 33, 104, 110, 131, 137, 162, 168, 173, 182, 185, 192–195, 215
Professional training, 204, 212–213
Program-based consultation model, 183, 187
Protective factors
overview, 27
poverty, 127
resilience and, 125
social competence, 45, 46, 53, 60, 84, 89, 190, 209
Psychoanalytical theory, 9
Psychodynamic theory, 146–148
Psychological risk factors, 96
Psychosocial characteristics, 165
Psychotherapy, 164–167

R

Reactivity
negative, 73
positive, 73
Reciprocal connections, 28–29
Reciprocal exchange, 44
Reflective functioning, 51, 52
Reflective practice, 182
Reflective supervision, 192, 193
Regulation
affect, 206
behavior, 15, 28
emotional, 3, 4, 28, 29, 174, 190
sensory, 15, 28
Relational context, 101–118
infant and early childhood mental health in, 101–118
Relational imperative, 102
infant and early childhood mental health in, 102
Relationships
bridge between theory and intervention, 101
caregiving relationship, 7, 128, 171
infant-caregiver relationship, 117, 149, 161, 171, 203
Representation, 114, 147
Research findings, 1, 88, 94, 115, 159, 182, 184, 196–198, 211
Research methodologies
computational techniques, 6
cross-cultural, 10, 54–60, 102, 106, 107, 109–111
emotional development, 13
empathy, 7, 16, 24, 31, 36
infant and early childhood mental health, 54–60
qualitative, 15, 55, 95, 131, 173
quantitative, 46
resilience, 131–135
social development, 8, 30, 36, 54, 74, 84, 101, 215
theory of mind, 28, 35–36, 47
Research strategies
behavioral paradigms, 30
caregiver reports, 73, 208
confirmatory statistical analysis, 74
cross-sectional, 29, 46, 132
developmentally appropriate tasks, 37, 45, 104
inter-observer reliability, 31
interviews, 32, 45, 46, 52, 173
laboratory, 25, 30, 46, 54, 58, 139, 163, 166
longitudinal, 5, 29, 33, 46, 71, 82–84, 90, 91, 105, 107, 108, 131–137, 151, 160–162
natural settings, 25, 174
observations, 30, 31, 45, 46, 52, 54, 55, 91
parental reports, 54, 95
questionnaires, 31–33, 46, 54, 55, 95, 162, 167
regression analysis, 74, 118, 133, 134, 175
Resilience, 131
applications of resilience research, 137–138
in children, 125–140
community, 129–131
in families, 125–140
implications for intervention, 72, 138–140
in a relational context, 128–129
Risk
additive model, 83
child depression and, 85, 87
conceptualization of risk, 82–84
cultural lens, 60
identifying risk factors, 84–86
infant and early childhood mental health in, 81–97
infant caregiver relationship and, 161
maternal depression and, 96
parental depression and, 87
in a relational context, 128–129
research methodologies for studying risk, 87–90
risk factors in developing countries, 96–97
statistical models to explain risk, 89–90
stress reactivity and, 89
vulnerability, 60, 73, 89

S

Sameroff's transactional model, 2, 150–152
Screening, 206, 216
Secure attachment, 6, 14, 26, 59, 94, 110, 148, 150, 165–167, 175, 212
Security, 9, 15, 75, 111, 127, 128, 145, 160, 170, 174, 175
Self-awareness, 36
Self-concept, 23, 149
Self-confidence, 132, 168
Self-control, 53
Self-esteem, 33, 53, 128, 129
Self-recognition, 36, 37
Self-regulation, 23, 32, 34, 53, 153, 206, 208
Sense of self, 6, 7, 15–16, 23, 28, 29, 36, 49, 149
Sensitive periods of development for behavior, 14
Sensitivity, 33, 59, 74, 75, 94, 105–112, 115, 127, 153, 161, 167, 174, 175, 196, 198
Sensory processing, 154
  dysfunction, 154
Serotonin, 72, 73, 75
Shared genetic vulnerability models, 74
  single parenthood, 86, 132
Social and cultural contexts in infant and early childhood mental health, 43–60
Social and emotional development in infant and early childhood mental health, 23–38
Social cognition in infants, 114–117
Social competence, 46, 60, 84, 89, 190, 209
Social development, 13
  assessment, 37, 47
  overview, 29
Social functioning, 46
Socialization, 4, 15, 43–50, 54–57, 59, 60, 82, 111
  home culture, 48–50
Social reciprocity, 44
Social referencing, 35, 44
Still face paradigm, 115
Strange situation procedure, 58, 59, 106
Strengths based focus, 137
Stress
  coping models and, 93
  CPP and, 164–167
  development and, 166, 187, 209
  during infancy, 164
  early experiences and, 13
  maternal depression, 94
  neural plasticity, 102
  stress diathesis models, 72–74
Structural equation modeling (SEM), 89
Substance abuse
  effects of, 60, 117
  foster care, 88
  intervention and, 159, 165, 171, 172, 189
  overview, 86
  parental, 60, 86, 171
  predictors of, 211
  rick factors, 27
Supervision
  overview, 192
  professional, 209
  training for, 212

T

Temperament
  caregiver reports, 73, 208
  continuity of, 32
  emotional development and, 27, 31–37
  family functioning and, 84
  insecure attachment, 94, 212
  maternal depression, 135, 136
  neurobiology of, 203
  questionnaires, 32, 33
  risk factors, 27, 84, 85, 88, 89, 91, 150
  stability of, 133
Temper tantrums, 37, 51
Theoretical models of infant mental health, 10–14
Theories of development
  Als' synactive theory of development, 153
  Ayres' sensory integration, 154–155
  Bagnato's convergent model, 153
  Brazelton's Touchpoints, 150, 155
Theory of mind
  foundations of, 36–37
  underpinnings of, 35–36
Toddlers, 26, 30, 37, 38, 48, 55, 57, 85, 103, 108, 115, 127, 148, 154, 159, 165, 203, 205–209, 213, 214
Touchpoints intervention, 155–156
Training, 214
  ethical considerations, 182
  goals for, 167, 212
  professional, 164, 181, 182, 204, 212–213
Transactional model of development, 10, 11
Transitions, 37, 46, 101, 118, 188
Transmitter gene, 73
Trauma, 60, 89, 95, 96, 159, 161, 166, 167, 181, 189, 206, 209

Treatment
overview, 163–164
planning, 103, 167, 172

U

Understanding social behavior in the early years, 44–48

V

Vulnerabilities, 16, 101, 109, 128, 172, 173, 191, 192, 206

W

Wondering not knowing, 191

Z

Zero to Three
cultural factors, 160
defining mental health, 8
diagnostic system, 103–105, 152
early experiences and, 204

MIX
Papier aus verantwortungsvollen Quellen
Paper from responsible sources
FSC® C105338

If you have any concerns about our products,
you can contact us on
ProductSafety@springernature.com

In case Publisher is established outside the EU,
the EU authorized representative is:
Springer Nature Customer Service Center GmbH
Europaplatz 3, 69115 Heidelberg, Germany

Printed by Libri Plureos GmbH
in Hamburg, Germany